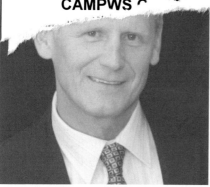

Professor George Jelinek is an

He

at

...tern Aust-
ralia, University of Melbourne, and Monash University. He was the first Professor of Emergency Medicine in Australasia and founding editor of the journal *Emergency Medicine Australasia*. He has given many public lectures and retreats for people with MS in Australia and New Zealand.

Professor George Jelinek's website: www.takingcontrolofmultiplesclerosis.org

Responses from medical practitioners and people with multiple sclerosis:

'Through George Jelinek's advice I have learned how to take my vulnerable nervous system and nurture it back to a life free from MS. Jelinek's work has given me back my health and my confidence to live my life to the full again. I am a busy General Practitioner, mother of four, hiker, equestrian, gardener, with a zest for life and thrilled to have it back again.

As a doctor I am grateful to have Jelinek's expert review of the research around MS. There is so much information and mis-information that one gets lost in the mire. To be able to say to the newly diagnosed or the gradually more debilitated, 'yes we can help' is medically exciting and such a relief.

I have had MS for 10 years now, the first four in denial with episodes every one or two years, the last six years since starting the Jelinek diet and lifestyle plan have become rapidly episode free, with my health and energy restored. I cannot recommend this book highly enough to anyone whose life is affected by multiple sclerosis.'

'Professor Jelinek is inspirational in empowering patients to take responsibility for the management of their disease. His holistic approach encouraging patients to consider more than just pharmaceutical treatment for the disease has proven itself as the modern approach to the management of multiple sclerosis.'

Clinical Professor Peter Silbert, MBBS, FRACP,
State Director of Neurology in Western Australia;
Head of Department of Neurology, Royal Perth Hospital

'People who have been diagnosed with MS are often vulnerable and open to ideas which offer false hope. Our Society recognises that George Jelinek's work provides important, genuine hope.

People diagnosed with the condition often feel stripped of control over their lives and future. This book is a wonderful resource that will help to redress the balance and give people the opportunity to thrive despite their diagnosis. Every person diagnosed with multiple sclerosis should receive a copy as a reference work and a motivational tool, encouraging them to take sensible steps to minimise their symptoms and maximise their enjoyment of life.'

Gary McMahon, General Manager,
MS Society of Auckland and North Shore, New Zealand

OVERCOMING
MULTIPLE
SCLEROSIS

AN EVIDENCE-BASED
GUIDE TO **RECOVERY**

PROFESSOR GEORGE JELINEK

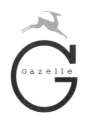

Gazelle

This edition first published in the United Kingdom and Continental Europe in 2010

First published by Allen & Unwin Book Publishers, Australia, 2010

Impala Books
a division of Gazelle Book services Limited
White Cross Mills
Hightown
Lancaster
LA1 4XS
England

Phone   +44 (0)1524 68765
Fax   +44 (0)1524 63232

email sales@gazellebooks.co.uk
Web www.gazellebooks.co.uk

ISBN 978 1 85586 111 4

Typeset by Midland Typesetters, Australia
Printed by South Wind Productions, Singapore

For Eva Jelinek

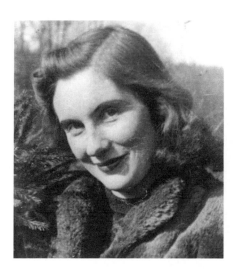

CONTENTS

TABLES AND FIGURES

TABLES

FIGURES

FOREWORD

Professor George Jelinek brings to this work an extraordinary and ideal combination. As a Professor of Emergency Medicine and editor of a medical journal, he has a long and very solid grounding in medical science. But then he became affected by MS. A patient. A whole new view. A whole new experience. A whole new imperative.

George responded to this imperative by scouring the medical literature, the Internet and the popular press. He was aided in his search by relatives, colleagues and other people dealing with MS.

The result of George's search is exquisite. In my opinion he has produced what can fairly be described as a definitive work on MS, a summation of the current understanding of the causes, effects and treatment options for MS. And all of this presented in a way that will be satisfying to anyone whose life is directly touched by MS, as well as a professional audience.

George's previous book, *Taking Control of Multiple Sclerosis*, rapidly established its importance. It changed the way medicine is being practised. It positively transformed the experiences of people dealing with the potentially devastating disease MS. Now this new book completely updates our knowledge and is available to an even wider audience.

It is wonderful to be able to assert these benefits. Medical history will look back on this book and give it a major place in the advancement of the treatment and management of MS.

For those of us who have been involved and been able to witness this progression, it has been truly wonderful. What Professor George Jelinek has done with this new book is to completely review and update something that has been working well enough already to transform lives.

What we have now is a major literature review which in all probability contains more detail, more scope, than other more formal texts on MS. Yet with George's humanity and capacity to communicate, the book remains easily accessible, in fact highly relevant to anyone with MS; while it is also essential reading for health professionals including GPs and neurologists.

For those people who have used George's books since the first printing, and for those who have attended the residential programs that George and I have run with my wife Ruth, a GP, and our other Foundation staff, the experience has been truly remarkable. Early data from the research analysis quantifies the gains, yet the human experience is even more obvious.

People regain hope. They realise that this new hope is real. That what they do will make a difference. That science solidly supports their hope—their hope that with the correct management, medically and especially personally, MS can be stabilised. We have the good fortune to meet these people later, now commonly some years later, and they are radiant. Increasingly we are receiving reports of multiple lesions clearing from MRI scans. While these are still early days, ongoing research is needed, and will be followed through to establish the true scope of what is possible.

But there is no doubt. For anyone diagnosed with MS, *Overcoming Multiple Sclerosis* is essential reading. It could save untold misery. It could positively transform many more lives. Enjoy it. Benefit from it. And be grateful Professor George Jelinek used his own experience of MS to research the disease and write this major book.

This is the most exciting book I have read in some time. Everyone affected by MS, either directly or indirectly, needs to read it. All medical staff need to read it. George Jelinek, as doctor, scientist and MS survivor, has written a comprehensive, definitive work that will save many lives, improve the health and wellbeing of many affected by MS, and is sure to add to the growing recognition of the value of a more holistic approach in medicine generally.

Ian Gawler OAM
April 2009

PREFACE

As with any journey, the beginning is often associated with much emotion, hope for the future, and great resolve. It was in that spirit that the first book *Taking Control of Multiple Sclerosis* was written. As time has gone by, and I have remained well and still firmly focused on my goal, I have had time to re-evaluate the information I initially collected and presented to people with MS. I have not changed my views on the core principles of staying well after a diagnosis of MS. Lifestyle change is the most important issue as it is with most chronic diseases. Diet, sunlight, exercise, meditation, preventing depression, resolution of difficult emotional issues. These are the keys.

What has changed is that the medical literature supporting these principles has grown enormously. My initial PubMed search on MS yielded around 19,000 references. The same search now yields twice that number. There is now high quality medical research evidence in support of a low saturated fat diet, sunlight and vitamin D, exercise, the negative effect of stress and depression, and so on. This has enabled me to present my synthesis of the literature in a much more evidence-based way, and for people with MS to be more certain of the science behind the decisions they make about lifestyle and medication choices.

The medical profession demands evidence before making recommendations to patients. In this new book, I have sought to systematically lay out the evidence in a clear, comprehensible format, so that what is fact and what is opinion can be clearly differentiated. And to make it possible for people being offered potentially toxic drugs to differentiate sophisticated marketing from science. The number of references has grown from 186 in the second edition to nearly 700 in this book; they are from highly reputable sources and the bulk of them are very recent. The good news for people with MS is that there is now a very large body of evidence making the case that it is possible to be well after a diagnosis of MS. There is every reason for people now diagnosed with MS to be optimistic about the future.

George Jelinek
April 2009

ACKNOWLEDGMENTS

I thank my wife Sandra; I am a very lucky man to have found her. I am very grateful for the help of my family, friends and colleagues who have supported me through good and bad times. Thanks to Sean, Michael, Pia, Ruby and Johnny, Suzette, Gina, Iva and Pete, and my wonderful friends Ian Hislop, Mike Galvin, Glenn McLagan, Dania Lynch, Jan and Mike Ramage, Aled and Rochelle Williams, Tracey Weiland, Graham Reilly, Amanda Paxton, Penny Tolhurst, Janet Fletcher, and Ian and Ruth Gawler. Thanks also to Wal Pisciotta, and to the hundreds of people who have been through the MS retreats I have run in Western Australia, the Australian Capital Territory, Victoria and New Zealand, who regularly keep in touch and send their support and their good stories. I also thank my friend and colleague, Dr Mike Cadogan, whose advice about how to clearly and concisely present data have I hope resulted in a more accessible book for people with MS. Thanks also to Dr Peter Silbert, whose comments on the manuscript have been very helpful in ensuring my recommendations are evidence-based.

And finally I thank my mother, Eva Jelinek. The year 2008 was a very important one for me. I was into my tenth year since diagnosis and was still relapse-free; and I was aware during the year that I had now lived half my life without my mother. I was a 27-year-old doctor three years out of medical school when she died. And in 2008, 27 years later, I was still learning how hard it was to live without the people we love, how final death is.

That my mother had become so incapable of any real enjoyment of life because of her illness, that she felt there was no other choice than to take her own life, is something that has become a driving force in my life. I hope that I can make enough of a difference to the lives of others with MS that people don't have to face this awful choice. Perhaps I stuck my neck out writing the first book three months into the illness, and very publicly declaring there was a way to stay well after a diagnosis of MS. My good health is clearly no accident and cannot be explained away as 'benign MS'. It certainly must make even the most sceptical seriously consider the evidence I present. And so I thank my mother, not only for everything she did for me as I was growing up, but for providing the driving force behind my own health, and behind the continuing good health of countless people with MS worldwide who have adopted this approach to life.

—GJ

PROLOGUE

Time is the only comforter for the loss of a mother

Jane Welsh Carlyle

I leant over and kissed her on the cheek. She was already cold. Strangely, I couldn't feel sad. I felt only overwhelming relief. Relief that the suffering had finally stopped. Relief that Mum wouldn't have to fight any more.

So this is how it ends, I thought. The insidious tentacles of multiple sclerosis had taken sixteen years to pull her down, but they couldn't beat her in the end. Mum had chosen to take her own life rather than get any worse, rather than be completely degraded.

She looked so peaceful. I had kissed her goodnight the previous night, not knowing that would be the last time I would see her alive. What must she have been going through? To have been so brave right to the end, to have not let on as she said goodnight to the most precious parts of her life for the last time. I felt my eyes misting, but no tears would come. We had all known this was coming for a long time. Most of us had already grieved while she was alive. But now it was real. The image of me sitting there alone on her bed will stay with me forever.

How could I know that eighteen years later I would be sitting in a neurologist's office some 7 kilometres away, listening but not listening as he was trying to tell me I had MS? I would not let myself hear what he was saying. It was a lovely Sunday afternoon in Perth. The West Coast Eagles were playing just down the road. The sun was shining. Why is he going on and on about MS, I thought. If he doesn't know why my leg has gone numb he should just say so. When it did hit me, all the memories of Mum came flooding back. I relived the gradual deterioration, the descent into paralysis, the indignity of urinary catheters and bedpans, the loneliness and frustration. And it was going to happen again. To me.

I don't know when I resolved that it wouldn't. Things just seemed to lead me down a path where answers kept turning up, real answers. Now, after a decade relapse-free, I know I'll be okay.

This is my story. I wish it could have been Mum's.

PART I

BACKGROUND

1

ABOUT MY MOTHER, MS AND ME

Do not give up HOPE

Dorothy Miller Cole

Mum and Dad had difficult lives. I understand that better now that they are both gone, and I am a parent. Dad was born in Prague in the newly created Czechoslovakia on the day World War I ended. Every year the government sent him and the few others born on that day a special certificate commemorating the event. Dad was very proud of that.

His was a farming family. Dad used to regale us as kids with stories of his childhood. We used to beg him to tell us all the tales, as we sat waiting to pick up Mum from Graylands Mental Hospital where she worked as a nurse. He used to deliberately take us early, so much did he love telling the stories. Who knows if they were true or not? We didn't care. Dad's father was six foot nine, with hands so badly disfigured by warts that he always wore gloves (see what I mean?). He was a tough disciplinarian, but you could sense that he loved his children and pampered them. It seemed that Dad was always getting into trouble. The time he tried to get back into class after playing hookey by climbing down the chimney. Falling and covering himself in soot, and jumping out of the fireplace in the classroom yelling 'Boo!' like a ghost.

Somewhere in his childhood Dad found time to learn a range of musical instruments. And to paint. He was a very creative man. One of my favourite childhood memories is listening to the sound of the piano accordion rolling through the house. Dad would be transfixed by the music at these moments. He couldn't speak. He just lived the music. My children have reaped the rewards of his genes. After starting and then pulling out of engineering, my son is now studying musical composition at university, writing and recording his own work, and teaching music to high school students.

Mum was different. She was born into an aristocratic family. Some time ago I visited the house in Pardubice where she grew up. It is now a school administration building with three storeys of secretaries typing away. No one stopped us as my sister and I wandered through, but we got some strange looks from the women at the old typewriters. When Mum married for the first time, the whole town turned up to the society wedding of the year. Mum started studying medicine. But then the war came. Nothing was to be the same again.

Mum and Dad met in a refugee camp. One thing you had to say about Dad was that he had the gift of the gab, and was a charmer if he wanted to be. Mum often wondered in later years why she took up with Dad. Suffice to say they were very different, and often not understanding or appreciative of each other's differences. Their marriage lasted but was not a happy one. Dad was more in love with Mum than the other way around. She never valued the strengths he had; mostly she couldn't even see them. Dad felt rejected. But they stayed together, as so many did in those days, for the sake of the kids.

They lost their first born, the older brother I never met, at six months of age, to pneumonia, in a refugee camp fleeing the communists. When faced with the big decision about which boat to get on out of Italy, with my older sister now in tow as a baby, they favoured Australia over Argentina because Australians spoke English. All the decisions that have led to me being here right now have happened as they should have. I'm only realising these important things now. That's just one of the gifts this illness has brought me.

One of Dad's favourite stories was that my older sister Iva was under-weight and couldn't legally get on the boat to Australia. Dad made her a dress out of curtain material he found, but then sewed some lead into the ribbons in her hair to get her up to the required weight. Judge for yourself whether this is true. I never knew.

And so to Australia. The Northam refugee camp. Learning English. Trying to find work. Dad did everything. He built houses, he painted them, he painted signs, he did window dressing for the big stores, anything that involved some creativity. He told us how in those days people would think he was stupid because his English was so poor and they would refuse to pay. 'Bloody new Australians!' But Dad would get the last laugh by sneaking back in the dead of night and painting their front door jet black while they slept.

Times were tough. One daughter turned into two, then two sons, then another girl, before they finally stopped. Seven hungry mouths to feed and never enough money. Never any regular income. Mum eventually pushed Dad into accepting a job as a clerk at Perth Dental Hospital, a steady job he kept until retirement. It wasn't fun or highly paid, but the money was regular. Mum qualified as a mental health nurse. She used to work night shifts so that she could be there in the daytime to look after the kids while Dad worked. The overriding priority for my parents, as it was for most other migrant families, was to set their kids up for the sort of lives they never had. And they succeeded. It would have been hard enough. But then along came MS.

MY MOTHER

How old was I when Mum got MS? I don't know. My youngest sister Suzette says it was when Mum was 40, which would have made it 1963. I was only nine then. It seems to me that Mum was 42 or 43. One night Mum was on her way to night shift at the hospital. She was no more than 500 metres down Scarborough Beach Road when a drunk driver turned in front of her. She was driving an old Morris Minor which had a doorknob for a gearstick handle. Seatbelts didn't exist. She flew through the windscreen and badly lacerated her face and head. Dad used to tell us that he got the call from a friend who saw it happen from a nearby phone box and raced down there. The ambulance officers couldn't get her out so Dad ripped the door off. He said he didn't know where the strength came from.

I heard all the hushed voices in the kitchen and got up to investigate. You can always tell when there's bad news, even as a kid. My brother Peter and I slept in the enclosed back verandah. We had not long graduated from bunk beds. I came back to the bedroom and Peter told me to stop making a noise. In the distance was the pitiful wail of an ambulance. I said, 'That ambulance is for Mum' and started crying. I reckon I was eleven and Pete was eight. That's when it started.

A few months later Mum started dropping things. As a kid all those things just sort of pass you by. Soon there were doctors' appointments, and tests. Mum even had her own neurologist. The real significance of what was happening didn't sink in. Children just go on having a good time, no matter what else is going on.

The next year I won a scholarship to Scotch College. My parents' dreams had come true. They were able to see me properly educated, without destroying the family financially. Without the scholarship a private school would never have even been considered. The first day at Scotch was the loneliest day of my life. Standing there in a large quadrangle, with my maroon school cap tightly held in two sweaty hands in front of me, knowing only two boys who were sons of friends in the whole school. I never wanted this.

Meanwhile, Mum started to deteriorate. At first it was just stumbling a bit. We always used to holiday in Denmark in the south-west of Western Australia with the family whose kids I knew at Scotch College. They were Czech too. I remember lying in wait for Mum when we were all going for a walk on the beach, jumping out from behind a sand hill and pushing her over. Then not letting her get up, with both of us laughing uncontrollably. We didn't know how bad it was going to get.

I can't remember when she went into a wheelchair. Modifications started appearing around the house: shower rails, showering chair, ramp up the front stairs, the car was modified. By now I was starting to grow up, and it was starting to mean something. And then I began university.

Why did I choose medicine? A little amateur psychology is enough to see what forces pushed me in that direction. And Mum was no amateur psychologist. She was an expert. Just as Mum had guided other decisions I had made in my life before, I was again unaware of her directing me to fulfil her adolescent ambitions. But her motivation was, I am sure, good. Mum was a curious mixture of sensitivity, intelligence and the kind of sarcastic cynicism that you get in some mental health nurses. She was also a great manipulator. Suffice to say I started medicine without ever really knowing why, although deep down a little hint of wanting to find a cure for MS occasionally bubbled to the surface.

Almost immediately I discovered a world I had only dimly glimpsed before. University was fantastic. Parties, independence, music, alcohol. It took a while for my previously very high marks to suffer, but suffer they did. Soon I had moved out of home, and in with what Mum would have thought was definitely the wrong crowd. But did the good times roll? I lasted one week at a residential university college before being expelled after a woman was seen leaving my room late at night. Luckily Mum and Dad were away on holidays in Tasmania at the time, and I managed to get myself into another college and concoct a fitting story for my parents. This was probably the last holiday Mum was capable of going on.

Forklifts were needed at the airport to get Mum into the plane. She said she felt quite regal with all the fanfare and attention. But it was a huge struggle. More and more often at this stage, when I'd come home for the night, I would catch Mum looking at me from her wheelchair with a tear in her eye. You knew when she had that look, that the big things in life were going through her mind. Loss, separation, death, the burden she was. The burden was her recurring theme; she was adamant she wouldn't be a burden to anyone. It was one of my first thoughts when I was told I had MS too.

MY DIAGNOSIS

I could see his lips moving but I couldn't hear anything. It was a beautiful late Sunday afternoon in Perth. The light was coming through the leaves from a low angle, firing them up with late autumn colour. In an instant, the whole world had changed. I was not to know it but I would never feel the same way about life again, and my orderly, seemingly successful life would soon fall apart.

'It's not the worst thing I could be telling you right now.' I heard it as if in some sort of dream. It certainly felt like the worst. We were suddenly talking about a magnetic resonance imaging scan that night at the hospital. He was ringing the radiologist. All I could think of was my family. I kept thinking to myself that my daughter was only seven. Only seven. All the plans I had, all the aspirations. Suddenly a big hand had reached into my life and taken away my future. And inexorably altered theirs.

On the outside I was calm and grateful that he had taken so much of his valuable Sunday afternoon to see me and make the diagnosis. Inside, I was just numb. Why hadn't I realised that I had MS? I now know that it is many times more common in family members, but somehow, with

Mum having had it, I had just assumed that lightning wouldn't strike twice. Not me.

We had got back from a wonderful week at Rottnest Island for the kids' school holidays. The first morning back at work, I noticed the shoelace on my left shoe kept falling down into my shoe. But every time I looked for it, it was no longer there. As the day wore on, the feeling of something there got more and more marked. By next day it was a feeling of numbness, like having been to the dentist, over all the toes of my foot. By now I was starting to remark on it. How odd it was. By the next day it had spread up the outside of my lower leg. I was getting nervous. Being an emergency physician, I am not prone to panicking. I started thinking about all the possibilities. A slipped disk? I had had back problems for years, but swimming regularly had fixed that. Some unusual peripheral neuropathy? I let it go for another day, but by the Thursday I knew I was in trouble. I chaired a conference session that afternoon for the national meeting of the College of Psychiatrists, and introduced one speaker completely out of order, so preoccupied was I. I hadn't ever made quite so public a mistake before. I was working late in the emergency department that night, and I just couldn't ignore it any more. I was taking over the evening shift from one of my colleagues and thought I would just casually mention it to him and maybe get him to look at me. I trusted his judgment. But it was not to be. Every time I was about to say something, someone would walk into the office. When we were eventually alone, I started, and the phone rang. That was the end of that.

So I worked hard that night, although I found it difficult to concentrate. The numbness was progressing pretty rapidly and by 11 p.m. I was numb all the way up the leg, and around my backside. I hardly slept that night. Next morning I had another colleague from ED look at me. However, I 'sabotaged' the diagnosis by telling him I thought it was a slipped disk. Being junior to me, naturally that's what he thought as well. So I spent an anxious hour or two waiting in X-ray while another friend tried to squeeze me into the burgeoning Friday queue for the MRI.

To my surprise, there was nothing there. But what you find depends on where you look, and they looked for a slipped disk and missed the MS lesion two levels higher. I found this really puzzling. Was I imagining it? I had long before promised that we would visit my father-in-law in the country over the weekend, so although it was already late in the day off we went. But to say I was distracted over the weekend would be an understatement. I was really worried. The amazing thing though is that MS never once entered my head. I feel embarrassed now that, as an emergency physician, I did not consider this differential diagnosis. We drove back on the Sunday, and I literally sprinted into the house and phoned a neurologist I worked with. I was so grateful that he could see me in his consulting rooms straightaway.

After seeing him, an MRI scan was booked for 6 p.m. I needed to tell my wife in person so I thought I would drive the 5 kilometres home before the MRI. But the Eagles had just finished playing and as I pulled out into the stream of traffic coming from the ground I realised I was not going to get home and back in time. So, sitting in the gathering gloom in the hospital carpark, I dialled home on the mobile. It sounded like someone else saying it. 'He thinks I've got MS.'

THE FIRST FEW DAYS

The first few days were awful. Should the kids be told? Should I tell anybody? What about the financial implications of not being able to work? The boys had only just started at an expensive private school. There were just no answers.

I realised that I had to face this, though. My initial reaction of not telling anyone just wouldn't work. How could I deal with this illness without acknowledging to the world that I had it? Keeping it a secret was impossible. I realised I had to start somewhere. Over the course of the day I resolved to tell my brother and sisters. First, though, I had an appointment at the hospital to get my first day of high-dose intravenous steroids. I wasn't prepared for how difficult that would be. Now the nurse putting in the IV line wanted to know how long I'd had MS. I found myself forced to talk about it. Those first few sessions of steroid therapy were awful. There was just no way to avoid the diagnosis. You could feel the pity in their eyes. Professor of Emergency Medicine at the university, young family, everything to look forward to. You could see how they would go home at night thinking 'Thank God it's not me'. At that stage, I still had no inner strength. I had nothing to hang on to. I felt like a man sentenced to a merciless, gradual destruction from which there was no escape.

That evening, it was hard to organise telling my brother and sisters all together. I ended up having to tell Iva over the phone. While she drove to Gina's, I picked up Suz and met her there. Peter lives about 200 kilometres south in Bunbury, and he wasn't home when I tried him by phone.

Sitting in Gina's dining room, crying. In between sobs, saying 'I don't want to be a burden, I don't want to be sick, I don't want people to have to look after me'. In the background Russell, Gina's husband, walking around, head bowed. He'd never seen me like this. I could see how he was hurting too.

All my life I had been strong and independent. It is becoming clear to me that this is a common characteristic of many people with MS. I couldn't imagine asking for or needing other people's help just to get around day to day. It was tough on everyone. We all hugged and cried over and over again until we were all cried out. And finally I got hold of Pete. I had hoped I could get hold of him earlier, so that he could go through the grief with all of us. I knew it would be harder for him on his own, especially if we didn't all do it together. There were no marvellous insights. No answers. All of us just thought it was catastrophically unfair, but that was all.

I left to drive home, feeling really empty but calm. I now realise how important this immediate expression of grief was, and how it led me so quickly to start finding answers in myself and get some feeling of control over the disease. Feeling so calm allowed me to then start thinking logically and without fear. This memory is quite vivid. Driving down the Mitchell Freeway, starting to piece together something. I had been trained really well in appreciating the effects of emotions on illness by one of my great mentors in medicine, Dr Ian Hislop. Ian had been a physician at Fremantle Hospital, and had since retired. I had worked for him as an intern in 1979. That's why I started thinking and wondering, as I was driving down the freeway, why this illness had happened to me just when it did. Why did I have this illness? What emotional needs was it serving for me to get ill just then? Was my subconscious knocking on the door of my seemingly well ordered life trying to tell me something was wrong?

Ian had taught us that the timing of illness is no coincidence. I had had a really tough two years in a new job, and maybe now that things were starting to settle down I was in a 'let go' phase, and had allowed myself to get sick. Perhaps getting sick was my way of getting people to love me and look after me. All these things started going through my head. I resolved to get in touch with Ian. I didn't realise it, but I was beginning to tackle MS.

IAN HISLOP

Ian Hislop was considered something of a dissident by some of the more conservative elements within the medical profession. But not by me. As an intern, I was dimly aware that many of the other consultants only tolerated his 'maverick' ideas about the effects of emotion on illness. I never took any convincing, though. From the moment I saw him on a ward round, what he was doing and teaching struck a resonant chord inside me, and I knew without question he was right.

One of the earliest patients we saw was a woman of around Mum's age at the time, say early fifties. She had been diagnosed with cervical cancer and it was incurable. I remember we walked into her hospital room, the whole show, consultant, registrar, intern, students, nurses all in tow. Ian did what many consultants rarely do, but he did quite often. He sat on the edge of the bed and held her hand. Within minutes they were discussing what it was about dying that she feared most. As she wept and talked about her fear of losing control after a lifetime of being dignified and proud, I fought back tears. I had never seen medicine like this. It was an influence which completely changed the way I practised.

Ian started taking a small group of interns and residents at lunch times, discussing the effects of feelings, emotions and grief on medical illness. There were never any journal articles to support his view, or textbook chapters. But everything he taught us was so obviously right, there was no need for verification. We learnt that when patients say they have been sick for a year, to ask what happened a year ago; when symptoms are sometimes baffling, to ask what else is happening in the patient's life; when therapies fail, to ask if there may be a reason why the patient needs to remain sick. The lessons have stayed with me through-out my career. The emergency department may seem a strange place to practise such medicine, but I have lost count of the number of times a patient has come in with chest pain only to go home with a referral to a clinical psychologist. Sometimes the nurses think it's akin to witchcraft. 'But I thought she was having palpitations,' they say.

I left Fremantle Hospital in 1997 to take up the Chair in Emergency Medicine at Sir Charles Gairdner Hospital. In my farewell speech, I made mention of three people who had profoundly influenced my career. Although I had not seen Ian in perhaps ten years at that stage, he was one of them. Funnily enough a mutual friend who was at my farewell rang

Ian, unbeknown to me, to tell him what I had said. It seemed no surprise to him when I rang him to tell him I had MS.

Ian's response was to say that we needed to talk. A day or two later he came around. We sat quietly outside in a corner, under a tree fern, at a small table. By now, everything in my life seemed to have slowed down to a crawl. I was acutely aware of every flicker of sunlight coming through the fern fronds, of every glistening patch of gold on the ripples in the pool. Time seemed to have little meaning.

In his calm and measured way he led me through the feelings I was experiencing. Every time I got to mentioning Mum I found it almost impossible to speak without becoming tearful. It was clear that I was seeing my own illness and future through the filter of Mum's disease and history. Until I could separate myself from those feelings a little, I was not going to get anywhere.

Ian listened quietly, occasionally interjecting with something to prompt me. He only said a little more when I started wondering if somehow I had brought this illness on myself as some sort of punishment. Ian was quick to stop that line of thinking. He told me about the three nurses who had gone to Europe together as students in their teens. Within three weeks of each other, in their thirties, they all got MS. It was a powerful message. There are factors we can control, and there are those we cannot. My heredity ensured I would have the 'right' pre-condition to get MS. Why it happened when it did might have been something more in my control.

Finally he gave me some assessment of what he thought I could do. First and foremost, he said, put yourself first. He suggested I take a long time off work in order to start doing some work on myself. This was great advice, but really difficult for me. I had just the day before told my colleagues I would be back in two weeks. For such a great challenge to one's life, two weeks is simply not doing it justice. Ian was suggesting that perhaps I may not want to go back to work at all. That I should consider all possibilities. I knew he was right. I was at a crossroads. Anything was possible.

I wasn't to know it but the simple process of trying to put myself first was to start a chain reaction of events that led my outwardly appearing 'perfect' life to seemingly fall apart, to head in directions I had never anticipated, to cause seismic shocks in the lives of my immediate family and many of my friends. As I write this I feel I am beginning to emerge from a long period of inner turmoil, trying to understand the lessons life is teaching me. Continuing to trust in this process of having faith in myself and my feelings and going where they lead me has been extremely difficult at times. I am discovering much weakness where I thought there was strength, reliving and investigating issues which I thought I had long ago dealt with.

Ian also asked if I had ever tried meditation. In fact, I had begun meditating when I was 21. I had taken a course in transcendental meditation while taking a year off medicine to tour around Europe. The week living with my teacher and her family on a farm in Switzerland was fantastic. I had stopped meditating when I took up the Chair, as I felt I didn't have enough time. Funny isn't it? That's when I needed it the most.

Finally he asked a question that was to start me on a greater journey than confronting MS. He wanted to know if I had ever thought much about the spirit. I searched for an answer. I soon realised that this was an extremely important part of my life, one that I was aware of but had put to one side because of the demands of the rest of my life. It was a simple question. Within the question lay the beginnings of a whole new journey in life for me. I hadn't yet realised it, but this was another of the gifts I was to get from MS.

THE SEARCH BEGINS

The first week of getting daily high-dose steroids was difficult but wonderful in its own way. The physical part of it didn't bother me much. I can put up with discomfort easily if I know it's doing me some good. But it was like someone was educating me about how much more suffering and heartache there was in the world than mine. The third day I met Barry.

Barry was dying of cancer. He had cancer in his liver and now in his back and hip and really found sitting there next to me getting his chemo very difficult. Barry had owned the Retravision shop in a little country town and was just the sort of bloke you'd expect. He was talkative and vivacious and loved life. In fact, anyone would have thought I was the one dying of cancer and he was the one facing many more years of happiness and life. Barry had played in a band in his town when he was young; I think he said they were called the Premiers. They had a bit of a twangy sound and he was the lead guitarist and sang. That hour, listening to the stories of the great times they'd had, filled me with joy.

We had a lot in common. We knew a lot of the same songs. We both enjoyed that wonderful feeling of entertaining people. We were similar, but there was a big difference: Barry was dying. Barry taught me gratitude for what I have. He was the first in a series of teachers that MS has thrown in my path. He also taught me about living in the moment, a lesson I have to keep re-learning to stay focused. Barry had a joy and spirit that even his imminent death couldn't touch. I went home that day a much wiser person for meeting him.

Saturday morning arrived and I had finished my steroids. Now I was doing what the neurologist had termed 'doing nothing' and waiting. He had said that if I was still okay in six months we should repeat the MRI to see if there were any new 'silent' lesions. I wasn't sure I liked the idea. If there were new lesions, surely finding out about them would just knock my optimism and confidence. The steroids, though, had done their job. There is ample evidence in the literature that high-dose steroids used in intermittent fashion for flare-ups or relapses greatly improve recovery from each individual episode. It is not so clear whether steroids make much difference long term in terms of progression. I still felt high as a kite from the mental effects of the drugs, but my leg was much better. I still had numbness and pins and needles but in a smaller area, and I still had a bit of trouble telling where my leg was in space unless I was looking at it.

What I really wanted to do was feel normal again. For years I had been very active and physically fit. I ran at least once a week and swam 1500 metres every other day, with one day a week rest on average. That Saturday I woke up and set myself a goal. I was going to go for a run.

I got myself ready and drove down to my favourite running area in bush and parkland at Perry Lakes. Years earlier, *The West* magazine in the local daily newspaper had done a piece on me, in a series headed 'My Favourite Place'. There had been a picture of me running through Perry Lakes, with Sean and Mike as five- and three-year-olds riding along next to me. It really was my favourite place.

The first few steps were like those of a baby learning to walk again, but I felt a rush of excitement go through me as I started to realise I could do it. I was euphoric. I ran and ran and ran. I wanted the whole world to see me running. By the end I was punching the air with my arms. I couldn't believe it. I had done it. I had run for 30 minutes and done some 5 or 6 kilometres.

Now, this may not have been so sensible an idea after five days of steroids. I got home and showered and had that wonderful post-run exhaustion feeling. But I paid a price. I could hardly walk for a few days. My legs ached. Most other parts of me did too. But I could not contain my delight. I knew that until the next attack, I would be able to keep up my fitness and all the happiness that brought me. It was a small victory, but a start.

My brother Pete went home on Sunday. I was following Ian's advice and had let everyone at work know that I would not be back and that my leave was indefinite. I refused to put a finger on how long. I needed to marshal every resource I had to start this process. On Ian Hislop's advice, I had bought a copy of Carolyn Myss' wonderful book *Anatomy of the Spirit* and was starting to explore mine.

The thing that started my search was a small, insignificant email from Pete, about Tuesday. I haven't kept it, because I didn't realise its significance then. It said something like: 'A friend's wife reckons you ought to try gamma linolenic acid. She's taken it for ten years and hasn't had a relapse. There was something in the medical journals about it a few years ago.' A message like that tends to wake you up when you feel there's no hope.

Luckily I am on the Internet at home and can plug into Medline, a medical database of all the papers published in the major international medical journals. Of the 15,000 or so biomedical journals published worldwide, only about 5000 are good enough to make it into Medline. You can search for key words or subjects and cross-reference things. It's a great tool and one with which I was very familiar in my day-to-day work. I fired up Medline and plugged in the key words 'gamma-linolenic acid', then cross-referenced it with multiple sclerosis. A few abstracts of papers came up from the 1980s. I was a bit surprised to see that, yes, there did seem to be a small benefit for patients with MS who took gamma-linolenic acid. In one of the papers there was a bit about linoleic acid deficiency in MS, and it referred to another paper on patients getting better with linoleic acid supplements.

My search had begun in earnest.

LIFE AFTER MUM

Mum died in the early hours of the morning on 30 August 1981, a month after her 58th birthday. She took a carefully calculated overdose of barbiturates. It was her third suicide 'attempt'. I knew she had been bitterly disappointed at being found the first two times. I can't remember where Dad was this time. She had somehow planned it so that no one would be home. She knew exactly what she was doing.

The second time she had tried, I was working in the intensive care unit at Fremantle Hospital at the end of my intern year. It must have been 1979. I got the call while at work late at night. Next morning I met the family in the ICU of a big teaching hospital 15 kilometres up the road. It was to be the first of several times in my life when I was suddenly on the other side of the desk from the doctor. These are always defining moments for doctors.

I remember walking into the ICU. Familiar with all the gadgets. Only hours before, joking with nurses just like these as we enjoyed the desperate camaraderie that comes with constant exposure to death and dying. But suddenly the tears would not stop. Mum on the end of a tube from a ventilator. Eyes puffy. Semiconscious and squeezing my hand. I realised how awful this environment was. How devoid of anything comforting or reassuring.

Mum recovered quickly. She used to say afterwards that the doctors were quite cross with her for being so silly, and were looking at prescribing better antidepressants. I knew this wasn't some gesture or passing phase of depression. She needed to get out, and she was going to. From then on it became a waiting game.

In 1981, I was in my third year as a resident medical officer at Fremantle Hospital. I wasn't a very good doctor. I hadn't enjoyed being a medical student. The endless hours of rote learning and rehashing fact after fact, to pass ridiculously difficult examinations. What a waste. Intelligent, eager young adults spending six years being ground down, losing all their natural inquisitiveness, the need to understand people and sickness, which had led them into becoming doctors. So as an intern, and then a resident, I prided myself on not opening a book, on not reading a journal, on not attending a clinical meeting. Yet I couldn't resist the rather unfashionable teaching of Ian Hislop. It required sacrificing lunch hours, but something in me resonated with what he was teaching.

These first few years determine what sort of doctors we become. Senior physicians are sometimes unaware of just what an important influence they have on young doctors and students. As in all walks of life, medicine is made up of the cynical, the judgmental, and the deeply compassionate and sensitive. Somehow the endless exposure to suffering and death can toughen the softest hearts over the years. Yet some retain their deep humanity. These are the outstanding physicians. Ian Hislop was one of them. It took many years for me to realise just how important an influence he had been.

Midway through my third year as a resident, I had decided to go overseas the following year. I didn't have any career plans. It was to be the first of several times in my life when I threw my future to the wind, to see where it would land. I never regretted doing that, and it always landed where it should. In my reading since I have started to come across the notion of surrender, over and over again. This has served me well over the years, without me knowing it. What a wonderful feeling it is to just throw away what you are doing and embark on something new, with no plans, no itinerary, and only fate to guide you.

Mum knew about my plans to leave. Several threads had come together for her in those last few years. Peter and I had graduated together from the University of Western Australia in 1979, Peter in Science, I in Medicine. Iva and Gina were settled, bringing up their families. Suzie was still a bit unsettled, but looked like staying with her long-time boyfriend and getting married. Mum had always had a few things she was holding on for. By 1981, there wasn't much left. She was beginning to plan her release. She could have held on to see me married, to see our kids, to see Peter marry, to see Suzie marry, and so on. But she was getting much worse. Everything was a huge struggle. The catheter strapped to the side of the wheelchair.

This was a woman described by her neurologist as almost 'regal'. It was too much to bear. I can remember the look in her eyes as I emptied and cleaned her catheter bag, or sprayed some local anaesthetic into her mouth to ease the pain from her 'trigeminal neuralgia'. When it was clear that I would be going soon that just about sealed things, as far as timing was concerned. At least that's how I saw it. I'm sure the others would see it differently.

After Mum died there was an awful emptiness for a long while. Dad was not the same. I had paid the mortgage on the house since graduating from medical school. I had always thought this was the very least I could do after all they had done for me. Despite that, Dad wanted to sell. I don't think he wanted to be around all the reminders any more. Life sort of went on, but with a gaping hole.

So I filled it by travelling for eighteen months, then working in London. Soon I was married, training in the speciality of anaesthesia, and had bought a house in Perth. Life had settled again. Much of the pain of all those years had been wallpapered over, but I realise now it had not really been dealt with. The first stirrings of disquiet came in my job. I had been working at the women's hospital in Perth as a registrar in anaesthesia for a few months. I couldn't really tell why, but little things were starting to get me down. I remember one night after working solidly all day without a break, I trudged past the serving window to the kitchen where they used to leave our meals. It was 11.30 p.m. I had been anaesthetising since 8 a.m. There were two neatly stacked meals with warmer covers on, one on top of the other, both stone cold. I just trudged past and jumped into bed. Within minutes of falling asleep, I was awoken for an epidural in the labour ward. The night just kept going like that. At about 5 a.m., as I lay in the on-call room beginning to drift off to sleep again, my pager went. This time it was a nurse on one of the wards. She wanted me to take out an epidural catheter so that a woman could have her morning shower.

I was overcome with unreasonable anger and resentment. I stormed off to the ward. I had never had difficulty relating to other staff over the years. I had made lots of friends, and wasn't one of those doctors who bullied nurses or paramedical staff. But that morning, I just lost it. When I had finished the nurse quite calmly said, 'Well, if you don't like it, why don't you just resign?' I could only stare at her. It was so obvious. I didn't weigh anything up. I didn't consider the pros or the cons. At times in your life like that, when it has built up to that point, you just do it. I threw my pager into the wall of the on-call room, and left the hospital. When I got home I rang the head of department, and told him I wasn't coming back.

Frankly I didn't have a clue what I would do next. In my confusion, I thought that I hated medicine. But it had really been anaesthesia which wasn't for me. It's a specialty that suits lots of doctors. But for me there was something missing. I just felt I wasn't getting any feedback. There were never any great successes, or grateful patients. There never seemed even a simple thank you. I wasn't getting any rewards.

So I made a few calls. I got some literature on becoming a teacher. This was something I had always felt I would be good at. I got some more on manipulative physiotherapy. And in the spirit of change, I decided to stop putting off having a family. Programming things in your life, timing things perfectly so that finances are right, work is right and so on, seems to be a modern epidemic. But the messages were loud and clear at that moment. There is no right time. How important it is to just go with things, to go where the feelings take you. Within days of resigning, Sean was conceived.

While I was trying to decide what to do next for a job, I visited my old friends down at Fremantle Hospital. Once again, a wise physician who ran the hospital, Dr Peter Smith, provided the necessary guidance. He knew me a lot better than I knew myself. 'I'll just park you in the emergency department for a while. You might find clinical medicine quite a change after anaesthesia for so long.' That was March 1985.

In August 1996, I answered an advertisement for the appointment of the first Professor of Emergency Medicine in Australasia, based at the University of Western Australia and Sir Charles Gairdner Hospital. Once again I was to throw my future to the wind. Unbeknown to me, I almost certainly had one or two MS lesions hiding quietly in 'silent' parts of my brain as I started the next phase of my professional life.

I started on 17 February 1997. A few people have since asked me whether I would have taken the job if I had known I had MS. The answer is certainly no. And yet I would have missed out enormously had I not taken it. Those early years establishing the academic specialty of emergency medicine in Australia proved to be the most rewarding and stimulating of my professional career. Until you challenge yourself, you never quite know what you are capable of. Mind you, the first few weeks at 'Charlies' were very lonely. No consultants, no registrars in training, no teaching program. I had been at Fremantle emergency department for twelve years. I had so many friends there. I missed the camaraderie and friendship enormously. But things worked out really well. As in the rest of my life, circumstances and events seem to get me to where I need to be, to learn the lessons I need to learn.

A little over two years after taking the post, I was to find myself with a whole new set of challenges when MS was diagnosed. The challenges were different, and I was not so well prepared as I was for my professional challenges. In hindsight, too, I had carried with me so many unresolved issues, and had really understood so little of their effects on me, as I busied myself with family and work. Perhaps anything less than MS would not have been a big enough shock to make me look hard at these things. I remember talking to a few friends after the diagnosis. For the previous challenges life had thrown at me, I could tackle them by studying, by getting prepared and working hard. But MS would be different. The challenges couldn't be met by study or passing exams or trying to fix the problem. Life was asking me to concentrate on other things now, things I had not paid enough attention to in the past.

The issue of taking control of the illness was the first I had to face, though. My professional background gave me some advantages. Without that experience, and without eighteen years' worth (since Mum's death) of genuine scientific advances in the management of MS to be sifted through, I could not have tackled in the same way the physical issues surrounding MS. Nor could I have written a book like this, which I hope can help others to effectively deal with this illness. But that is only part of the story. I have a lot of growing to do. There are very painful things about myself and my life I am now starting to face, and a whole new set of perspectives on life to absorb. As with previous changes, I have to trust myself, let go, and just go where they take me.

WRITING THE BOOK

I started writing this book on 21 July 1999. I know because it's written in my diary. I tried hard to resist writing it. Janet, my secretary at work at the time, who used to make many of the suggestions that turned out to be important in my life, said something about publishers for the book over coffee one morning. Inside, I had been bursting to write this. I was having trouble containing it. In my mind, I had the plan all mapped out. I knew exactly what I was going to say. I just had to find the time to let my fingers tap out on the keyboard the story that was fully formed inside my head.

But I felt that to begin writing it too early would be fraudulent. I had only had MS for just over three months. I couldn't prove that any of what I had been doing had been successful. It was unlikely that I would have had another attack in three months anyway, unless I had a particularly active form of the disease. I thought I should really put if off until I had been well for a year or so. I had my milestones worked out: three months, running the City to Surf 12-kilometre fun run in August, six months, a year, starting the book, etc. Of course things look very different now, writing this new book after a decade free of relapses.

So Janet suggested that maybe I should do a short sample for the publisher. I drafted up a letter to go to several publishers who looked like the right sort. I wrote the prologue in about five minutes. I didn't change a word. It felt like I wasn't writing; it was just the story coming out through my fingers. Within days I got positive faxes back from two publishers in response to just the one page prologue. By then, I had written two more chapters. I couldn't stop. I felt I had this knot in my stomach, which wouldn't be eased until I had finished. Every spare moment went into the book. Seven weeks and one day later it was finished, edited and ready to go.

Although I knew from the moment I started the book what I would write, one thing was not there. The ending. Perhaps this is a good thing. None of us knows how it will end. I wrote this book for people with MS. All over the world, every day, many, many people are walking out of the offices of neurologists with a diagnosis of MS. It is one of the emptiest feelings that can be experienced. I hoped that by writing this book there would be something for these people. MS is a treatable disease. When Mum died in 1981, there wasn't much you could do about MS. Professor Swank was patiently getting on with his work. His patients were doing extremely well, but most of the world didn't know about them yet. We were only just beginning to understand immunology.

The ensuing eighteen years saw an explosion of knowledge about the immune system, cytokines and eicosanoids, auto-immunity, and drugs which affect these. And as more time has gone by, the evidence base about MS has grown exponentially. We are very close to being able to manipulate the immune response. As doctors, though, we have been slow to embrace nutrition as a healing therapy. We have been equally slow to give credit to patients for their own healing. As patients, we have not always been aware of our own inner strengths in combating illness, and these have not always been encouraged by health professionals. We have at times found difficulty accessing the information we need in order to tackle illness. I hope this book addresses these issues. Above all, I trust this book provides hope for people with MS.

This is not the first book written about MS by George Jelinek. Dad's name was George. When Mum died, he wrote a book called *To Live is to Hope*. Strangely enough, although I have had a copy of it ever since, when I went to find it early after diagnosis it had vanished. I looked everywhere. Eventually, I asked Gina and Pete if they had copies. A copy from Gina arrived in the mail on Friday, and Pete arrived on Saturday with his. I felt I needed to read it again before I could finish this book.

When I did read it, I was overcome with sadness. But also helplessness. For about two days, I felt as if I was beaten again. Let me quote a couple of pieces from it. In reading this, keep in mind that Dad learnt

English at the age of 31 when he first came to Australia. I never cease to marvel at how well he used the language, despite it not being his native tongue.

> *Time was quickly passing by and her inability to safely manage the staircase increased. Knowing that every handicapped person must be encouraged to do as much as possible for themselves didn't eliminate our concern for what might happen if she were alone while I was at the office and the children at school. At such time, I very often asked myself a question: 'Why? Why couldn't we sell the house? Surely there are many houses suitable for the handicapped!' Yet, being certain that, at that time, my wife wouldn't agree to the sale of the house, I respected her wish to stay. Throughout my life, I did and still do believe in the free mind of the individual human, for this is the most treasured thing in the world. Any one of us must be given a chance of complete freedom of mind to take any direction one wishes.*
>
> *The days and weeks passed very quickly. My wife's inability to walk reached such a degree that finally she spoke out: 'I believe that all of us know the difference between a house and a home and I am sure that this house became our "home" quite a long time ago. At the same time it disturbs me to know that by staying here any longer all of you will never stop worrying about me. To eliminate all of this, why not sell the house? After all, who knows what will happen tomorrow and what way the world will go. How it will end and why we are here? I believe there is one story in the world. Humans are caught in their lives, in their thoughts, in their hungers and ambitions, in their avarice and cruelty and in their kindness and generosity too—in a net of good and evil. I think this is the only story we have and that it occurs at all levels of feeling and intelligence.*
>
> *'Yes,' she continued, 'we have only one story. All novels, all poetry are built on the never-ending contest in ourselves of good and evil. What a blessing it is that evil must constantly spawn, while good and virtue is immortal; evil must always find a new and fresh face, while virtue is venerable as nothing else in the world is. I have a lot of problems and yet, I am grateful! Grateful to you all, not only for your love and understanding, but mainly for the fact that we are still living as a family and if the sale of the house will help us—let's do it!'*
>
> *Within the next few weeks our house was sold and we moved into a much larger house.*

Months and years passed by and once again we were facing the inadequacy of the new house.

'No more selling,' we decided unanimously with my wife, 'this time we will call in the experts and see what could be done.' After a few consultations with various building contractors, a plan was made to construct a wooden platform covering the three steps on the front of our house, thus enabling my wife to drive her electric wheelchair from the house directly on the footpath leading to the street.

A small portable wooden platform was placed between the doorstep and the floor of the back patio and from then my wife didn't experience any difficulties in driving her chair onto the patio and barbecue area. Once again the shadows of multiple sclerosis were defeated and for a while the singing and guitar playing of our two sons echoed nearly every evening from our place to the tall trees bordering our back garden, while the gentle echo bounced back into the open windows.

But it was only the beginning. After twelve months the songs were no longer there. Not that they were forgotten. Music and songs, as well as dances, definitely mirror life and happiness. Our house was still full of life. Life in every variation, but happiness. The dark horror of multiple sclerosis was spreading its wings once again.

When I read this book, and saw the inexorable progression of MS in Mum, I wished there was something I could have done. But in the 1970s we simply didn't know enough. Once you had MS, you waited, passively, hoping it wouldn't be too bad. That is how I felt as I came out of the doctor's office when I was told. And I felt it again when I re-read Dad's book.

But it is no longer true, and with each passing year more and more research is being done. There is so much we can do. Yet people being told they have MS often go home feeling just like this, feeling like they have been given a sentence. But now there is hope. The key is to stop the disease progressing. Much scientific endeavour still focuses on healing damaged nerves, on remyelination. But realistically, we have some time to wait yet before these therapies may be available. What we do have right now are therapies which have either been 'proven' or hypothesised to slow the progression of MS. Nutrition, sunlight, meditation, exercise, positivity. They are all natural healers. We also have powerful drugs if these fail, or to use in conjunction. We now have real hope.

The foreword to my father's book was written by Mum's neurologist. He said:

This is the heart-rending story of a courageous woman who suffered deeply from the privations and humiliation of a severe chronic neurological disability. Much of her physical and mental torment was offset by her very supportive family and by many kindnesses shown to her by many people. Fortunately, most sufferers of multiple sclerosis are not so profoundly afflicted, even many years after its onset. One is heartened to know that severe chronic disability is still compatible with an enjoyment of life which can at times be supreme.

My book is about Mum, MS and me. It was Mum's story. But it has become mine. I don't know how it will end. In many respects, I am glad for that. While the life I had before MS may have seemed perfect to some, it was not. The process of sorting out the 'dis-ease' in my life that gave rise to MS has at times resulted in my life turning into chaos. MS has caused me to throw away security and comfort, to go where the winds have blown me. In some ways, it has woken me up. I think in many ways I needed it, although I have never felt such pain and loneliness as I did in the early years after diagnosis. But it has redefined some of my values. I have rediscovered some of the poignancy in simple moments. I have much to look forward to. I trust that you do too.

THREADS

And so Mum has come back into my life. All these years after her death. For the sake of my own survival, I have had to come face to face with agonies I have tried hard to bury and repress. The pain of reliving these things, and of deeply feeling things I have not felt since childhood, has been enormous. It is no longer a question of doing these things so that I can deal with MS. I now know that facing these things is fundamental to my whole life, to my growth and development. Without MS, I may never have faced these things.

My relationship with Mum was a very adult one. Even in the face of MS, she did not seek pity. I related to her no differently than if she did not have MS. I wonder what I would be like if I ended up as she did. The ensuing years have gradually seen Mum slip out of my life in many ways, as you would expect. But since I found I had MS, she has come back. Threads of her life have started to entwine with threads of mine again, in ways I never expected.

Her genetic make-up that was passed on to me contained many things. It contained the blueprint for an analytical mind, the capacity for deep reflection, a love of learning; it also contained the seeds of MS. I don't know how much that was responsible for me getting MS, and how much of it was my lifestyle. I feel that, probably, I didn't get the disease until I was 45 because many factors related to my diet and environment were quite favourable. But Mum and I looked very much alike. I think Peter and my sisters would agree. We were alike in many other ways as well. I know it is illogical but it seems sometimes that I got a big dose of her DNA. The 'soil' was perfect for MS to grow. Whatever, she had MS, and I have MS.

And now, a quarter of a century after she died, she is very much alive for me. The process I have been through since diagnosis has ensured that I have dreamt of her, spoken to her in my thoughts, walked along the beach with her, changed her catheter bag. At times, I have felt the pain so acutely, that I just wanted to stop and forget everything and hide. At others, I am grateful we could be reunited, even if it is for this reason.

There are other reasons as well. MS has forced me to confront a lot of the fears I have had since I was a little boy, fears that stemmed from my relationship with Mum but had nothing to do with MS. MS provided the spark for me to change my life, and now I am re-shaping it with a growing awareness of the influences my childhood has had on me. As I write this I am beginning to feel more secure in myself, with a growing trust that I will be okay.

Mum was buried in a place about as far removed from a cemetery as you can imagine. It is a tranquil parkland, full of Australian native trees and shrubs. Mum's ashes lie under a grass plant, a classic Australian native plant, with a twisted black trunk and spiky, brittle green shoots radiating out from the centre. Dad's ashes are next to hers. I took the kids up there once. My youngest, Pia, fell into the pond. I wrapped her in a blanket and took her, lip trembling, back home. A shivering, unhappy little three-year-old. Every now and then I sit down in front of Mum's spot, thinking and talking to her, seeking her wisdom and comfort.

I think about my own death a lot. What will I have been through before that happens? I can't tell. I go from times of great inner strength, seeing myself as a white-haired 70-year-old man, striding along the beach, skin golden brown, to times of weakness, fear and self-doubt, although these are less and less common with time.

Somehow, though, she is here for me now. Like the little boy I was, I feel her cradling my head on her shoulder, stroking my hair. The way she used to press her cheek against my forehead when I was sick, to see if I had a temperature. She is Mum again for me; the energy of her spirit which lives on in me literally guides my hand as I write this, even now as I come to the end of this particular journey, as I find answers that she could never have found. Somehow my getting MS is helping me to learn how to look after myself all these years after she died, helping me to eventually find my own inner peace and confidence after all this pain and difficulty.

2

ABOUT THE BOOK:
EVIDENCE, RESEARCH
AND STATISTICS

I would much rather know what sort of person has the disease than what sort of disease a person has

Hippocrates

My brother's innocent email message started me on a search. This culminated in my discovery of a whole host of ways in which the progression of MS could be slowed. In the next section of the book, I outline all the different forms of therapy I found in my search. The focus in MS really needs to be on early diagnosis and the institution of measures that will slow down or stop the progression of disability. Once disabled, although there are many therapies and aids that make life easier, at present the conventional medical teaching is that normal function cannot be restored. Hence my focus is on preventive treatment, although I believe that this conventional outlook is also pessimistic.

In any event, most of the recent breakthroughs in treatment of this disease have been therapies that have been shown to slow disease progression. As we develop more understanding of the immune basis of MS, and as the science of immunology grows, so we develop new ways of manipulating the immune system to our advantage. It is quite possible that people who elect to start on currently available therapies today will take them for only five to ten years, by which time we can expect major breakthroughs and newer, more specific immune system treatments.

LIFESTYLE CHANGE AND WELLNESS

My concentration, however, is on lifestyle change and wellness, and this is no accident. Although a specialist emergency physician with a typically conservative medical background, I have also experienced MS from a patient's perspective. Treatments look very different when you have to take them yourself. Side effects take on a new meaning. Giving yourself an injection each day compares rather unfavourably with taking a tablet, or changing your diet and getting some exercise. Studies which have not 'proven' the treatment to be beneficial but which suggest a major benefit look much more interesting when you actually have the disease, especially when the treatment has other health benefits as well.

I deliberately begin with less conventional yet more mainstream therapies, such as diet and sunlight. While the drug therapies of interferon, glatiramer, and other immune-modulating agents have been more accepted, the lifestyle changes provide other health benefits as well and are much more empowering. In some cases they have been studied in detail over much longer periods, and just as thoroughly. While modern medicine often concentrates on drug therapy, this is just an ancillary to genuine health. There is growing evidence that lifestyle change is in many cases more effective than drug therapy, particularly in Western degenerative diseases, of which MS is one.

Despite this effectiveness, lifestyle change is often not promoted. This is partly because drug therapies are often heavily promoted by pharmaceutical companies, who stand to do very well if their drugs are widely taken up, but also because, as doctors, we often underestimate the ability of patients to make healthy changes to their lifestyles.

> Lifestyle changes are generally the most effective therapies for chronic Western diseases, of which MS is one.

For instance, research published in *Diabetes Care* in 2006 showed that a low-fat vegan diet was not only better than the currently recommended diabetic diet, but also more effective than standard diabetes drugs.[1] Yet very few people with diabetes are on such diets, the vast majority taking the medications. A major 2007 review in the *British Medical Journal* showed that people with glucose intolerance who were about to develop diabetes were 50 per cent less likely to if they adopted lifestyle approaches to modify the disease including diet and exercise; in contrast, those who relied on drugs were only 30 per cent less likely to develop the disease.[2] On a trip to India, I noticed the *Times of India* reported that the largest-ever study on lifestyle interventions in coronary heart disease, the Abut Healthy Heart Trial, had shown that a low-fat vegetarian diet, combined with exercise and meditation, actually caused a reversal of coronary heart disease. Cholesterol also fell by 24 per cent and the amount of blood pumped out by the heart per beat increased by over 30 per cent.[3] Again, most people with coronary heart disease are on at least one medication, often with problematic side effects, without embracing lifestyle changes with proven substantial benefit.

One of the great values of these lifestyle changes, apart from positive side effects, is that they empower the individual and usually make you feel better. This was well demonstrated by Dean Ornish, showing the health benefits of comprehensive lifestyle change, first in heart disease[4] and then in prostate cancer,[5] but additionally reporting the improvements in quality of life for those making the lifestyle changes.[6] But it's obviously not just about feeling better; at two years after commencing the study, for instance, only 5 per cent of Ornish's patients with prostate cancer who had adopted the lifestyle approach had required conventional medical treatment for the cancer, compared with 27 per cent of those on standard therapy.[7]

PRESENTING THE EVIDENCE

In this book, I present a full discussion of all the potential therapies I have encountered in my search through the medical literature, not just those which have been 'proven' according to modern criteria. In the chapter on clinical studies into dietary fats, I go into what constitutes proof in science in more detail. This is a slippery concept at best, and is not as straightforward as it may seem. I also go through evidence from all levels of scientific endeavour, not just randomised controlled trials. It is sometimes easy to overlook basic science, laboratory and animal research, as well as many other study designs in human research. Overall, my goal is to assemble the most important evidence about what can be done to improve the outlook for people with MS and analyse it from a medical scientist's perspective, but also the perspective of a person with MS, and make it easily accessible for other people with MS. I hope that I will provide enough background on the evaluation of scientific literature to enable people of any background to make a thoughtful analysis of the evidence. In this electronic age, the evidence is much more easily accessible for all people than it ever has been.

I include references to the literature where possible. Some may wish to go to the original paper and read it in detail. Importantly, the scientific papers are not opinions published in the popular press: the articles come from the major reputable medical journals in the world, and represent a distillation of the most significant scientific thought and study on MS. It is important that you be the judge, though. For a therapy to work optimally, it helps to believe it will work and be prepared, in many cases, to make commitments to ensure it will work. This applies particularly to therapies involving major changes to lifestyle, such as dietary changes and exercise.

Some may feel it is too soon after diagnosis to go into the medical literature in any depth, and others may not feel like delving into it at all. For this reason, I start each chapter with a box that includes 'Summarising the evidence' and 'Evidence-based recommendations'. This may be enough for many people who don't want to go into all the science in detail. Some may wish to just skip the scientific background altogether, and go straight to my recommendations. So I have put the chapter 'Evidence-based lifestyle and therapy recommendations' at the end, and gone into detail here on the exact components of the Recovery Program. These are the synthesised guidelines of all the current evidence out there about how to recover from MS. If people just want to read this, then at some future time it will be worth going back and looking at the reasons behind these recommendations.

But my suggestion is to take the book step by step. Go through it systematically so that a clear picture can emerge of what MS is, how lifestyle factors affect its development and progression, and what results the many drug therapies that have been tried in MS have had in improving the outlook for people with MS. Then, having looked at all the evidence, go on to the summary of my recommendations and make up your own mind about which of these treatments you want to commit to. Understanding the evidence makes that commitment much easier to sustain. It is important to realise right at the outset that recovery from MS requires a sustained commitment over many decades, really the rest of your life.

I think it helps to go through the science before making any commitments on what to do but, equally, the section on the mind–body connection should not be missed. While this is supposedly less 'scientific', I make no apologies for presenting this in detail. A whole generation of doctors seems to have forgotten how important the patient is. Yet there is abundant medical literature on this, and many of the doctors of previous generations were well versed in this area. I believe the various components of the program complement each other in improving the chances of recovery. Dealing with emotional and spiritual problems is just as important in achieving balance and counteracting 'dis-ease' as optimising physical health through diet, sunshine and exercise.

Many neurologists who have read this book find it a good way of giving people the information they need to make informed choices about treatment. One of the participants at the first MS Residential Retreat Ian Gawler and I ran at the Gawler Foundation told the story of her neurologist, who brought the book in to her during a hospital visit when she was having a relapse. He said, 'You are not leaving hospital until you have read this.' Although some doctors get nervous about patients knowing too much, and about some patients becoming 'difficult' when they recommend therapies, in the end it is the patient's right to choose their therapy. If they feel they have made a decision based on all the information, they are more likely to continue with the treatment and to put themselves wholeheartedly into it. I hope that the days of people leaving their doctor's office feeling they have no options open to them are over.

I present evidence on all the major therapies that can slow down or halt the progression of MS. At the beginning of each chapter and at the end of the book I summarise what my recommendations are, based on this evidence. Any two medical scientists, analysing the same data, will not come up with identical conclusions. Some time ago, in my own department, we concluded a study which provided simple, definite answers. Yet we spent a considerable amount of time debating the significance of the findings. The conclusions were potentially quite different, and we chose the one that seemed most sensible to us as researchers. There is quite a bit of 'spin' that can be put on any body of medical evidence; I know people find this a difficult concept. We place an enormous amount of trust and confidence in our doctors. People are often surprised when I tell them that of ten specialists analysing the same medical studies, three or four may favour one treatment, three or four the other, and the rest may be undecided. Or that one in twenty neurologists will not ever prescribe steroids for an MS relapse, for example, because they don't believe they work. This is despite what appear to be unambiguous results of multiple clinical studies.

The recommendations I make are peculiarly my own. They are bound to differ from those of other doctors. What I bring to the process of analysis is an academic background, the experience of editing a major MEDLINE-indexed medical journal for twenty years, and around 30 years of clinical practice in medicine. Far more importantly, though, I have MS. I understand the process of considering the various treatment options for this disease from a very personal point of view. When I make a recommendation it is generally what I consider the best and safest for people with MS, given the available options and taking into account the evidence. I hope I have presented enough evidence and information for people to make their own choices. I also now have the experience of a decade of living with these lifestyle changes, and remaining relapse-free. What started as an abstract, scientific exercise of discovery is now being reinforced by personal experience of the success of the program.

In the chapter on the mind–body connection, I present an extraordinary doctor, Bernie Siegel. Like some of his cancer patients, when diagnosed with MS I set off analysing everything I could get my hands on, to work out what I could do about this disease. But I was fortunate. With my background and experience, I could access virtually everything ever written and studied about this illness. Further, I could analyse it scientifically. I can now, I hope, save many thousands of people newly diagnosed with MS the trouble and difficulty of attempting the same thing. I hope it helps.

INTERPRETING THE MEDICAL LITERATURE ON MS

Before I go into an analysis of the medical literature on MS, there are several ideas and terms to become familiar with. This will help when deciding whether the studies I present constitute any sort of proof for the various therapies which have been tried in MS. My experience helps me judge what sort of weight to attach to the various claims made about individual therapies. Rather than just taking my word for this, though, I want to provide a little background in the ways of interpreting the evidence base which medical scientists use.

Publishing research

Most medical research is published in reputable medical journals. To get a research paper into a journal, the authors must analyse the results of the study, then write it up to highlight what they consider the important findings and how these fit into what we know about a particular disease. Journals use a system known as peer review to decide the worth of these papers. Once received by the journal, papers, if of high enough quality, are sent to other experts (reviewers) in the field for their opinion. Most journals hide the identities of the authors from the reviewers, and vice versa. They feel that this ensures the reviewers won't be influenced by the prestige or position of the authors. Usually, only two experts review a paper, and send their comments back to the editor.

Incidentally, there is a growing body of literature on the process of peer review itself. Most agree that peer review is far from perfect, but that we have few alternatives. Personally, I am against anonymous peer review, and a lot of major journals have now abandoned it as a process. I feel that it allows reviewers licence to make unwarranted attacks on authors from a position of anonymity. Science is poorly served by secrecy. The journal I edited, *Emergency Medicine Australasia*, changed its policy at the end of 1998 from anonymous peer review to disclosing both the reviewers' and authors' identities. I outlined the reasons for this in an editorial in the journal entitled 'Lifting the veil on the editorial process'.[8] We analysed the effect of this policy of openness on the quality of the reviews, and found a trend towards better reviews once the process was open.

Once the reviews are returned, the editor is faced with deciding whether the paper is good enough to be published, on the basis of the reviewers' opinions, and if so whether it requires any modification. For instance, the reviewers may feel that the value of a particular therapy has been overstated, and is not supported by the results. The reviewers don't, however, check that the actual scientific data presented in a paper were real and not fabricated. They are not in a position to do so. The editor may ask the authors to tone down any views the reviewers feel are overstated and publish the revised version, or they may reject the paper entirely.

This system seems to work pretty well, by and large, with most bad pieces of research getting weeded out, and most overenthusiastic claims by researchers being toned down. Nevertheless, it is not perfect. The scientific community, and indeed all patients looking for new treatments for illness, are in the hands of the researchers and the reviewers. We are in a position where we must trust the honesty and integrity of researchers in collecting, analysing and reporting their data, and the fairness of reviewers in reviewing the submitted manuscripts.

Once a paper is published, the rest of the scientific community in that area of medicine then makes a judgment on the published research. Often a journal will commission another expert to write an editorial or a commentary to go with the paper in the same issue. This is intended to put the piece of research into the context of other research in the field, and present a balanced, impartial view of its worth.

Further, the journal is happy to take correspondence about these papers. Letters to the editor of the journal about a particular paper are then published, if of sufficient quality, in a future issue. Sometimes these may be very revealing, as other experts assess the quality of the medical evidence and pass their own comments. Until now, perhaps only the authors and perhaps a few of their colleagues, two other expert reviewers, and the editor have had a chance to critically analyse the paper, yet it is already in print with the tacit backing of a scientific journal behind it.

As far as finding these research papers goes, some are available free, in full, on the Internet. All the abstracts of these papers, that is 250-word summaries, are available electronically through PubMed (www.ncbi.nlm.nih.gov/Entrez), the electronic bibliographic database of the National Library of Medicine of the United States; it references the top 5200 or so of the world's estimated 15,000 medical journals. It is also possible to get paper copies of most of them from a medical library, and a friend or relative who is a nurse or doctor or who works in a paramedical field may be able to copy them. Most hospitals and the health departments in each area have medical libraries, and they may be accessible here.

The abstract is a short (250 words or less) summary of the paper that appears at the front of the article in the journal in which it is published. Abstracts should in theory provide all the information about a paper, but because they are short, and because some journals do not insist on them being very informative, they can occasionally omit a lot of detail. It is usually necessary to go to the original. Indeed, any major paper is best read in full. Often the devil is in the detail. Through PubMed, the original papers can be ordered over the Internet, but of course there is usually a charge.

Randomised Controlled Trials (RCTs)

Medical scientists, in assessing the value of medical evidence, have a pecking order for the strength of the evidence. Generally, at the top they place most weight on studies called randomised controlled trials, and on combined results of several RCTs, so-called meta-analyses. RCTs are where a new treatment is compared in a clinical study to either a known treatment or an inactive substance like salt water or sugar (called a 'placebo'). Patients are randomly allocated to groups receiving either the active treatment or inactive placebo (or other effective treatment if there is established effective treatment against which to compare the new therapy). This latter group, receiving the placebo or previously known effective treatment, is the control group. The results of therapy for the treatment group are compared against what happens to patients in the control group. This is done principally because people taking a therapy for some disease often get some benefit just because they feel that the therapy must be doing them some good (this is known as 'the placebo response'). By using a control group taking just an inactive placebo against which to compare those taking the active drug, this effect can be accounted for.

Incidentally, I have some difficulties with this approach, even though it has been taken up so wholeheartedly by the medical profession. It seems to me to have an underlying message that it is okay to 'trick' patients into getting some response, and to encourage secrecy. It also fails to make maximal use of this powerful response we all have to make ourselves better using our own resources. After all, the placebo or control group doesn't get the full placebo response they would if they were sure they were getting the real drug, because they know there is a 50|50 chance they are taking a placebo.

This method of setting up clinical trials eliminates the effects of bias of various sorts in affecting the outcome of treatment. Firstly it accounts for the placebo response, which should be similar in magnitude between the two groups: the treated group and the control (placebo) group. This assumption, though, may not be realistic, particularly where drugs have powerful side effects which ensure that patients know they are taking them, and hence are more likely get a real placebo response. I will talk about this more in the chapter on interferons, which are a typical example. Secondly, because patients are randomly allocated to the groups, researchers can't, for example, put the people with mild disease in the treatment group and serious disease in the control group, in order to show the treatment in the best light.

While RCTs remain the gold standard by which to assess the value of medical evidence, there are some problems with this technique. One issue is that, now that we have RCTs, many scientists have lost faith in the outcomes of other forms of research. RCTs are only one research methodology. In this book I refer to all sorts of other research, such as case-control studies, epidemiological studies, animal research and basic laboratory research, to name a few. While RCTs are considered the pinnacle of clinical research, they are not the be all and end all. For instance, the evidence that smoking causes cancer, which we all accept, was not from RCTs but from population-based epidemiological and case-control studies.

> Evidence-based medicine is not restricted to randomised trials and meta-analyses.

As one of the key figures in the development of evidence-based medicine has stated: 'Evidence-based medicine is not restricted to randomised trials and meta-analyses. It involves tracking down the best external evidence with which to answer our clinical questions . . . if no randomised trial has been carried out for our patient's predicament, we follow the trail to the next best external evidence and work from there.'[9] This will be particularly relevant when we come to the stunning body of research on diet in MS, a therapy with astounding potential for keeping people with MS well, but one that has been largely ignored by most doctors in the area because of a paucity of RCTs in the area.

Other specific problems with RCTs, particularly in MS, include the fact that patients may for instance find the therapy so difficult to comply with that they drop out of the study. This messes up the proposed groups for comparison, and raises all sorts of questions about why they dropped out. For instance, did they drop out because the disease became worse and they gave up on the therapy? This would have the effect of leaving in those patients who were going to remain well anyway, regardless of the therapy, making the therapy look better than it really is. This weakens the value of the evidence. Worse, many reviewers and hence journals are not strict about detailing exactly why people drop out of some of these RCTs and hence we cannot make a balanced judgment about the effectiveness of the therapy. Again, this has been criticised, particularly in the interferon studies in MS.

RCTs are typically of short duration because of the complexity of organising them. Using them as the gold standard can therefore ignore other important determinants of the value of scientific evidence. For instance, is a therapy studied over six months to be given the same weight as a study over twenty or 30 years? Long-term studies, by their nature, are stronger because short-term variations in patients' conditions that can occur as part of the natural history of the disease tend to be accounted for. This is particularly important for such a variable and chronically active disease as MS.

There is also the problem of patient numbers. Recruiting patients prepared to take part in these randomised studies is difficult due to the relatively small number of patients with the disease in any given area. This has plagued a lot of the RCTs in MS. If the numbers are small, it is more difficult to get a result that is statistically significant unless the difference between the treatments is very great. This leads on to the tricky area of statistics in clinical trials, an area understood poorly by most doctors, let alone people without medical training. Incidentally, this is one of the reasons why drug research is so dominant in medicine; drug companies have the funds and motivation to support very large, multi-centre studies, but are unlikely to fund studies on diet, exercise or meditation for which there is no financial gain.

Statistics and p values in medical research

Again, I am going to have to get a bit technical to enable an understanding of the statistics involved in these studies. The statistics we use in medicine in comparing two treatment groups are based on probability. It is really important to realise that we cannot actually prove one therapy is definitely better than another in clinical trials. While one group may have better results, that may have happened because of chance. We know for instance that a coin tossed in the air falls about 50 per cent of the time on heads and 50 per cent on tails. But if the number of tosses is small, it may, for example, fall three times in a row on heads. The chances of that happening are $2\times2\times2$ or 1 in 8. It is much less likely, though, that it will fall on heads six times in a row, the chances being 1 in 64, and so on.

In small trials, results may occur further and further away from what we expect to be a 50 per cent chance, like this, just by chance. All the good results might occur in one of the groups by chance. To work out how often the sort of difference in outcome we see between two groups would occur by chance alone, and not because there really is some benefit from the treatment we gave one of the groups, we use standard frequency statistical analysis. This tells us how significant a result is, and what the likelihood is that the difference we found occurred by chance.

Over and over again the medical literature reports a difference between two treatments followed, usually in brackets, by $p<0.05$ (p for probability), for example. What a p value of 0.05 represents is this: If there is actually no difference between say the treatment and the placebo (fake drug), then we would get a result showing such a large difference in favour of the treatment as we have shown in this particular study 1 in 20 times purely by chance. That is, effectively, the odds of this result occurring because the treatment works, and not by chance, are about 20:1.

We can then infer, though we can't prove, that the treatment actually works. We settle on a 1 in 20 figure by convention. But even if the treatment doesn't work at all, if we do the study 20 times, then by chance on one occasion it will appear to work. And, of course, the study may have been done by somebody without a difference being found, but as soon as someone actually finds a difference they are very likely to send it to a medical journal to publish as a new breakthrough. This is yet another confounding factor; it is called publication bias. Journals are more likely to publish papers which show a difference in favour of a treatment than studies showing no difference.

There is nothing magical about the number 0.05 itself. It is only convention. But it sometimes amazes people to know that scientists will completely ignore a study where the p value is $p<0.06$, but enthusiastically endorse one where the p value is <0.05. The difference is only that the probability of the difference occurring by chance in the former study was less than 6 in 100, and in the second study less than 5 in 100. It's interesting to see how rigidly people of science have been trained to think, isn't it?

A couple of things flow from this. The larger the number of patients in a study, the more likely it is that any difference in outcome between treatment and control groups will have a p value less than 0.05. Likewise, the smaller the difference between the groups, the bigger the number of patients needed to get a p value of <0.05. This can be pretty difficult in rare diseases, for instance. If there is a very big difference between the treatment and the control groups, that is if the therapy is highly effective, a statistically significant (p<0.05) difference is apparent with only a small number of patients.

One of the biggest studies in the medical literature, for example, the GUSTO study, looked at a comparison of one type of thrombolytic agent against another agent which was known to be effective, to see which was best. (Thrombolytics are used to 'unblock' clogged arteries to the heart in heart attacks.) Even though the difference between the two agents was tiny, and most would think insignificant in clinical practice because the researchers recruited over 40,000 patients for the study, the p value was less than 0.05, and so the results were said to be significant. As a result the study radically changed practice, with the new drug becoming the accepted treatment.

Thus, a statistically significant result, even if p<0.0001, does not say anything about the magnitude of the benefit, only about how likely such a difference was to occur by chance. With GUSTO the result was unlikely to have been a chance result, yet the magnitude of additional benefit over established treatment was very small, and possibly insignificant. This background knowledge is crucial to understanding the evidence behind some of the controversial treatments for MS.

The Kurtzke Expanded Disability Status Scale (EDSS)

It is worth going over this in a little detail too as most of the studies in MS use this system to determine whether people in the study get better or worse. The scale was devised by Kurtzke in 1983, based on the findings of neurological examination.[10] In most studies, so that there is no bias, neurologists who grade the patients are unaware of whether or not the patients are in the treatment or control group. This is called blinding. A double blind trial is one in which the patient doesn't know whether the substance he or she is taking is the active drug or the inactive placebo, or which of two therapies it is (if two therapies are being compared), and the neurologist doesn't know either. Hence the long-winded description randomised, double blind, placebo-controlled trial.

Kurtzke's EDSS scores eight functional systems from 0 for normal to 5 or 6 for maximal impairment. Based on these functional system scores and the person's ability to walk, the EDSS is determined. The EDSS goes in half point scores from 0.0 for normal to 10.0 for dead from MS. From 0.0–4.0, people are able to walk without assistance, and the

EDSS is derived from the functional system scores. From 4.0–7.5, the EDSS score is determined mainly by how far the person can walk and with what assistance. Essentially, point 6 on the scale represents walking with a cane, and this point is often used as an end-point in studies looking at progression of disability. From 7.5–10.0, the main determinant of EDSS is the person's ability to transfer from wheelchair to bed and to self-care.

While this scale is widely used in most MS studies, it is not used a lot in day-to-day medicine, and is a bit insensitive to changes in people's conditions, particularly once they have difficulty walking. Nonetheless it has stood the test of time.

General cautions about drug trials

It is worth making a few general remarks about drug company-sponsored clinical trials and drug therapies in MS. It is important for people with MS to keep an open mind, perhaps even a critical one, about the supposed benefits of many of the drugs that are widely prescribed in MS, indeed about many of the drugs that are widely prescribed in general. It is unfortunate, but MS is big business. It is a disease of young adults, and if drug companies can develop drugs that are expensive and need to be taken for life, they are in for a financial windfall. For instance, the worldwide market for the interferons in MS amounts to many billions of US dollars annually. This is staggering. When natalizumab (Tysabri) was fast-tracked onto the market by the Food and Drug Administration (FDA) in the United States, it stood to make around US$3 billion in its first year.

Virtually all of the RCTs for these drugs are sponsored by the drug companies who make them because of the expense of the drugs and of conducting such large trials. We know that the results of drug company-sponsored research are less reliable than those of independently conducted research, and that therapeutic claims tend to be exaggerated. For instance, it has been shown that drug company-sponsored research is four times as likely to be favourable to a company's product than independently conducted research;[11] authors of company-sponsored research are more than five times as likely to recommend the company drug as independent authors, regardless of results;[12] and researchers with industry connections are far more likely to favour company products. In one study of calcium channel-blocking drugs used in heart disease, 96 per cent of authors of papers favourable to the drug had financial ties to the company making it, versus 37 per cent of those critical of the drug.[13]

These sobering research findings may surprise some readers, and indeed they should. We should have more faith in our medical researchers. Worse still, the doctors conducting drug company-sponsored trials have a vested interest, often financial, in ensuring that the drugs are prescribed once they are released. A 2007 study published in the *New England Journal of Medicine* confirmed these strong financial links between medicine and the pharmaceutical industry.[14] In that US national survey, 94 per cent of physicians reported financial links with drug companies. Of these, over one-third received financial reimbursements for travel, etc., and 28 per cent received direct payment for lecturing or acting as consultants on behalf of the companies. Further, there was clear evidence that the drug industry focused on opinion leaders in the medical community, as they were the ones with the most influence on the prescribing patterns of their peers.

This is not a conspiracy theory, this is actually what happens in modern drug-focused medicine. A neurologist I know suggested to me that the best place to go to find the latest information on new drugs is the *Financial Times*, not the medical journals. This is because the drug companies' share prices are directly affected by such things as the reporting of unexpected side effects, and drug companies must disclose these things urgently to the Stock Exchange or risk serious financial consequences. For instance, the day the medical community found out about the unexpected deaths from natalizumab, the two sponsoring drug companies' share prices fell dramatically and it was front page news in the financial papers. To read more about the real problems faced by ordinary health care consumers because of the insidious influence of drug companies, I recommend *The Truth About the Drug Companies* by Dr Marcia Angell, former editor in chief of the *New England Journal of Medicine*.[15] Here she states, no doubt to the grave concern of many ordinary consumers of health care, 'In many drug-intensive medical specialties it is virtually impossible to find an expert who is not receiving payments from one or more drug companies.'

OVERVIEW

I have gone over the background knowledge required to be familiar with the terms and techniques used in modern medical research. Now to MS.

In the next chapter, I provide some background medical data about MS. I hope this helps in understanding the illness and the rationale behind some of the therapies. Then I explore the evidence, looking closely at the many studies and RCTs in MS.

3

ABOUT MS:
UNDERSTANDING THE ILLNESS

One of the most life-altering diagnoses a person can receive

T.N. Fawcett

Multiple sclerosis is a chronic, usually progressive disorder of the nervous system. It is the most common neurological disorder in young adults. It has a very uneven geographical distribution, being common in affluent so-called 'Western' industrialised countries, and also progressively more common in countries further and further away from the equator.

WHAT IS MS?

MS is a disease of the central nervous system (CNS). The CNS is the term used to describe the brain and spinal cord. MS is described as an inflammatory demyelinating condition. Taking the inflammatory part first, inflammation can best be thought of by picturing how angry a wound gets when it becomes infected. It may help to recall a cut or abrasion which has become infected. Typically, the wound gets hot, red, swollen and painful. Gaelen, in very early medical writings, first described the findings in inflammation as *rubor et calor, tumor et dolor*. This means

43

redness and heat, swelling and pain. He added *et functio laesa* which
translates as 'and loss of function'. So the inflamed part stops working
as well. These are the typical features of inflammation. At a microscopic
level, the immune system sends white cells to the area. These cells secrete
messenger chemicals which cause the inflammatory reaction, and they
dispose of bacteria, debris and foreign substances in the wound.

Demyelination refers to the myelin sheath around nerves. The CNS,
that is the brain and spinal cord, is predominantly fat. The type of fat that
is incorporated into the cells that make up the CNS depends on what we
eat. The membranes of cells are the outer envelopes which hold in the
cellular contents. They are made of a double layer of lipids (fats). It takes
some months, but after changing to a diet consisting of different fats there
are quite marked changes in cell membrane composition. It is important
to remember that our bodies are not static, unchanging structures like
a table or a rock. Deepak Chopra in his excellent little book of insights
Journey into Healing says, 'Just one year ago, 98 per cent of the atoms in
our bodies were not there. It's as if we live inside buildings whose bricks
are being systematically taken out and replaced.'[1]

> MS is an inflammatory, demyelinating condition.

Importantly, because of the different chemical properties of the fats,
that is their respective melting points, the cell membranes of people who
consume mainly unsaturated fats are more fluid and pliable than of those
who consume saturated fats. For people who eat mainly saturated fat cell
membranes are more rigid and inflexible, and more prone to degenerative changes.

Nerve cells in the CNS have many branches, which reach out and
travel to other nerve cells, so that they can communicate by transmitting
electrical impulses. These branches or axons are like telephone wires
connecting phones so that they can 'talk' to each other. They are coated
with a form of electrical insulating material called myelin. Myelin is
essentially the fatty coating around the axons which results from specialised cells (oligodendrocytes) wrapping themselves around and around
the axon, like continuous layers of an onion. This coating is fatty because
the membrane or outer coating of every cell is made up largely of fat, so
when the cell wraps itself around and around the axon the multiple layers
form a fatty sheath.

It is important to recognise as well that the signals which pass down the axons are not really electrical currents, but appear to be, due to the rapid movement in and out of the cells of charged particles called ions. These are the minerals we are very familiar with like sodium, potassium, calcium, magnesium and so on, and again, these largely come from the diet. So diet is crucial to nerve conduction. Demyelination occurs when some of this myelin is broken down; inflammatory demyelination means that the myelin is broken down as a consequence of inflammation of the area.

The typical sequence of events then, is that inflammation of a portion of the myelin sheath of a nerve in the CNS is followed by demyelination. This forms the so-called 'lesion' of MS. These lesions were often in the past called plaques, but this is a bit of a misnomer as it implies that something is coating the nerve. In these inflammatory lesions, white cells of the immune system gain access to the myelin sheath, which they usually can't do because of what is called the 'blood-brain barrier'. Further white cells are probably attracted by some of the chemical messengers released by these initial white cells. The demyelination is followed by some repair and scarring, as usually happens after an episode of inflammation. The functional result is that nerve impulses don't travel along the axon as well as they did before it was injured.

SYMPTOMS OF MS

What the person with MS experiences depends on what the affected nerve connects to. If it is a nerve axon in the spinal cord bringing sensory messages up from the legs, then the person might notice tingling or numbness. If it is carrying motor messages down to the leg muscles, there may be some weakness. If they are nerves inside the brain responsible for, say, the sense of balance, it may be impossible to walk without tipping over to one side. Because there is some swelling of the surrounding nervous tissue associated with this process of inflammation, nerve transmission through these nearby axons will also be affected. As the swelling subsides, these nerve cells which aren't seriously injured, but are not functioning because of inflammation and swelling, start to work again. So there is almost always some recovery for this reason alone. Also, some limited repair of damaged nerve cells takes place with some remyelination, particularly early in the disease, so the symptoms further settle to some degree. There is growing evidence now that remyelination occurs throughout the disease and is considerably more prominent than we have realised to date.[2]

Thus the area of numbness or tingling is likely to get smaller and the weakness is likely to improve over time, as the lesion heals and scars, and the nerves which are not actually injured but are not working well due to swelling recover. Recovery though is often incomplete and people are left with residual symptoms, although less severe than when the attack was at its peak, in the same part of the body. These residual symptoms typically wax and wane depending on numerous factors. Most important of these for most people with MS is the temperature. Nerves conduct less well the warmer they get. So heat tends to make these residual symptoms worse for most people. But dietary factors like the minerals in the diet are also important for day-to-day nerve conduction. An important point here is that although heat makes the nerves conduct more slowly and the symptoms worse, it is not actually damaging the nerves. So exercising is fine even if it makes symptoms temporarily worse.

Gradually, as more and more of these lesions occur in the CNS, more and more pathways are knocked out. Hence the person notices gradual decline in function. A lot of these lesions occur in 'silent' parts of the brain and so are not noticed. The ones we really notice occur in the spinal cord or in the nerves leading to the eye. Virtually all of these nerve fibres are essential for things like sensation, power, balance, vision and so on. Even a small lesion here is therefore usually noticed. It is a bit like the fact that we can tolerate a few problems in particular programs on a computer (the brain) without noticing too much, but if the cable (spinal cord) connecting to the monitor gets damaged we lose a lot.

A lot of research is now being done on how the CNS attempts to repair these lesions. The nervous system has an amazing capacity not only to regenerate so that impulses can now 'detour' around the damaged lesion, but also in the brain changes occur which involve recruitment of new nerve cells and pathways to compensate for what is missing.[3] When there are only a few lesions, the CNS is extremely good at this regeneration and compensation, even if there isn't much remyelination. However, if the process continues, these compensatory mechanisms become overwhelmed and progressive disability occurs. Hence my focus on stabilising the disease early and preventing further damage after initial diagnosis.

Optic neuritis

For many people, the first attack of MS will affect the eyes. Optic neuritis is the term for inflammation of the optic nerve, the major nerve carrying visual information from the retinas behind the eyes to the brain. Optic neuritis is a common cause of relatively sudden loss of vision in one eye in young people.[4] People who develop optic neuritis have a 40–50 per cent chance of developing MS in the next fifteen years.[5, 6] The best predictor of the risk of subsequent MS for someone who develops optic neuritis is the presence or absence of other lesions in the brain on MRI at the time of the attack.[6] About 25 per cent of people with no lesions at the time of the attack go on to get MS, but if there is one or more lesions the risk is about 75 per cent. Women are also more likely than men to go on to develop MS after an attack of optic neuritis. The presence of spinal cord lesions at the time of the initial attack appears to be the most important predictor of subsequent disability.[7]

Optic neuritis is the first presentation of MS for about 15–20 per cent of people with MS.[8] Between a third and a half of all people with MS develop optic neuritis at some point in the illness.[8] Even for those people with MS, the long-term outlook for vision after an attack of optic neuritis is good, with 72 per cent having normal vision in at least one eye and two-thirds having normal vision in both at fifteen years.[9]

Many neurologists argue that people developing optic neuritis who have MRI changes suggesting a greater likelihood of developing MS should start on one of the disease-modifying therapies like glatiramer or interferon immediately.[10, 11] Such therapy has been shown to delay or prevent the onset of MS substantially. I would equally argue that rapidly adopting the Recovery Program is a priority for anyone diagnosed with optic neuritis. There is every reason to believe that this is likely to prevent the onset of definite MS. The role of steroids in optic neuritis is less clear. While intravenous steroids are commonly prescribed to speed up resolution of symptoms, they don't seem to affect the long-term outcome for vision.[12]

HOW COMMON IS MS?

In the United Kingdom it occurs in approximately 1 in 800 people, affecting around 90,000 people, and in northern Europe approximately 1 in 1000. In the United States, there are between 250,000 and

350,000 people with MS, and it has been estimated that there are about 2.5 million people with MS worldwide. There is evidence that the disease is becoming more common. A US study from 2007 showed that MS had become 50 per cent more prevalent there over the previous 25 years.[13]

In Australia there are around 20,000 people with the illness and there is a marked increase in incidence the further one is away from the equator. In far north Queensland, for instance, the disease affects about 12 people per 100,000, rising to about 36 in New South Wales, and peaking at around 76 people per 100,000 in Tasmania. This effect of MS being more common the further one gets from the equator applies from country to country as well as within countries.

It is very likely that the incidence of the disease is increasing. A 1922 review from the United States showed that the incidence had increased over the preceding twenty years.[14] Swank, in his *Multiple Sclerosis Diet Book*, cites a 1952 report which indicated that the incidence of MS had doubled in Europe early in the twentieth century, and other data from his own health system in Montreal document a 50 per cent increase from 1935 to 1958.[15] More recently a 2005 study from Sardinia, a high risk area for MS, showed that the incidence of MS on the island had increased more than fivefold over the 30 years to 1999.[16] There are now data from several countries including Japan, Canada and Ireland to show that MS incidence is increasing.[17, 18, 19] Similar increases are being noticed around the world. Data from the MS Society of Western Australia indicate that MS had a prevalence rate of about 30 per 100,000 in 1981; 25 years later the rate had skyrocketed to 114 per 100,000.[20]

> MS is common, particularly further from the equator, and its incidence is increasing.

***

MS is a 'modern' disease. Textbooks are not definite about when it appeared but it seems that we first got descriptions of the disease in the mid 1800s. Swank says the first case recorded in the literature was that of Augustus D'Este, who suffered an attack at the age of 28, followed by remission, at the beginning of the nineteenth century. He then documented in his diary a series of relapses and remissions which, to those now familiar with MS, is characteristic of the disease. Swank points out that by the turn of the twentieth century, the disease was commonly recognised throughout Europe.

For many diseases we get really good descriptions going back into antiquity if they have been around that long. Despite often having very little with which to treat patients, the doctors of previous ages practised the art of medicine extremely well. They described patient's signs and symptoms beautifully. Many would argue that today's doctors are very poor at this aspect of medicine. Thus we have detailed descriptions of pneumonia and stroke and so on, going back to the earliest records. Syndromes consistent with what we know to be MS have only been described, though, over the last 150 to 200 years or so.

Any disease that, like MS or coronary heart disease, has appeared only in recent times and increased rapidly in incidence is very likely to be caused or at least precipitated by lifestyle changes that the human race has made due to the industrial and technological revolutions. Most of these lifestyle changes centre around diet and exercise. A really good account of the changes in foods and diet over recent years is provided by Dr Simopoulos in *The Omega Plan*.[21] She also details much of the current knowledge of fats in the genesis of modern degenerative diseases.

Dr Simopoulos shows us graphically how the fats in human diets have changed over the centuries. She illustrates the sudden dramatic changes to the balance of dietary fats which occurred for the first time in human history around the beginning of the 1800s, with a sharp and sustained rise in the proportion of saturated animal fats in the human diet. The fact that MS is first recorded around this time is no coincidence. Later I present abundant evidence about the pro-inflammatory effect of saturated fats in the diet, and the anti-inflammatory effect of unsaturated fats. The fact that a range of other auto-immune diseases is also on the increase should come as no surprise to us.

Sex and age distribution

MS typically affects people in their twenties or thirties but no age is immune. With better diagnostic tests these days, MS has been found in very young children and in the elderly. Experts have estimated that as many as 20,000 children in the United States may have the disease but are not yet diagnosed. Children have been diagnosed with MS as young as four years old. Women have always been affected more commonly than men, in a ratio of around 3:2, but the ratio is changing towards a much greater female preponderance now of the order of 3:1.

A major study from Canadian Collaborative Study Group in 2006 showed that the sex ratio of females to males with the disease in over 27,000 Canadian people with MS had changed significantly over the previous 50 years.[22] The ratio was now over 3.2 women for every man with MS. This is supported by a 2007 French study.[23] The significance of these findings is twofold. First, it implies that incidence of the disease is increasing, but more importantly it shows that environmental factors play the major part in the risk of getting the disease and, therefore, that many cases are preventable with changes to these factors. We shall later see that these factors mostly relate to lifestyles we have adopted in Western society.

Genetics of MS

MS is more common in family members of people with MS. I was unaware of this until I was diagnosed with MS. Some authorities say it is up to 80 times more common in first-degree relatives like brothers and sisters or children. We now know that identical twins have 300 times the risk of other people of getting MS if the other twin has the disease. It has long been taught that for ten pairs of identical twins in which one of each pair gets MS then three of the other twins will get the disease, that is, a 30 per cent risk.

> MS is a disease that runs in families.

A very large Danish study in 2005 clarified this further.[24] This study of 13,286 people with MS showed that amongst identical twins the risk was 24 per cent, and for non-identical twins the risk was 3 per cent. A first-degree relative such as the son of a mother with MS has 20 to 40 times the risk of getting the disease than someone without such a relative.[25]

There has now been from Canada a very substantial research effort expanding our knowledge in this area. The Canadian Collaborative Study Group has published a number of groundbreaking papers on various aspects of the family risks of getting MS. Initial studies published in 1995 showed that the increased risk of MS in a family was due to genetic factors, that is, factors passed from parent to child, not factors in the shared family environment.[26] The researchers screened 15,000 people with MS with questionnaires, and compared the risk of MS in genetically related family members to that in family members who had been adopted, and therefore were not genetically related. Adopted family members had no higher risk than the general population of getting MS. This is reassuring for people who may worry about 'catching' MS by living with someone with MS. It is clear that this does not happen.

More recently this has been confirmed by the same group in Canada, who evaluated MS risk in 687 step-siblings of 19,746 MS index cases to determine whether any transmissible factor in a family's micro-environment might enable one to 'catch' MS.[27] They found the risk of MS in these step-siblings to be indistinguishable from that of the general population. So it is clear now that there is no transmissibility other than genetic from one affected individual to another in this high MS prevalence area of Canada. So environment influences MS risk at a population level, not a family level.

The step-sibling research suggested that the majority of the risk comes from the mother having MS, at approximately twice the risk of getting MS as if the father has MS.[28] This has been contradicted by US research showing that men with MS pass on the disease twice as often to their children as women.[29] A very large Canadian study examined this question carefully in response to this discrepancy, and found there was equal transmission of MS from affected fathers versus affected mothers.[30] A follow-up study of the actual genes involved in determining suscep-tibility to MS showed that, as expected, MS is not inherited as a result of a single gene, like diseases such as cystic fibrosis or muscular dystrophy.[31] The susceptibility to MS is the result of the interaction of several genes, probably over 100 genes, each with small effects.[32, 33] Hence predicting its occurrence in offspring is not possible at present.

A key area of interest for many people is estimating the increased risk of getting MS that a brother or sister of someone with the disease has. I know that my own brother and sisters were understandably concerned about this when I was diagnosed. The Canadian Group has shown that the risk is higher if a parent also has or had MS, if the disease occurred at an earlier age, and if the sibling for whom we are estimating the risk of MS is female.[34] In my case, my sisters are therefore at comparatively high risk because of their sex, and the fact that Mum had MS, but the risk is a little lower because MS came on in me at a later age. If it had come on in my twenties, their risk would have been about as high as it could get, around a 1 in 10 chance (using the Canadian data). My brother's risk is about half that of my sisters.

To put this into perspective I have made a table of the risks, using the data from the British Columbia study (Table 1). This is Canadian data, so the rates may be different from those in other areas. Nevertheless, the relative risks should still be roughly the same, and can be compared to the normal baseline risk for the general population in Canada. This is a lifetime risk of getting MS of about 1–2 per 1000, or around five times the risk in Australia, depending on location.

Table 1: Risks of getting MS (per 100) for family of people with MS

	Risk for sister	Risk for brother
No parent with MS		
Brother has MS	2.3	1.5
Sister has MS	2.7	0.6

It should be noted that the risk to siblings was three to four times higher than this if a parent also had MS. The risk was five times higher if the brother or sister got MS at age twenty years or less, compared to whether the brother or sister was 40 years or more when they got MS. Thus for sisters of someone with MS, where a parent has had it as well, the risk is as high as 8.1 per cent, and even higher if the patient's MS came on under twenty.

So there is no doubt that genetics plays an important part in susceptibility to developing MS. Interestingly, there is evidence that once an individual has the right genetic make-up to develop MS, one of the factors which can reduce the risk of it developing is childhood exposure to a wide range of infectious diseases.[35] It is felt that this exposure makes the immune system more tolerant of challenges to it later in life.

TYPES OF MS

MS is said to occur in four main forms, but it is still uncertain whether the underlying process is different in these or whether there are more than four distinct types. Up to 20 per cent of patients are said to have benign MS, but most authorities put this figure at around 6 per cent.

This means that they suffer one or two attacks, but either that is all or they have only very occasional further episodes, and remain active. Often these are people whose first attack was of visual disturbance, or other sensory symptoms. Researchers have suggested, however, that we probably overestimate the number of people who have benign disease because we don't account for subtle problems like cognitive disturbance, fatigue, and social and psychological disturbances.[36]

At the other end of the spectrum is primary progressive MS. This is said to occur in about 10 to 15 per cent of cases. In this form of MS, people, often middle-aged men, from the first attack progress relentlessly downhill, usually without obvious attacks or remissions.[37] The other 65 to 70 per cent or so of people with MS begin with typical relapsing-remitting MS. This means that they have an attack, followed by some recovery, partial or sometimes total, then a period in which they have no further attacks. This period may be called a remission, because the symptoms remit. Remission is a bad term, though, because it implies that the disease is not active during this period. We know it usually is. This period is then followed by another attack, or relapse.

Most of these patients end up after some years of relapsing-remitting disease progressing to secondary progressive MS. This is the typical later stage of relapsing-remitting MS, where patients again progress relentlessly downhill, presumably due to continued accumulation of lesion upon lesion. Evidence is coming to light now that, even during periods of so-called remission, damage continues to occur to the CNS. Even though attacks may not be obvious to the person with MS, there may be progressive loss of brain tissue. This may become evident in subtle ways, such as the development of memory problems. The obvious attacks are only the tip of the iceberg, and this is one reason why it is so important to get started with therapies to slow down or stop the disease as early as possible.

DIAGNOSIS

The diagnosis of MS used to be a real hit-and-miss affair. I know when Mum was diagnosed, it took some years before the neurologists were sure she had MS. Doctors then used lumbar puncture findings, which weren't specific for the disease, but were highly suggestive, to confirm a clinical picture of someone with several relapses and remissions of neurological symptoms. In a lumbar puncture, a fine needle is inserted into the lower back between two vertebrae, into the area surrounding the spinal cord. From here, cerebrospinal fluid (CSF) is withdrawn and analysed to determine its composition. Even when computerised tomography (CT) scans became available in the 1980s, the lesions of MS were too small to be seen and this test couldn't be used to help diagnosis.

The diagnostic breakthrough came with the development of magnetic resonance imaging (MRI) scanning. MRI is an imaging method which, unlike CT, doesn't use X-rays or other forms of radiation. It uses powerful magnets and sensors to detect minute magnetic fields within cells, so it can be used again and again without any radiation risk to the patient. Mind you, it can be extremely claustrophobic being inside one of these machines. Some people just won't go back a second time. It is possible, though, to ask for a short-acting sedative to make these scans more tolerable. The scans produced enable us to see tiny defects in the CNS. The lesions of MS usually show up even if they are very small, although some will not. MRI is said to show lesions in 95 per cent of people with clinically definite MS.[38] MRI isn't definitive though. Some other diseases produce lesions that look like MS on MRI. It needs to be used in conjunction with the doctor's clinical diagnosis, that is assessment of features of the patient's symptoms, as well as findings on clinical examination.

The MRI breakthrough has led to much more sophisticated clinical trials of therapies for MS. Now, with MRI, for the first time we can be sure of exactly how much the disease has progressed, rather than having to rely on the not so accurate clinical picture of signs and symptoms as assessed by a doctor. This is particularly important given that most of the damage that is occurring can't be detected by clinical examination by the doctor. In turn, though, this has created its own problems. As will be seen later, we may show that a particular therapy decreases the number of new lesions, yet we may not see any difference in the person clinically.[39] This occurred with many of the interferon studies. At least with earlier studies we were using the patient as the yardstick, not what the scan looked like.

Nevertheless, large studies correlating MRI findings with clinical course have now shown that people with MS have significant atrophy (shrinkage) of both white and grey matter in the brain.[40] Secondary progressive patients have more atrophy than relapsing-remitting patients and a higher lesion load. Lesion load and atrophy in this study significantly predicted EDSS score, and grey matter atrophy was the most significant MRI predictor of final disability.

The advent of MRI, although making the diagnosis of MS easier, para-doxically has caused some difficulties. Multiple sclerosis is two or more attacks of scarring in the CNS. It is, by definition, multiple. Previously, people might have had one episode of neurological disturbance, and the doctor may have thought 'This might be MS' but had to wait until a second attack to be more certain. With MRI, we can see the typical lesion often on the first attack. Because it is an isolated lesion, the doctor may call it 'transverse myelitis' if it is in the spinal cord, or some other term. With the MRI though it is now often possible to see evidence of other lesions which perhaps didn't cause any symptoms, thus providing some evidence that the disease is 'multiple'.

Being told the diagnosis

Many doctors feel that to tell the patient they have MS on the basis of one lesion is unfair. They feel it would unnecessarily worry the patient. I'm not sure this is a sensible approach. Until patients become aware that they have MS, they can't begin to do anything about it. Now if the view of the doctor is that this doesn't matter, because there is nothing that can be done about it anyway, then it is denying the patient a chance to take control of the illness. In any event, there is a whole range of things which can be done that have either been shown to work or look highly promising. Patients need to know what is likely to be wrong with them, and what they can start doing about it. For all of these therapies, there is growing evidence that the earlier the treatment is started, the better the outcome.

It is important to note, though, that people who have a single episode of transverse myelitis, often called a clinically isolated syndrome (CIS), but have no lesions on brain MRI, have a very low rate of progression to definite MS, at least over a five-year period.[41] Having lesions on initial brain MRI at the time of the episode of CIS makes the development of definite MS much more likely. Elian and Dean, in *The Lancet* in 1985, showed that people overwhelmingly want to be told they have MS after diagnosis.[42] Only 6 out of 167 surveyed MS patients preferred not to be told. More recently a very large Greek study reported that of 1200 people with MS, 91 per cent favoured being told immediately, yet only 44 per cent had.[43] For 27 per cent it took longer than three years to be told.

Most people with MS wish to be told the diagnosis.

Likewise the guidelines for the management of MS issued by the UK National Health Service National Institute for Health and Clinical Excellence (NICE) recommend that 'if a diagnosis of transverse myelitis is made, the individual should be informed that one of the possible causes is MS'.[44] While the diagnosis of MS is 'considered one of the most life-altering diagnoses a person can receive',[45] it is important for the person to know what they are up against. As one newly diagnosed person with MS noted, 'the potential challenges of the journey ahead have to be viewed with realism, optimism, and meaning',[45] and this journey can't begin until people know what they are facing.

A qualitative study in 2007 reported that all 23 people interviewed with MS reported the moment of diagnosis as powerfully evocative and unforgettable.[46] Its effect on partners too should not be underestimated, with one study reporting feelings of helplessness and isolation.[47] Unfortunately, very poor levels of support and information were sometimes given, and this is something I am commonly told by people with MS.

I was fortunate. The neurologist, because of my medical background I suspect, and the fact that we were colleagues and friends, was very frank with me. Initially when he thought that the spinal cord lesion was the only lesion I had, he said that it was probably the first lesion of MS, even though many doctors would have called it transverse myelitis. I really appreciated this, and I think most people would. Within days I was actively seeking out ways of helping myself, and starting to take control of the illness.

THE COURSE OF MS

MS is essentially a progressive condition. It is uncommon for people with MS not to progress to disability over time. The rate at which this happens has been the subject of much conjecture and mythology, but recent studies have clarified this considerably, particularly now that the introduction of the disease-modifying drugs, interferon and glatiramer, appears to have changed the course of the disease for many people. A large study of the natural history of the condition has shown that a relapsing course is followed by chronic progression in around 80 per cent of cases within 20 years.[48] While there is considerable individual variation in the rate of progression, this process is relatively typical in most patients and seems likely to be degenerative in nature.

Primary progressive MS (PPMS) appears to proceed to disability faster than other forms, although again there is considerable variation. One large study showed that a quarter of patients with PPMS needed a walking cane by 7.3 years after diagnosis; in contrast a quarter still didn't need one at 25 years.[49]

> If nothing is done about it, the great majority of people with MS steadily progress to disability over time.

A recent study suggested that disability progression in MS is actually slower than previously reported.[50] It showed that in a group of 2837 patients with all forms of MS, only 21 per cent needed a cane fifteen years after disease onset, and by age 50, 28 per cent required a cane. These figures are considerably more optimistic than those from many earlier studies, and may reflect the effect MRI has in making the diagnosis in people with subtle clinical features and in making the diagnosis earlier. It should be noted that a very large review has shown that MRI is not particularly accurate at diagnosing MS, and tends to lead to over-diagnosis and over-treatment.[51] The study on disability progression did, however, show that men progressed 38 per cent more quickly than women.

Another US study reported similar findings.[52] In following 115 patients in one county, they noted that the median time from diagnosis to EDSS score of 3 was seventeen years, and to a score of 6 was 24 years. Twenty years after onset, only 25 per cent of those with relapsing-remitting MS had EDSS scores of 3 or more. The median time from diagnosis to EDSS score of 6 for the secondary progressive groups was ten years and for the primary progressive group was three years. Once an EDSS score of 3 was reached, progression of disability was more likely and more rapid. This study again suggests that the progression to disability in MS is not as rapid as previously thought, but does support the importance of stabilising the illness as early as possible after diagnosis to avoid later progression of disability.

A further large study of 1844 patients suggested that MS is really one disease with progressive illness, whether primary or secondary, essentially following the same course.[53, 54] It concluded that for most people with MS, disability landmarks were reached at about the same age. For instance, patients required a cane on average at about the age of 63, give or take a couple of years, regardless of the initial course. It also noted, as in previous studies, that women reached these milestones later than men. The authors suggested that age-related degeneration may be an important mediator of this progression in people with MS.

This is quite positive for people with MS because we know that a number of lifestyle modifications affect the ageing process and its associated degeneration. For instance, daily walking and regular gardening were found in a large Australian study to prevent age-related dementia.[55] We also know that regular long-term supplementation with certain vitamins prevents some degenerative changes in the body. For instance, an Australian study found that long-term supplementation with vitamins from the B group, folate and B12, prevented the development of cortical cataracts in the eye.[56]

PROGNOSIS

One of the difficulties with MS from a medical point of view is that at present we have no way of determining into which group any particular person with MS falls, from the point of view of prognosis. This is both good and bad. Those who are going to have a rapid downhill course won't know about it until it happens, but equally those who needn't worry may do. Although the statistics tell us that women tend to do better than men, and the older people are when diagnosed the more likely they are to go downhill, these are only generalisations, and don't apply to any individual case. I'm glad of that, because the statistics put me in the group with the worst prognosis.

> It is not possible to give an accurate prognosis at the time of diagnosis.

One of the things that has really been missing from MS research has been case-control comparison of these groups in terms of risk factors. It would be extremely important to know, for example, if the group who had benign disease approached things differently, changed their diet or modified their lifestyles, compared with the group who deteriorated rapidly. I can find no such studies in the literature, despite the huge amount studied and written about this disease. Surely, it would be useful to have this information, so that people with MS could make modifications to try to change their risk of deterioration.

The medical literature makes the observation that the only way to predict how someone will go is to observe the progress of the disease. Those with more severe early attacks with poor recovery are more likely to continue in that pattern.[57] An Australian study has found that people have a worse prognosis if they are older at the onset of the disease, have a progressive disease course, have symptoms at onset which are multiple, motor or balance, and have a short time to their first relapse.[58] One of the few constant findings in the MS literature is that the 'sooner to cane, sooner to wheelchair'.[49]

There are many myths about the long-term outlook for people with MS. It used to be said that people with MS did not have a shortened life span compared with the general population, and that no one dies of MS. In fact, it is clear that people with MS die considerably earlier than those without the disease, at least if they do nothing about the illness. This can be seen quite clearly later when I present findings from Swank's work on diet and graphs showing how large groups of people with MS have fared over time.

More recently, a 2004 Danish study analysing a registry of people diagnosed in that country with MS since 1948 showed that people with MS die around ten years earlier than the general population.[59] They also showed that over half (56%) died from MS. An encouraging feature was that the excess death rate for those with MS compared with the general population fell by the end of the study to about half the rate it was in the mid 1900s. It is likely this represents the fact the diagnosis is being made earlier and in more people these days, and the effect of the newer disease-modifying drugs.

Another registry study, this time from Wales in 2008, showed that the average age at death for women with MS was 65.3 years, and 65.2 for men.[60] This is considerably less than might be expected in the general population. Again cause of death was related to MS in nearly 58 per cent of people. In over a quarter there was no mention of MS on the death certificate, which may explain why it is so commonly underestimated as contributing to death.

One group of patients who seem to have quite a benign early course is those whose first symptoms are visual, that is those who get optic neuritis.[61] This group of people seem to develop only mild disability over the ten years after the diagnosis of optic neuritis.

THE CAUSES OF MS

There are many theories as to what causes MS. I will go into them in considerably more detail as I deal with each therapy which has been tried. Most of the theories revolve around a problem with the immune system, which is tricked into initiating immune attacks on its own nervous tissue. In effect, somehow the immune system seems to 'see' the myelin in the CNS as a foreign invader and, like overcoming an infection, it tries to get rid of it by attacking it. This is called auto-immunity. A virus or viruses may somehow trigger the process in susceptible people. Alternatively, the immune system may be tricked in a process called molecular mimickry, where part of some foreign molecule looks just like part of myelin. The immune system may mount an immune reaction against this molecule, and later be tricked into doing the same against myelin, seeing it as foreign. A number of different molecules have been suggested as mimicking myelin, including dairy protein[62, 63] and gut bacteria.[64]

In addition to auto-immunity being a cause of MS, there has been a lot of discussion about MS also being a degenerative disease, like Parkinson's disease and Alzheimer's disease.[65, 66, 67] Recently, renewed emphasis has been placed on the MS-initiating role of diet, particularly fats. These may be involved because of their role in production of immune system chemicals, and the integrity of cell membranes. There has also been a lot of interest in the proteins in cow's milk, which look in part like myelin to the immune system. And there is now a lot of speculation about the effects of lack of sunlight, given the unusual geographical distribution of the disease. A number of other factors have been proposed including exposure to organic solvents (one study found painters had about twice the risk of other workers[68]), dental amalgam, heavy metals, and others, but the evidence for these is far from compelling.

Poser, a world authority on MS, has more recently proposed a plausible theory about how these various factors may cause MS to develop in susceptible people.[69] He proposes a systemic condition called the multiple sclerosis trait (MST) which basically results from a challenge to the immune system of a genetically susceptible person that doesn't cause damage to the nervous system and may never evolve into full blown MS. However, that individual is now primed so that if a certain environmental event then occurs, it can turn the trait into MS. This event could be any of the lifestyle factors I discuss in this book, including viral infection, vaccination, exposure to food antigens like cow's milk, inadequate sun exposure, and so on. The person may then develop symptoms of MS, remain symptom-free, or perhaps even only have lesions on MRI with no noticeable effects for the patient.

> MS is triggered by multiple environmental agents in genetically susceptible people.

A study published in 2006 lent considerable weight to this hypothesis. Italian researchers performed MRI scans on 296 first-degree relatives of people with MS and people without MS.[70] They chose those with MS from families where there was no recorded MS (sporadic cases) and where there was a history of MS (familial cases). All of these people had no symptoms of MS and had not been diagnosed with MS. Surprisingly, they found that 10 per cent of relatives of familial cases had MRI brain lesions indistinguishable from MS. In the relatives of sporadic cases, 4 per cent of people had such lesions. In people who were not related to someone with MS there were no lesions suggestive of MS.

This may be frightening news for people with MS when they contemplate the potential for their close relatives to have MS lesions, but it strongly suggests that there is a susceptibility conferred by genetic make-up that requires the right set of environmental circumstances to develop into actual MS. The potential therefore exists, for parents worried about their children getting MS, that making lifestyle changes such as those discussed in this book can significantly affect their chances of developing MS. Canadian expert in the genetics of MS Professor George Ebers actually estimates, on the basis of his research, that modifiable environmental factors hold the key to preventing some 80 per cent of cases of MS.[71] For me, it also raises the intriguing possibility that, by reversing the various lifestyle factors which turned this MS trait into MS, it may be possible to somehow revert to this 'carrier' state, with a few MS lesions, but have no progression to further illness.

In mid-2009, another interesting theory emerged. Scientists measuring venous blood flow from the brain noted that in people with MS, but not in other people, there was some abnormality in this flow.[72] This seemed in keeping with early anatomical observations that MS lesions tended to occur around the venous system in the brain. This may be a particularly important lead to follow, as there is potential for surgical manipulation of these veins if these observations are correct and venous blood flow does play a causative role in MS. Considerably more research is required, however, before we have a good understanding of this issue.

OVERVIEW

MS is a chronic, progressively disabling disease which is still regarded as incurable. Nevertheless, there are now many treatments, including lifestyle changes and other non-drug therapies, and drug therapies that have been shown to slow disease progression, some quite dramatically. It is extremely important for people with MS to tackle this disease early, because much of the damage occurs without us being aware of it. To date, there has been little success in trying to reverse established neurological problems, although that is clearly possible for some people. For people who are diagnosed early, and make some of the changes I outline in coming chapters, the future should be bright.

I will now go through in detail the evidence behind the many life-style changes, and drug and non-drug therapies that can slow or stop the progression of MS. My focus is on lifestyle changes for two reasons. Firstly, the evidence suggests that lifestyle changes offer the greatest potential for remaining well with MS, just as in many other degenerative diseases. But, lifestyle changes have a variety of additional benefits. They are inexpensive compared with drugs. They require no prescription or medical intervention. They are likely to result in many other health benefits. They are empowering, because they entail doing something for yourself. And finally, they enhance hope and positivity. This compares very favourably with drugs, many of which have serious side effects and only modest benefits.

It seems that an interplay between the genetic susceptibility of an individual and environmental factors results in MS developing. The ratio seems to be about 30 per cent genetic and 70 per cent environmental. I will go through the environmental factors in the next few chapters, starting with diet as it is probably the most important change that can modify the progression of the illness. My search of Medline started with gamma linolenic acid but soon branched into other dietary fats. I will now go through what I found and where it led me.

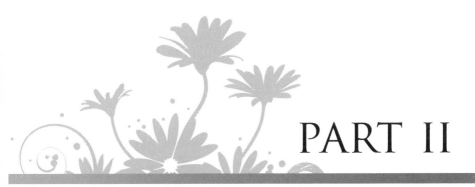

PART II

CONSIDERING THE EVIDENCE

4

DIETARY FATS: EVIDENCE OF IMMUNE SYSTEM EFFECTS

. . . beneficial effects of dietary omega 3s may be of use as a therapy for disorders which involve an inappropriately activated immune response

P.C. Calder

TYPES OF FATS

An overview of the various different types of fat in our diet might be helpful before looking at the evidence of their effect on MS.

Saturated fats are those fats found principally in animals, but also in large quantities in coconut and palm oils. The term saturated is a technical one meaning that all of the carbon atoms in the long chains of these fats, often described as the carbon backbone, are connected to each other with single bonds. When the carbon chains of these fats have all the hydrogen atoms they can hold, they are said to be saturated with hydrogen, or simply saturated fats. These fats have high melting points and so are typically solid or nearly solid at room temperature, except for coconut and palm oils.

If there is one double bond present between any two carbon atoms, the fat is monounsaturated. The typical example of this sort of fat is oleic

SUMMARISING THE EVIDENCE

- The immune system is in balance between exciting the immune response (Th1 response) and dampening it down (Th2 response).
  - MS is an inflammatory disease characterised by an overactive Th1 response towards components of the body's own brain and spinal cord.
- Fatty acids are the basic building blocks for the chemicals the immune system uses in these responses.
  - Saturated (animal) fats and omega 6 (vegetable) fatty acids tip the balance towards the Th1 response.
  - Omega 3 fatty acids (fish and flaxseed oils) tip the balance towards the Th2 response.
  - Monounsaturated fats (olive oil) are immune neutral.
- MS is not just about auto-immunity; degeneration plays a significant role.
  - Unsaturated fatty acids (omega 3, omega 6 and monounsaturated) combat degeneration.
  - Eating fewer calories also protects against degeneration.

EVIDENCE-BASED RECOMMENDATIONS

- Dietary omega 3 fatty acids can be used to suppress auto-immune disease.
- Dietary unsaturated fatty acids can be used to protect against degenerative disease.

acid in olive oil. These fats have lower melting points and so are liquid at room temperature, but will solidify a little or go cloudy in the fridge. If there is more than one double bond present in the backbone, the fat is polyunsaturated. These fats have the lowest melting points and are liquid at room temperature and in the fridge. Many of these polyunsaturated fatty acids are what we call essential fatty acids. That is, they are essential for normal bodily function, but cannot be manufactured in the body. They must be taken in the diet. They can be thought of in the same way as vitamins.

There are two principal types of polyunsaturated fats, those with the first double bond at the third carbon from the omega end of the chain, that is omega-3 or n-3 fatty acids, and those with the first double bond at the sixth carbon from the omega end, that is omega-6 or n-6 fatty acids. The omega-3 fatty acids are typified by fish oil and flaxseed oil, and the omega-6s by all the cooking oils with which we are familiar, namely sunflower oil, safflower oil, corn oil and so on. Later I show that these polyunsaturated 'cooking' oils are very poor foods and should be avoided altogether in cooking. The monounsaturated fats are sometimes called omega-9 fats because their only double bond is at the ninth carbon from the omega end.

We now know that the melting points of these fats determine one of their important properties, that is their stickiness and flexibility when they are incorporated into the cell membranes of bodily cells. It is important to remember here that body cells are surrounded by an envelope, the cell membrane, that is made up of fats. Our bodily cells are not static objects, they are constantly being remade. Depending on where they are in the body they may be rapidly being remade, like in the gut or the skin, or only very slowly being remade, like in bone and cartilage. But the fats which make up the outer layer of these cells come from the diet when they are remade.

> The way fats act in the body depends to a large extent on the simple chemistry of their melting points.

If the fats in the diet are mainly saturated, then the cells behave accordingly. That is, their membranes will be hard and inflexible and tend to stick together. This one fact is really at the heart of the current epidemic in Western countries of diseases due to cells sticking together; diseases due to clots, like heart attacks, strokes and deep venous thrombosis, are all the result of this increased stickiness. And tissues and organs made up of these hard and inflexible cells themselves become hard and inflexible.

So the big blood vessels coming out of the heart, for instance, become very rigid, in a process called atherosclerosis, or hardening of the arteries. So when the heart pumps out blood, the pressure rises much higher than if the arteries were soft and flexible. Hence high blood pressure (hypertension) results. If polyunsaturated fats were the main fats in the diet, the tissues would be soft and pliable instead, and so less likely to clot or result in high blood pressure. Hard cells are also more prone to degeneration, and we will later see that degeneration is now known to be a key part of the development and progression of MS.

But there is another important part of the story with unsaturated fats. Fats form the basic building blocks of the immune system chemicals. A diet high in monounsaturated fats is essentially neutral for the immune system. One high in omega-6s results in immune chemicals which promote the inflammatory response, and one high in omega-3s results in chemicals which suppress the inflammatory response.

There is widespread agreement that MS is a disease involving inappropriate activation of the immune system. It follows then that modulation of the immune system with various dietary and lifestyle changes, and drugs, may modify the course of MS. To better understand how these therapies might work in MS, it is important to first understand a little bit about what the immune system is, how it works and what goes wrong in MS.

THE IMMUNE SYSTEM

The immune system is made up of a complex mixture of cells that together protect the body against foreign invaders and toxins as well as stopping the development of internal cancers. The cells have individual functions like secreting antibodies, engulfing foreign viruses, or making and secreting chemicals that either promote inflammation or suppress it. The cells are all derived from the bone marrow. B cells come directly from the bone marrow to the bloodstream, where they secrete antibodies that attach themselves to foreign proteins or toxins to neutralise them. T cells are first processed by the thymus gland and differentiate into a number of sub-types.

To oversimplify things, essentially their job is to initiate or turn off the immune response and to secrete chemicals (cytokines, eicosanoids and leukotrienes) which either whip up (T helper 1 or Th1 response) or dampen down (T helper 2 or Th2 response) the immune response. The Th2 cells are also known as suppressor cells. There is usually a balance between these responses, so that the immune system can set up an inflammatory response when it needs to get rid of a foreign invader, but also switch it off or suppress it so that it doesn't continue unabated when no longer needed.

The Th1/Th2 hypothesis revolves around the patterns of chemicals released by these two cell types, and how they modulate immune responses. Mossman and Coffman initially proposed that mouse T-helper cells could be classified based on the chemicals they secreted.[1] Th1 cells rely on interferon-gamma, interleukin–2 and interleukin–12. Th2 cells rely on interleukin–4 and sometimes interleukin–5.

Immunity and auto-immunity

The immune system is designed to protect us from outside challenges to our bodies, whether from bacteria or viruses, foreign substances, poisons and so on. MS appears to be at least triggered by auto-immunity. The term auto-immune is used to describe a range of diseases where the immune system is fooled into recognising its own body's substances as foreign and starts attacking them. Examples of auto-immune diseases include systemic lupus erythematosus (SLE) and rheumatoid arthritis. In MS the immune system seems to recognise part of the myelin (fatty) sheath of nerves as foreign, and starts attacking it.

It is now recognised that MS is typified by the balance between Th1 and Th2 responses shifting to a predominantly Th1 response.[2] This is a critical concept in MS. It fits nicely with the central thrust of this book, that balance is the key, and that there is a range of things we can do to shift that balance. In MS, we need to re-balance the immune system more towards a Th2 type response. Researchers have found that a number of lifestyle changes in the twentieth and 21st centuries, particularly surrounding diet and exercise, have tended to shift people in Western societies to a predominantly Th1 response, making them more susceptible to auto-immune disease. For instance, infection with intestinal worms was once very common, and is still quite common in developing countries. Investigators have shown that such infestations, probably because of their continual challenge to the immune system, result in a chronic state of Th2 predominance. People with such infestations seem to be protected against the auto-immune diseases MS, diabetes and rheumatoid arthritis.[3]

MS has been reproduced in experimental animals by injecting them with their own myelin base protein. The animals then develop a relapsing-remitting disease similar to MS and progress to paralysis. This disease in animals is called experimental auto-immune encephalomyelitis (EAE). It does not occur naturally in these animals, only under these

experimental conditions and only in animals specially bred to be susceptible to the disease. The animal model of EAE is quite useful as it enables
us to test a variety of therapies before potentially subjecting patients to
the agents. What works in animal models of MS, though, does not always
work in humans, but at least it gives us an idea of what therapies may be
promising, leading to further work. This is how, for example, glatiramer
was first found to be effective in MS.

Despite many years of intensive research, however, MS still defies
complete understanding and treatment remains suboptimal. The prevailing theory is that MS is immune mediated and that EAE is a suitable
model. EAE, however, may not be an adequate model as it represents
more a model of acute CNS inflammation than the counterpart of MS.
Researchers are currently reconsidering the utilisation of EAE, especially
when this model is used to define therapy. This may in fact be helpful
as it will also force us to examine MS without the restraints imposed by
EAE, examining what it actually is rather than what it looks like.

Immune system messenger chemicals

The immune system produces a range of chemicals which act as messengers, promoting or suppressing inflammation, for instance, or attracting
or otherwise affecting other immune cells. There is a bewildering array
of these chemicals but mostly they belong to the classes of cytokines and
eicosanoids. Cytokines are soluble proteins which are produced by cells
in response to certain stimuli. They include such chemicals as tumour
necrosis factor (TNF), the interleukins (ILs), and the interferons (IFNs).
Interferons are now being used in the treatment of MS.

Some of these cytokines promote inflammation, that is they are
part of the Th1 response, and some suppress it (Th2 response). Recent
research has shown that people with MS who are challenged with myelin
base protein secrete more of the Th1 type cytokines than people without
MS.[2] What is really interesting is that many of the chemical messengers
are made from essential fatty acids. Eicosanoids are a class of unsaturated
fatty acids derived from dietary essential fatty acids. They include prostaglandins, leukotrienes, and thromboxanes. They are a bit like hormones
but act only in the local area in which they are produced. Again they can
promote or suppress inflammation.

In recent years there has been a great advance in our understanding
of these pathways, and the effects of these messengers. From the point

of view of people with MS, it is important to realise that omega-3 and omega-6 fatty acids are converted into messenger chemicals which act in different, often opposing ways. This is in addition to their effects of altering the structure and behaviour of cell membranes, making them more fluid and flexible. Eating more of one or the other types of poly-unsaturated fats therefore can shift the immune response more towards a Th1 or Th2 response.[4]

Omega-3 versus omega-6 fatty acids and the immune messengers

The pathways in the body for these fatty acids are quite complex. A simple plan of this is presented in Table 2. Artemis Simopoulos in her book *The Omega Plan* (*The Omega Diet* in the United States) describes these pathways in more detail and the interested reader is referred there for further information.[5] Table 2 shows that the essential fatty acids alpha-linolenic acid (omega-3) and linoleic acid (omega-6) are converted in the body to intermediate fatty acids, which are then converted into a range of eicosanoids. Our understanding of the importance of these chemicals has leapt in recent years. The eicosanoids have very different functions in the body. Research now has shown that the omega-3 group of eicosanoids slows down inflammation and suppresses the growth of tumours. The omega-6 group does the opposite.

Dr Simopoulos' book presents evidence that the typical Western diet is heavily over-balanced towards omega-6 fats. By cutting down on omega-6 and increasing omega-3 consumption, Simopoulos points out that not only are auto-immune diseases improved, but many of the typical Western degenerative diseases are dramatically improved as well. These include diseases such as coronary heart disease and cancer. These are the unexpected beneficial side effects we can get from cutting out saturated fats and supplementing with fish and flaxseed oils. Not only are we likely to live longer and not be so disabled from MS, but it is a comfort to know that we are less likely to get the other degenerative diseases one gets with ageing in our society.

Omega-3 fatty acids have been shown to decrease production of messengers which promote inflammation, and increase those which settle inflammation down, moving the immune system to a Th2 state. Omega-6 fatty acids seem to do the opposite (Th1), although the effects are a little variable. Prostaglandin E2 (PGE2) is an eicosanoid which has been shown to promote inflammation. It is produced in higher quantities when

Table 2: Pathways in the body for the omega-3 and omega-6 fatty acids

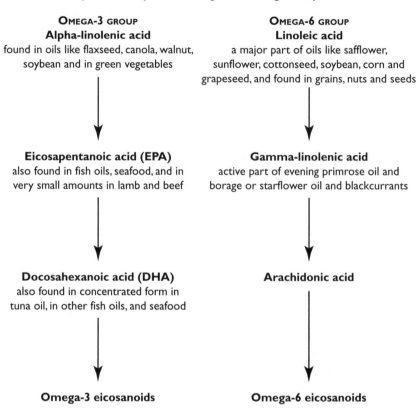

OMEGA-3 GROUP	OMEGA-6 GROUP
Alpha-linolenic acid	**Linoleic acid**
found in oils like flaxseed, canola, walnut, soybean and in green vegetables	a major part of oils like safflower, sunflower, cottonseed, soybean, corn and grapeseed, and found in grains, nuts and seeds
Eicosapentanoic acid (EPA)	**Gamma-linolenic acid**
also found in fish oils, seafood, and in very small amounts in lamb and beef	active part of evening primrose oil and borage or starflower oil and blackcurrants
Docosahexanoic acid (DHA)	**Arachidonic acid**
also found in concentrated form in tuna oil, in other fish oils, and seafood	
Omega-3 eicosanoids	**Omega-6 eicosanoids**

omega-6 fatty acids are eaten, and is suppressed by omega-3 fatty acids, steroids, aspirin and various anti-inflammatory drugs. Leukotriene B4 (LTB4) similarly promotes inflammation, and has been shown to be involved in a host of inflammatory conditions such as asthma, ulcerative colitis, rheumatoid arthritis and others. Eating omega-6 fatty acids enhances production of this eicosanoid; omega-3 fatty acids compete with omega-6 fatty acids for key enzymes which reduce its production.

> Dietary fat intake markedly affects the function of the immune system.

The effect of essential fatty acid intake on these eicosanoids has been studied in great detail in people with MS. Gallai and co-workers showed that there was a marked decrease in the chemicals which promote inflammation after only four weeks' supplementation with fish oils.[6] IL–1beta,

IL–2, IFN-gamma and TNF-alpha were all significantly decreased. The decreases were even more pronounced after three and then six months. The pro-inflammatory eicosanoids PGE2 and LTB4 were also decreased. This is important because these chemicals have been shown to be involved in causing relapses in MS patients.[7, 8] The patients in this study were taking quite large doses, of the order of 5g a day, of EPA plus DHA. In most fish oil capsules, only 30 per cent of the oil is EPA and DHA, so about 16 or 17 of the 1000mg capsules a day is equivalent.

The authors noted that to get a similar level of suppression of the immune system as they had achieved with fish oil, one would have to use standard agents used in chemotherapy such as steroids and cyclo- sporine A. These powerful drugs have many toxic effects, particularly with long-term use. In the chapters on steroids and other therapies affect- ing the immune system I show that some of these drugs have been used successfully in treating MS. How much better all round if we can achieve the same effect through diet.

Calder has summarised the effect of taking various doses of essen- tial fatty acids on the production of many of these chemicals.[4] He notes that omega-3 fatty acid supplementation reduces the production of IL–1alpha, IL–1beta and TNF. These cytokines have all been implicated in causing auto-immune diseases. The effects are achieved with relatively high doses of omega-3 fatty acids, of the order of 1–3g a day of EPA and DHA, although these are lower than in Gallai's study. Here we also find evidence that corn oil, an omega-6 fatty acid, increases levels of the pro-inflammatory TNF.

> Omega-3 fatty acids suppress inflammation.

Researchers are now starting to put this basic science into practice. A paper published in 2007 in *Journal of the American Medical Association* from the University of Colorado examined the effects of differing amounts of omega-3 and -6 in diets of children over a year old who were at increased risk of developing type 1 diabetes.[9] This type of diabetes is the auto- immune type, and is very similar to MS as a disease except that the target of auto-immunity is the insulin-secreting cells of the pancreas rather than the myelin sheaths of nerve cells in the brain. In this study, they showed clearly that infants with higher amounts of omega-3 fatty acids in their diets were 55 per cent less likely to develop auto-immunity to their pancreatic cells as evidenced by development of one of the three measured auto-antibodies to pancreatic cells; for children with at least two of these three measured antibodies, that is those at highest risk of developing diabetes, the risk was reduced by 77 per cent for those consuming larger amounts of omega-3s. This association was confirmed by showing that, in a subset of this group of children who had fatty acid composition of their red blood cells measured, those with higher amounts of omega-3s in their membranes had a lower risk of developing auto-immunity to pancreatic cells.

We have seen that we can change the balance of fats in the membranes of our bodily cells by reducing saturated fats and increasing the polyunsaturated essential fatty acids. The fats get taken up into the cells of the nervous system, making nerves more pliable and more resistant to immune attack. They also get taken up into the immune cells themselves, and every other cell of the body, improving their function, reducing degeneration and decreasing cancerous change. In addition, by changing the balance to favour the omega-3s over the omega-6 fatty acids we eat, the production of pro-inflammatory omega-6 eicosanoids is altered, thus diminishing inflammatory attacks. So while I believe there is probably little difference between omega-3 and omega-6 fatty acids in terms of membrane pliability and function, the suppression of immune system activation achieved by omega-3 fatty acids makes them the supplements to concentrate on in replacing saturated fats.

We have evidence for other inflammatory and auto-immune diseases which have much more easily monitored clinical effects, such as fibromyalgia and rheumatoid arthritis, that a low saturated fat, vegan diet is effective, at least in part by altering the balance of unsaturated to saturated fats.[10, 11] Another study examined the effect of a fish, olive oil and vegetable based Mediterranean diet on the clinical effects of rheumatoid arthritis.[12] The diet resulted in improvements in measures of disease activity and also quality of life. Of interest, the authors noted that the patients who did best had a higher intake of omega-3 compared with omega-6 fats.[13] We know from other studies that the Mediterranean diet causes a general dampening down of inflammation.[14]

Low saturated (animal) fat diets suppress inflammation.

A comprehensive review of this literature on fats in rheumatoid arthritis concluded that supplementation with omega-3 fatty acids improved clinical features of rheumatoid arthritis and, although difficult for some patients to adhere to, vegan diets and fasting were also of benefit.[15] The authors pointed out that such 'dietary manipulation provides a means by which patients can regain a sense of control over their disease'. Rheumatologists are clearly very aware of the importance of this sense of control for people facing many years of living with a chronic disease. The issue is also vital for people with MS.

McCarty proposes a number of theories why vegan diets plus fish oil and vitamin D may be of wide-ranging benefit to people's health, largely through their effects on the immune system,[16, 17] and UK scientists have added new experimental evidence for the benefits of fish oil in regulating inflammation.[18] Das has also published extensively on the anti-inflammatory effects of fish-based Mediterranean type diets.[14, 19, 20]

Types of omega-3 fatty acids

Fish oils are the omega-3 fatty acids which most people think of in this context and much of the work in the medical literature has been done with fish oil supplementation. However, there are plant omega-3s as well. Alpha-linolenic acid is the plant form, and this is found in abundance in linseeds (otherwise known as flaxseed) and their oil extracts, canola or rapeseed oil, and some nuts, mainly walnuts and pecans, and their extracted oils. As can be seen from Table 2, the plant omega-3s are converted in the body to the fish form (EPA and DHA). Many authorities say that this is not always an efficient mechanism, and is blocked by saturated fats and the absence of certain vitamins and minerals. Possibly less than 10 per cent of alpha-linolenic acid gets into the EPA and DHA forms. For this reason many people prefer to get these substances directly from fish oil and bypass the conversion in the body.

I have hunted for scientific references to support this fact, and can find little. So it may well be that the plant form, typically taken as flaxseed oil, is just as good as fish oil in its immune effects. Certainly all the medical literature on trials using flaxseed oil seems to show just as impressive results as those with fish oil. It is probably a question of personal choice. Later I will show how one scientist has calculated this conversion, suggesting that flaxseed oil may be sufficient on its own.

All of these substances, because they are full of unsaturated (that is double) bonds in the carbon backbone, are very prone to oxidation in air or heat. Once eaten and taken up into cell membranes they may be similarly prone to oxidation, in a process known as lipid peroxidation. More on that later.

THE ROLE OF IMMUNITY VERSUS DEGENERATION IN MS

Having examined the immune system in detail, and its role in MS, there is a growing view that MS is not just about the immune system.[21] Degeneration is also likely to be a key mechanism in MS,[22] particularly in progressive phases of the disease. A degenerative disease is a disease in which the function or structure of the affected tissues or organs progressively worsens over time, due to normal bodily wear and tear or lifestyle choices such as exercise or diet. Some examples include Alzheimer's disease, motor neurone disease, cancer, diabetes, heart disease, inflammatory bowel disease, Parkinson's disease and osteoarthritis.

The growing evidence of a degenerative component to MS means that many lifestyle interventions such as diet and exercise which are known to be helpful in other degenerative diseases will also be of benefit to people with MS, and provides further rationale for why they are effective in MS.

MS is both auto-immune and degenerative in nature.

The evidence that MS is not just an immune system disorder but also a degenerative disorder is extensive. For instance, there is currently much research into the contribution of plasma homocysteine (a chemical measured in blood) to various degenerative disorders, including coronary heart disease and atherosclerosis, but also to a variety of degenerative diseases of the nervous system.[23] It has been found that plasma homocysteine is also elevated in MS[24] and that its level correlates with the degree of cognitive and motor impairment.[25] It has also been noted that people with MS who are depressed have high homocysteine levels.[26]

Others have documented clear evidence of nervous system damage on MRI in people with high homocysteine levels and low folate levels.[27] It is well known now that high folate intake tends to lower homocysteine levels.[28] Indeed, Swedish researchers have shown that supplementation with vitamin B12 and folate of people who have raised homocysteine levels and mild cognitive impairment appears to strengthen the blood-brain barrier and slow the decline in cognitive function.[29]

There is also MRI evidence that the process of degeneration of nerve cells begins very early in MS and is not just a feature of the progressive phases of the illness.[30, 31] These authors found that damage to the CNS is very widespread in MS and is not just confined to the 'lesions' that are seen on standard MRI. They felt that the concept of MS as a focal, demyelinating disease needs to be re-examined, and that we should now regard it as a diffuse disease of the CNS with a major degenerative component. This is supported by German neuropathologists, who have pointed out that damage to the CNS is widespread in MS, is degenerative in nature, and not just confined to demyelinating lesions.[32, 33] The accumulating loss of nervous tissue does seem to be what ultimately leads the disease to become progressive.

British researchers have shown that a drug which produces very significant immune system suppression results in quite substantial benefit when given early in the illness when the disease is relapsing-remitting, but no benefit once the disease is progressive.[34] This lends further support to the concept that while the disease probably has a degenerative component all along, it is largely immune-mediated early on, and later mainly degenerative, once secondary progressive disease has occurred. Another study of the effect of interferon given early to people likely to progress to MS showed quite a disparity between the number of new lesions and the loss of brain volume.[30] This suggests that the immune-mediated inflammation and the neurodegeneration in MS are separate processes right from the beginning of the disease. Indeed, there is now much opinion that the distinction between immune and degenerative diseases of the nervous system is becoming blurred, and that both processes probably contribute to many neurological diseases, typified by MS.[35]

Polyunsaturated fats have been shown to be useful in degenerative diseases of the nervous system, and degenerative disease in general.[36] For instance, they have been shown in RCTs to be beneficial in Huntington's disease.[37] They are also helpful in preventing the memory loss and deterioration in mental function that accompanies ageing and nervous system degeneration,[38, 39, 40] and they appear to lower the risk of Parkinson's disease, another neurodegenerative disease.[41] DHA, one of the omega-3 fatty acids in fish oil, has been shown to be powerfully neuroprotective and prevent degeneration in a rat model of brain injury.[42, 43] Additionally, a diet high in saturated fats has been shown to aggravate the effects of brain trauma.[44]

Dietary unsaturated fats are helpful in preventing degeneration.

A dietary change which has been known for a long time to prolong life and protect particularly against degenerative disease is to eat fewer calories. It is well known that Western society is overweight. This predisposes us to many degenerative diseases including heart disease, diabetes and arthritis. By eating fewer calories health and longevity can be dramatically improved.[45] Further, it has been suggested that just restricting calories every second day, and then eating as much as desired the other day, has the same health benefits.[46] Animal work has shown that acute starvation caused a shift to a Th2 cytokine pattern in animals with EAE, delayed onset of the disease, and resulted in milder clinical symptoms in the animals.[47]

OVERVIEW

It is clear that omega-3 fatty acids shift the immune balance towards a Th2 response, although both omega-3s and omega-6s are likely to be helpful in combating degeneration because of their membrane effects. Monounsaturated fats, which are neutral in their effects on the immune system, are also of benefit, presumably by their effect on membranes as well. It is important now to see how all this knowledge translates into effects on the disease when we look at the health of whole populations of people who consume particular diets involving more or less of these fats and, later, when diet is used as a therapy for people with MS.

5

DIETARY FATS: EVIDENCE FROM POPULATION STUDIES

The truth is that human physiology sustains health best when its intake of meat fat and proteins is small or nonexistent

Deepak Chopra

While RCTs are considered the strongest level of medical evidence there are many other types of evidence, all contributing to our knowledge and understanding of mechanisms and therapies in disease. Epidemiology, the study of the incidence and distribution of diseases, and their prevention, can also provide important information in establishing the causes and possible treatments of MS. The larger the study, the stronger such evidence is. These data are often used to infer the causes of disease, and guide what we should be studying in RCTs.

THE BELGIAN SCHOOL OF PUBLIC HEALTH STUDY

A very significant paper published in the *American Journal of Epidemiology* in 1995 provided important evidence of the effects of dietary fats in MS.[1] The study from the School of Public Health in Belgium is the largest yet reported of MS incidence, with MS mortality data from 36

SUMMARISING THE EVIDENCE

- Epidemiological studies have consistently shown that MS is more common where saturated fat consumption is high, and less common where fish consumption is high.
- Many epidemiological studies have now confirmed the close association of cow's milk consumption and the incidence of MS.
  - Laboratory data strongly support this link of cow's milk consumption to MS.
- Case control studies have revealed a protective role for vegetarian diets and an increased risk of MS with high calorie intake and animal-based diets.

EVIDENCE-BASED RECOMMENDATIONS

- Major population-based studies clearly implicate saturated fat in MS causation.
- Cow's milk is also clearly implicated.
- These large studies indicate that vegetable and fish-based diets have a protective effect.

---

countries from 1983–1989. Using data from the United Nations Food and Agriculture Organisation on fat consumption in these countries, they assessed the impact of diets with differing amounts of animal, fish and unsaturated fats on MS mortality. Mortality, or the rate that people were dying from MS, was used as a measure of the prevalence of MS in those countries, as it was an easy statistic to obtain. Most countries do not have accurate data on how prevalent MS is, as it is not a disease which must be notified to health authorities. Most countries do, however, have accurate statistics on causes of death.

> MS is more common in countries where people eat more animal fat.

The findings fit neatly with our knowledge of the immune system and anti-degenerative effects of dietary fats. Essentially, researchers found that the higher the saturated fat consumption the higher the MS mortality, and the higher the animal fat consumption the higher the mortality. After taking away the amount of fish oil consumed from the animal fat consumption, the final figure too was related directly to mortality (see Table 3). In Table 3, I list countries in descending order according to mortality (among women). I have removed some of the smaller countries to make the table a little easier to follow.

Those populations with high fish oil consumption had lower MS mortality, unless it was overbalanced by very large animal fat consumption, as in the case of Denmark. The p values for these associations were between 0.001 and 0.01 depending on which was being assessed. These findings were very unlikely to have been due to chance. Further, the researchers found that the higher the ratio of polyunsaturated to saturated fats, the lower the mortality, and similarly with the unsaturated to saturated fat ratio. The p values here were 0.001 to <0.05.

While these are not the results of clinical trials, the evidence, from very large populations in a large number of countries, is very strong. Animal and saturated fats do play some role in the development of MS, and these effects are to some extent counteracted by fish oil and other poly- and mono-unsaturated fats, in keeping with the evidence presented in the previous chapter.

EARLIER EPIDEMIOLOGICAL STUDIES

While this is the largest population data thus far analysed, it supports much previous work done in the 1950s to 1970s, including the original work by Swank. After he initially proposed his theory in 1950, follow-up work showed the intriguing finding that MS was less common in coastal Norway, where fish consumption was high, than in inland areas of Norway which were dependent on dairy diets.[2] These findings were supported by a large population study by Knox published in 1977.[3] Analysing mortality data from twenty countries, he also suggested a causal relationship between total fat intake and MS.

Another study in 1974 found that people who were fed cow's milk as children had a higher incidence of MS than those breast fed. It was postulated that this was because of the low linoleic acid (an essential fatty acid) content of cow's milk compared with human milk.[4] Another interesting study looked at people of similar Danish genetic backgrounds living in the Faroe and Shetland Islands.[5] Those on the Faroe Islands maintained a fishing lifestyle with high fish consumption, that is a diet high in omega-3 fatty acids. Those on the Shetland Islands adopted the agricultural diet of their English counterparts. The Faroe Islanders had a low incidence of MS, whereas the Shetlanders had a high incidence.

Extraordinarily, most of this work has lain dormant, and little systematic research has been done in the area. I feel this is a reflection of modern medicine's desire to give the patient a drug or other treatment rather than relying on patients taking control themselves by altering their diets.

Table 3: Multiple sclerosis—fat consumption 1979–1981 by country, listed in order of highest to lowest MS mortality

Country	SFA (%E)	MUFA (%E)	PUFA (%E)	P/S	U/S	AF – FO (%E)	VO (%E)	FO (%E)
Denmark	16.6	16.9	5.9	0.36	1.37	33.4	9.2	1.07
United Kingdom	14.7	14.6	6.5	0.44	1.44	27.2	12.1	0.19
Switzerland	16.7	14.6	6.9	0.41	1.28	29.1	13.0	0.21
Poland	12.8	10.7	4.2	0.33	1.16	23.6	6.6	0.31
Czechoslovakia	13.2	12.2	4.5	0.34	1.26	24,5	8.5	0.19
Norway	15.1	13.5	6.9	0.46	1.35	24.6	14.0	0.56
East Germany	14.6	12.6	4.9	0.34	1.20	26.3	9.2	0.24
Netherlands	17.3	17.6	6.9	0.40	1.41	31.8	13.6	0.15
West Germany	14.1	14.1	6.6	0.47	1.48	26.0	12.1	0.27
Sweden	16.5	16.1	6.1	0.37	1.34	29.9	12.0	0.89
Belgium	16.0	15.9	7.0	0.44	1.43	30.1	12.4	0.24
New Zealand	17.8	13.2	4.3	0.24	0.99	32.7	6.9	0.13
Austria	14.1	14.4	7.4	0.52	1.55	25.5	17.8	0.18
Canada	14.5	16.7	6.8	0.47	1.61	27.8	13.7	0.27
United States	13.9	15.3	8.6	0.62	1.72	25.0	16.4	0.20
France	14.6	14.4	7.0	0.49	1.48	27.8	12.0	0.31
Finland	16.9	13.2	4.6	0.27	1.06	30.3	7.5	0.64
Romania	8.7	8.4	6.7	0.78	1.74	16.7	9.6	0.16
Yugoslavia	8.6	8.8	6.3	0.73	1.75	16.6	9.3	0.08
Australia	12.1	11.0	4.7	0.38	1.30	25.0	11.7	0.25
Italy	9.9	14.6	6.3	0.64	2.11	17.4	16.4	0.20

Bulgaria	8.1	7.9	8.7	1.07	2.04	14.4	12.8	0.12
Greece	9.4	17.3	5.1	0.54	2.39	14.4	20.7	0.20
Malta	10.0	8.8	6.3	0.63	1.51	17.6	14.9	0.60
Argentina	10.4	11.0	7.4	0.71	1.76	20.9	11.1	0.08
Cuba	7.0	6.1	3.8	0.54	1.42	13.5	5.6	0.39
Portugal	7.7	10.9	7.6	0.99	2.41	13.1	15.4	0.42
Spain	9.5	14.6	7.6	0.80	2.34	16.7	17.9	0.44
Israel	9.2	10.4	9.0	0.98	2.11	12.9	18.8	0.27
Japan	6.5	8.8	7.1	1.09	2.44	9.5	13.2	2.78
South Korea	3.4	3.8	3.1	0.91	2.03	5.2	6.5	0.47
Hong Kong	10.0	15.2	7.4	0.74	2.25	20.1	16.1	0.85
Singapore	7.4	8.1	5.1	0.69	1.79	13.9	9.0	0.74
Mean	12.3	12.4	6.2	0.56	1.61	22.4	12.0	0.44

Abbreviations

%E = per cent of total energy including alcohol

SFA = saturated fatty acids

MUFA = mono-unsaturated fatty acids

PUFA = polyunsaturated fatty acids

P/S ratio of PUFA to SFA

U/S ratio of unsaturated fatty acids (PUFA plus MUFA) to SFA

AF – FO = animal fat minus fish oil

VO = vegetable oil

FO = fish oil

(Modified from Esparaza et al.[1], courtesy Oxford University Press.)

MOUNTING EVIDENCE ON THE COW'S MILK– MS CONNECTION

There has been a long-standing opinion that cow's milk consumption has a role to play in the development of MS, and indeed other auto-immune diseases like type 1 (insulin-dependent) diabetes. Recent high quality epidemiological work strongly reinforces those views.[6, 7] These researchers found a very high correlation between cow's milk consumption and MS all around the world. But stunning laboratory work from Germany and Canada now provides a possible explanation of why this may be so.[8, 9] A number of cow's milk proteins have now been shown to be targeted by the immune cells of people with MS. Further injecting them into experimental animals has caused lesions to appear in the central nervous systems of the animals. Other researchers have demonstrated how certain proteins in cow's milk mimic part of myelin oligodendrocyte glycoprotein, the part of myelin thought to initiate the auto-immune reaction in MS.[10]

> There is a strong link between cow's milk consumption and MS.

There seems to be a link to diabetes here, with similar suggestions now being made for cow's milk being involved in its causation. Indeed, medical researchers are now so concerned about this that a worldwide study has begun in which children are being kept off cow's milk to see whether diabetes can be prevented.[11] This involves a major collaborative international study group of 78 clinical centres in fifteen countries, with the aim of recruiting 2032 children into the study. This study was in part triggered by an RCT from the University of Helsinki that studied 242 newborn infants who had a first-degree relative with type 1 diabetes and the genetic predisposition to diabetes.[12] They found that avoiding cow's milk formula provided significant protection from developing the auto-immunity associated with diabetes compared with the infants who did get cow's milk.

Another study into the degenerative neurological disorder Parkinson's disease found that people who consumed more dairy products had two to three times the risk of getting the disease.[13] This result is very likely to be correct as it involved over 135,000 men and women in the United States, and used stringent methods for collecting data on food consumption. The researchers speculated that dairy products may have a generally toxic effect on nervous tissue.

While the evidence is still not conclusive it is mounting by the day, and it has been strong enough for me to drop from my diet all cow's milk products since I wrote the first book. Fortunately there are some very good alternatives, such as soy yoghurt, although finding a tasty one can be tricky. I don't regard cow's milk as a very healthy food at all, in fact. It is worth noting that up to 1 in 5 Australian adults of British descent, 2 in 5 of Mediterranean descent, and 4 in 5 of Aboriginal or Asian descent have lactose intolerance, and can get quite ill taking milk products. This can be in the form of mild or more severe bloating, flatulence, stomach cramps and diarrhoea. Soy and rice milks don't contain lactose. There are lots of good reasons not to drink cow's milk.

The evidence is quite nicely laid out in Campbell's best-selling book *The China Study*.[14] Campbell, a world renowned nutrition researcher, argues from a very large base of accumulated medical evidence that the best diet for overall human health is a wholefood, plant-based diet. For people with MS the book is interesting reading, as he shows the links between animal fat and protein, and particularly cow's milk, with MS and a range of other Western diseases.

EVIDENCE FROM CASE-CONTROL STUDIES

There are other methods in epidemiology to assess what risk factors individuals have for certain diseases. So-called case-control studies involve researchers recruiting a certain number of patients with a given disease, in this case MS, and randomly choosing a similar number of people without that disease carefully matched to be very close to the disease group in terms of sex, age and so on. Both groups are then carefully questioned about various lifestyle factors of interest.

For instance if the theory is that sunlight prevents MS, the researchers may ask the individuals to document carefully the exact amount of time they have spent in the sun over a period leading up to the study. They then take all those cases who are in the top 25 per cent of time spent in the sun and all those in the bottom 25 per cent and compare how many in each of those groups have MS. It may show for instance that of 100 patients who spent more than two hours a day in the sun (the top 25 per cent of values), 20 had MS, and all the rest were the matched controls. Of the 100 patients that spent less than 15 minutes a day in the sun (the bottom 25 per cent values), 80 had MS. This means that a person is four times more likely to have MS after spending only a small amount of time in the sun. In case-control studies, this is expressed as an odds ratio. That is the odds of getting MS for those with low sunlight exposure is 4:1, or an odds ratio of 4.0.

This is quite useful information. While it doesn't prove cause and effect, it does pinpoint possible risk factors. For instance, people who drink bottled mineral water may have an odds ratio of 0.5 for MS; that is, they are half as likely to have MS as those not drinking it. But this may reflect just greater health consciousness on the part of the mineral water drinkers, and generally healthier lifestyles, rather than anything in particular about the mineral water. So the results need to be interpreted with caution.

Nevertheless, where such results support evidence from clinical trials and animal studies, they can add weight to theories about the cause of disease.

Such case-control studies have been performed in MS in several countries. The most comprehensive comes from Montreal in Canada, published in 1998.[15] The authors compared various factors amongst 197 people with MS to 202 matched people without MS. Dietary information was collected with a 164-item food frequency questionnaire in a face-to-face interview, so the figures they used are likely to be fairly accurate. They found positive associations, that is higher risk of MS, for increased amount of food intake overall and for increased animal fat intake, with roughly a doubling of risk for every extra 900 calories of food and 33g of animal fat intake. Nutrients shown to be protective included vegetable protein, dietary fibre, cereal fibre, vitamin C, thiamin, riboflavin, calcium and potassium. I have listed some of their findings in Table 4 so that the reader may look up particular foods of interest. The underlined values are variables for which the p value was less than 0.05, that is, the results were felt to be statistically significant. If an odds ratio is less than 1, it means that the particular nutrient has some protective effect. If it is greater than 1, it is associated with *that much* higher risk of MS. For instance, if the odds ratio is 2, this means double the risk of MS.

Table 4: Risk of MS per unit of daily nutrient intakes, Montreal 1992–1995

Variable	Unit[a]	Odds ratio	P
All subjects (197 cases/202 controls)			
Energy, kcal	897	2.03	0.02
Protein, g	37	0.52	
Carbohydrates, g	115	0.73	
Total fat, g	44	1.71	
Saturated fat, g	17	1.88	
Oleic acid, g	18.15	1.12	
Linoleic acid, g	6.64	0.73	
Animal fat, g	32.64	1.99	0.02
Vegetable fat, g	22.33	0.84	
Animal protein, g	21.6	0.93	
Vegetable protein, g	14.3	0.38	0.02
Dietary fibre, g	12.19	0.54	0.05

Vegetable fibre, g	4.75	0.84	
Fruit fibre, g	4.81	0.93	
Cereal fibre, g	5.57	0.57	0.02
Vitamin A, IU	5882	0.88	
Retinol, IU	1491	1.11	
Beta carotene, IU	3849	0.86	
Vitamin E, mg	13.24	0.78	
Vitamin C, mg	162	0.58	0.008
Thiamin, mg	0.66	0.24	0.005
Riboflavin, mg	1.3	0.33	0.003
Niacin, mg	8.87	1.67	
Calcuim, mg	633	0.39	0.002
Iron, mg	6.88	0.40	
Potassium, mg	1670	0.29	0.03
Total sugar, g	60.35	0.75	
Alcohol, g	10.4	1.01	

[a]Unit = for nutrients, units are the difference between upper and lower quartile (25%) cut points for all controls.

(Modified from Ghadirian[15].)

Overall, the study lent weight to a protective role for vegetarian type diets and an increased risk with high total energy and animal food intake. It should be noted that this does not constitute proof of cause and effect, but the data clearly lends weight to the accumulating evidence we have seen of the causative role of animal fats in MS.

Another case-control study from the United States had very similar findings and conclusions.[16] The author went back to data from the US veteran series from World War II and geographically compared this with a range of socio-geographic variables which had been recorded from around that period. Apart from the effects of latitude (that is, distance from the equator), about which I shall talk more later, two main factors emerged in the incidence of MS. The first was typified by indicators of higher affluence, with increased risk of MS associated with higher meat consumption in particular. The second reflected further dietary variables, in particular a diet low in fish and high in dairy products.

A smaller study from Croatia again showed similar findings.[17] Forty-six MS patients were compared with 92 matched control patients. Participants were given a 51-question survey about their dietary habits.

Patients consuming more full-fat milk were over twenty times more likely to have MS than those not, with similar results for those consuming potatoes with lard and fresh or smoked meat. A 1996 case-control study from Moscow again found that the most significant risk factor was a predominant meat versus vegetable-based diet.[18]

THE US NURSES HEALTH STUDY

One of the few pieces of evidence to emerge recently which contradicts these findings from epidemiological and case-control studies is from the US Nurses Health Study.[19] This is a very important long-term piece of research in which scientists have studied a large group of nurses for many years, carefully documenting a range of lifestyle factors and then observing what illnesses the nurses have developed. The study failed to confirm the results of the studies I have presented previously. Nurses consuming the lowest amount of saturated fat in the study essentially developed MS at the same rate as those consuming the most satu-rated fat. It is difficult to come up with an explanation of this finding, although to date it is an isolated finding and goes against most of the other available evidence.

The study is very large and carefully conducted and I would have expected it to show a difference between the groups if saturated fat played the role we think it does. Swank's work, to be discussed in detail in the next chapter, does however show that the intake of saturated fat needs to be absolutely minimal to be effective in slowing the progression of MS. It is quite likely that nurses in the lowest intake category did not have low enough saturated fat consumption for us to see a difference. It is not possible from the data presented in the study to determine whether this was so or not. We know that saturated fat consumption is extremely high and going up in the United States, and it would come as no surprise if the nurses in the lowest fat consumption category still had intakes many times higher than Swank's recommended levels. After all, poor dieters who did so badly in Swank's study had reduced their saturated fat intake by around 75 per cent.

OVERVIEW

Overall, these results should be assessed in combination with the work reported in the previous chapter. Together, they leave me in no doubt that, regardless of what it is that triggers MS in susceptible individuals, immune balance is protective and the disease is less likely to be triggered if saturated fat consumption is low, or balanced by fish and unsaturated fats. Many prominent scientists are now arguing this, and suggesting it be further explored.[20, 21, 22] What we need to explore now is what happens once a person has the disease. Does diet modify the course of the illness when it is used as a treatment?

6

DIETARY FATS: EVIDENCE FROM CLINICAL STUDIES

Food is the chief of all things. It is therefore said to be medicine for all diseases of the body

Taittiraya Upanishad

A very coherent picture of the effect of dietary fat in MS development and progression emerges from many papers in reputable medical journals. There is substantial literature on the effects of dietary fats on the immune system and the distribution of MS worldwide and how it relates to diet, particularly fat consumption. The most important piece of the jigsaw, though, is what happens when you apply this knowledge to people with the disease and see what happens when diet is used as therapy for MS, that is, in clinical studies.

The most significant part of this story is the fascinating lifelong work of Professor Roy Laver Swank of the Swank Multiple Sclerosis Clinic in Portland, Oregon, in the United States. Professor Swank's interest in the fat hypothesis started with his publication in 1950 about the way MS distribution around the world seemed to follow the consumption patterns of saturated fats.[1]

SUMMARISING THE EVIDENCE

• There is good evidence from clinical studies that diet plays a major role in the initiation and progression of MS.
  – The key aggravating factor appears to be high saturated-fat consumption.
• Intervention studies where people with MS have maintained very low saturated-fat diets have consistently shown significant reductions in relapse rates and slowing of disease progression.
  – The major work is that of Roy Swank, Professor of Neurology in Oregon, who followed 144 patients for 34 years; those who stuck to the low saturated-fat diet had dramatically better outcomes.
• Basic science research in the laboratory has confirmed that people with MS have more saturated fat in their cell membranes and less polyunsaturated fat.
• RCTs have shown that essential fatty acid supplements can also slow the progression of the disease.

EVIDENCE-BASED RECOMMENDATIONS

• A very low saturated-fat diet seems the optimal diet to facilitate MS recovery; in practice, this is a plant-based wholefood diet.
• This diet should be supplemented with essential fatty acids 17–23g/day, either in supplements or food (fish); current knowledge of fats and oils suggests that these should be omega-3 fatty acids.

PROFESSOR SWANK'S LOW SATURATED-FAT STUDY

Professor Swank made the observation that the incidence of MS seemed to follow the consumption of saturated fat, particularly dairy products, and was lower wherever fish consumption (with its high omega-3 fat content) was high. Much of this work is reported in various papers in the medical literature. The best summary, though, is from Swank and Dugan's book, *The Multiple Sclerosis Diet Book*.[2] Here Swank shows graphically how the consumption of fat in Western countries such as the United States jumped in the twentieth century. In 1909, people in the United States consumed on average 125g per day of fat. By 1948 this had risen to 141g. By 1972 this figure had leapt to 150g. In Western Europe the rate of increase was even higher. Worse, the percentage of all calories in the diet in the United States coming from fat had jumped in this period to over 40 per cent. This is in comparison to an estimated 15 per cent some 200 years ago.

Swank went on to show that the daily fat intake in countries where this was known seemed to correlate with how common MS was. He produced a table of high MS incidence countries and low MS incidence countries, and their fat intakes, from which I have modified Table 5. Swank drew several conclusions from this and other data he presented about dietary fat intake. He felt that the dietary change from unsaturated to saturated fats which has accompanied industrialisation in most Western countries was involved with the causation of MS.

Table 5: Daily fat intake by country according to incidence of MS

MS common	Daily fat intake (g)	MS uncommon	Daily fat intake (g)
USA	121	Cuba	49
Canada	118	Italy	60
UK	122	South Africa	50
Scandinavia	130	Japan	25
Germany	111	Brazil	52
Switzerland	105	Mexico	43

(Modified from Swank and Dugan.)

This may have remained just that, an interesting observation. However, Professor Swank then began a quite remarkable study. Why this study has not attracted the attention it deserves is hard to understand.

Beginning in 1949, he enrolled 150 MS patients in his study and commenced them on a very low saturated-fat diet.[3] He then followed them with meticulous examination and recording of their dietary fat consumption for the extraordinary period of 34 years. There was no control group who had normal diets, however, we have data on relapse rates in MS from many other studies and many of the patients were unable to stick to the diet, allowing comparison between those who did and those who did not. The study was supported by grants from the MS Society of Canada, the Montreal Neurological Institute, the Department of Health and Welfare of Canada, the MS Society of Portland and other grants. For its time, this was a major piece of medical research.

A number of papers resulted from this study. One of the most important was published in one of the world's premier medical journals, *The Lancet*, in 1990,[3] and another in *Nutrition* in 1991.[4] For those of us with MS, these results are worth going through in detail. They give enormous hope to people with MS.

The paper in *The Lancet* reported results for 144 of the patients. Of these, 72 patients were able to stick to the diet (good dieters), that is, they consumed less than 20g/day of saturated fat. The other 72 could not keep fat consumption below 20g/day. I will detail the requirements of the diet and my recommendations in a later chapter. The patients' neurological disability was graded using a neurological disability scale devised by Swank, which goes from 0 (essentially unimpaired) to 6 (deceased). Point 4 on the scale represents wheelchair needed, and point 5 confined to bed and chair (see Table 6). I previously described Kurtzke's EDSS. Swank's scale essentially used 2 points on Kurtzke's scale to every 1 point on his.

Table 6: Swank's disability scale

0 = normal performance and normal neurological findings
1 = normal performance physically and mentally, neurological signs present
2 = mildly impaired physical performance but ambulant, neurological signs present, able to work part time or full time, occasionally variable memory impairment
3 = severely impaired performance but ambulant, able to work (usually part time), neurological impairment usually widespread, variable memory impairment frequently present
4 = wheelchair needed, memory often impaired
5 = confined to bed and chair
6 = deceased

(Modified, with permission, from Swank and Dugan[3].)

The results were dramatic. Regardless of level of disability at entry to the trial, good dieters did not deteriorate significantly. Good dieters who were at level 1 on entry had an average final grade of 1.9 34 years later. Good dieters at level 2 had a final level of 3.6, and those at level 3 or worse a final level of 4. The results were best for those who started with minimum disability, with 95 per cent surviving and still physically active 34 years later, excluding those who died from non-MS diseases. I think all people with MS would hope that they ultimately die from a non-MS related disease. It is important to note, however, that the benefits occurred in all three groups, and that even people with significant disability were shown to markedly slow the progression of the disease if they could stick to the diet.

> A 34-year study by Professor Swank showed dramatic slowing of disease progression with a very low saturated-fat diet.

The picture for poor dieters was terrible, much in line with results we have seen from other series of MS patients whose conditions have been monitored over time. Poor dieters with minimum disability at entry ended with an average grade of 5.3, that is, wheelchair and bed bound. Those with moderate disability ended up at 5.3 also, and those with severe disability at 5.6. Only 7 per cent of patients who did not stick to the diet remained active. The death rate amongst the poor dieters was extremely high: 58 of the 72 were dead by 34 years, 45 from MS-related causes (see Table 7). The statistics were very strong. The p values were generally of the order of $p<0.0001$ to <0.0005 for most of the differences between good and poor dieters. That is, the difference was extremely unlikely to have occurred by chance. It is rare to see p values so low in any medical publications. Because they are so important I have reproduced the main features of these results below, with some details omitted.

Table 7: Results for patients in Swank's saturated fat study

	Good dieters		Poor dieters	
Minimum disability (grade 1)				
Number (M:F)	23	(14:9)	6	(3:3)
Mean duration of MS (years)	31		25.9	
Before trial	2.4		3.5	
Diet period	28.6		23.8	
Average final neurological grade (change)	1.9	(0.9)	5.3	(4.3)
Deaths				
All other causes	5	(21%)	5	(83%)
MS only	1	(5%)	4	(80%)

Mean lipid intake		
Fats	17.1	35.7
Oils	16.3	11.0
Moderate disability (grade 2)		
Number (M:F)	25 (9:16)	33 (16:17)
Mean duration of MS (years)	32.0	28.0
Before trial	4.9	5.3
Diet period	27.1	22.7
Average final neurological grade (change)	3.6 (1.6)	5.3 (3.4)
Deaths		
All other causes	10 (40%)	25 (76%)
MS only	8 (34%)	16 (66%)
Lipid intake		
Fat	15.4	46.1
Oils	18.2	10.2
Severe disability (grades 3–5, average 3.21)		
Number (M:F)	24 (7:17)	33 (17:16)
Mean duration of MS (years)	33.8	29.9
Before trial	6.2	10.4
Diet period	27.6	19.5
Average final neurological grade (change)	4.0 (0.8)	5.6 (2.4)
Deaths		
All other causes	8 (33%)	28 (84%)
MS only	5 (21%)	25 (75%)
Lipid intake		
Fat	15.8	36.5
Oils	18.1	10.5

(Reproduced, with permission, from Swank and Dugan[2].)

Swank's paper in *Nutrition* is equally impressive, describing 150 patients.[4] These were essentially the same patients with some additional patients found for follow-up. Again patients treated early did best but, whatever the disability level at entry, deterioration was markedly less than those who could not stick to the diet. Some of the graphs below from that paper present the evidence in quite startling fashion. Figure 1 shows the dramatic fall in relapse rate after commencement of the diet, from around 1 relapse per year pre-diet to about 0.05 per year once stable on the diet. It should be noted that although the fall in relapse rate occurred quite quickly, down to 0.3 relapses per year within a year, patients did not achieve complete stability for around five years. This is an important point for those tempted to 'try the diet' and give up because nothing seems to be happening.

Figure 1: Relapse rate (number per year) before and after going on low-fat diet

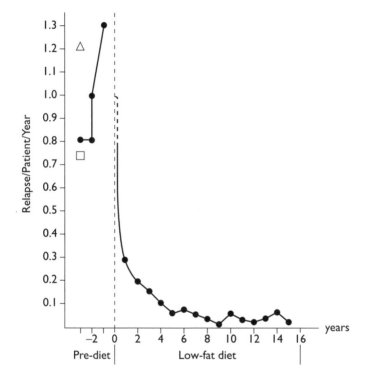

(Reprinted with permission from Elsevier Science, from Swank[4].)

Figure 2 is worth examining in some detail. It shows that regardless of the level of disability on commencement of the diet, for those who adhered to the diet there was minimal deterioration over the course of the study. For those who did not adhere to the diet, the death rate was extremely high (78–91% depending on initial level of disability). There are two important things to learn from the graph. Firstly, this gives great hope to people who already have some disability. There is real hope of stabilising the illness no matter how advanced it is. Secondly, and most importantly, those who could not stick to the diet and deteriorated actually reduced their saturated fat consumption very significantly (to

29–32g/day: this is a huge change compared with the average American intake of around 150g/day), but this was not enough. It is clear that close enough is not enough; the diet is really an all-or-nothing change.

Figure 2: The effects of fat consumption on early, mildly disabled (0, 1, 2; solid line), and late seriously disabled (3, 4, 5; broken line) patients in the Swank study

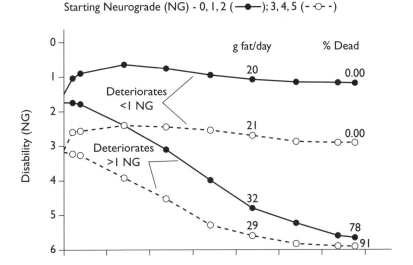

(Reprinted with permission from Elsevier Science, from Swank[4].)

FIFTY YEAR FOLLOW-UP OF SWANK'S PATIENTS

Swank continued to follow up the surviving patients of his original study. His most recent publication, in 2003, about these patients makes fascinating reading, and provides a little more insight into the original work.[5] For instance, Swank notes that the patients who adhered to the diet actually consumed 16g of saturated fat per day on average, whereas those who did not adhere to the diet consumed 38g/day. Even for the 'poor dieters' this was a marked reduction from the average 125g/day they were consuming prior to the study. It reinforces the message that the diet is an all-or-nothing issue. Just lowering saturated fat consumption, even by two-thirds as the poor dieters did, is not enough to make a difference to the progression of the disease. Saturated fat must really be completely avoided if possible.

The 63 patients surviving at the end of the 34-year study were then followed up after a period of 50 years by the time of this review.

Not surprisingly, the great majority of the surviving 63 patients (47) had adhered to the diet; there were only sixteen survivors who had not adhered to the diet. For the next fifteen years after the original study they were not seen by Swank, but he attempted to contact them at the end of this period. Fifteen patients were able to be contacted, interviewed and evaluated, thirteen from Toronto, one from Portland, Oregon and one from Montreal. All fifteen had remained on the low saturated-fat diet for 50 years. The ages ranged from 72 to 84. Of the fifteen, thirteen were essentially physically normal and walked without difficulty. The other two required assistance with walking. Swank concluded that if people with MS can rigorously follow the diet, with no more than 10–15g of saturated fat per day, they can expect to 'survive and be ambulant and otherwise normal to an advanced age'.

An editorial on this follow-up study by Swank in the same journal attempted to provide a biochemical explanation of why the diet should work in MS.[6] It concluded with the intriguing question: 'The big question is: If their results are so stunningly impressive, why haven't other physicians, neurologists, or centers adopted this method of treatment?' Swank has his theories on why the diet hasn't been widely taken up by the profession, which can be read at www.drmcdougall.com/res_swank.html in an interview with Dr McDougall.

WHY HAS THIS BEEN IGNORED?

This quite unique piece of research has been largely ignored. We must question why. Most neurologists when they inform patients of the diagnosis of MS do not tell them about diet. Yet treatment with interferon, about which I shall talk more later, is discussed with most patients. I feel this just indicates the fundamental thrust of medical research. Medicine has always sought cures. The lure of a 'magic' injection, which can be given to patients to fix their illnesses, is very strong.

We probably have the antibiotic revolution of the mid-twentieth century to thank for that. Before that, the medical literature is full of descriptions of patient factors in the resolution of illness. Once antibiotics came along, medical treatment could be pictured as a war against disease, focusing on externally administered 'cures'. Things that the patient could do seemed less important. The patient became much more of a passive recipient of the magic cure. I will discuss this further in talking about the spiritual dimension of illness, the mind–body connection, the effects of optimism and psychoneuroimmunology. It has been well shown that passive patients are not survivors.

CRITICISMS OF THE PAPER

Suffice to say that this startling piece of research, where the patient is empowered to make the changes to lifestyle that may result in success- fully delaying the progression of this insidious disease, has been ignored. The statistics show us that these very large differences in disease progres- sion did not occur by chance.

One could be critical of this research, saying it was not an RCT. There may have been factors other than diet which caused the results. Patients who could stick to the diet may have been different in terms of moti- vation, optimism and how they tackled the illness in other ways. Perhaps patients who had relapses thought there was no point sticking to the diet. I take the other view: what Swank has shown us is that if we are strong enough and determined enough to stick to the diet, we can stop the disease progressing. If that is for reasons other than the diet, does it matter? Mind you, I don't believe for one second that it is.

To criticise the research on the grounds that it was not an RCT is really a bit silly. RCTs did not exist at the time Swank started his work. It was obviously not possible to undertake an RCT. Swank used the appro- priate research methodology of his time. He studied a cohort of people after instituting a medical intervention and meticulously followed their clinical course with regular review by experienced specialist clinicians. This was the correct method for its time.

There is now a huge worldwide interest in a group of drugs called statins, which in the laboratory and in limited human studies seem to significantly benefit people with MS. The statins seem to work in a similar way to Swank's diet. They are used already in medicine to lower the levels of 'bad' fats in the blood and seem to also have an immune effect, just as the diet does. Of course, being pharmaceutical drugs they are much more likely to attract research funding, and to be marketed strongly if proven to be effective. The fact that they have potentially toxic side effects whereas the diet does not seems to be ignored. One wonders about modern medicine sometimes. Interestingly, experts in the area have suggested that polyun- saturated fatty acids and statins achieve their benefits in a similar way.[7]

There seems to be a real preoccupation in medicine currently with providing drug solutions to problems caused by poor lifestyles. In many cases, the drugs bring their own problems. One 80-year-old lady I treated recently in the emergency department complained to me that the cure she was receiving for her cancer was worse than the disease, and I couldn't help but agree with her. She couldn't eat because of thrush in the mouth, couldn't go to the toilet without pain because of thrush in her rectum, had no hair, was vomiting and kept getting infections.

As we have previously seen, another problem is that often the drug therapies are not as effective as lifestyle changes, yet modern medicine promotes them above the lifestyle changes. This is partly because of financial considerations, but also because there is a widespread feeling within the medical profession that people just aren't capable of making major lifestyle changes.

I have previously given the examples of diabetes, heart disease and prostate cancer. As another example, scientists recently suggested that everyone should be taking a 'polypill' which contains several of the drugs currently in use for treating or preventing cardiovascular disease.[8] They hypothesised, on the basis of published medical evidence, that heart disease rates could be cut by 88 per cent and stroke by 80 per cent if everyone over 55 took one of these 'all-in-one' pills. Towards the end of their paper they did admit, though, that with this wonder drug, 8–15 per cent of people would experience side effects.

Somewhat tongue-in-cheek but nevertheless accurate, Dutch researchers proposed a safer, cheaper and tastier alternative, the polymeal.[9] This would utilise all the elements of diet currently known to reduce the risk of cardiovascular disease. Their research findings showed that if everyone ate a diet rich in wine, fish, dark chocolate, fruits, vegetables, garlic and almonds, cardiovascular disease events would be reduced by 76 per cent. This is very close to what I am recommending in this book, minus the chocolate, which is unfortunately full of saturated fat, counteracting the benefits of its rich antioxidants. And, of course, the only side effects of this diet would be positive, with beneficial effects for a whole range of diseases from MS to arthritis and depression.

There has only been one major criticism of Swank's work published that I can find.[10] The authors argued that the neurological assessments of the patients, that is, determining how they progressed, were not blinded. This means that the investigators knew which patients were sticking to the diet when they tested them to see how the disease had progressed.

While this may have introduced some bias into the assessment, it is very hard to argue that there is bias in assessing whether someone is bed-bound or confined to a wheelchair (or dead!), as most of the poor dieters were.

Another criticism is that the good dieters had more cases of short duration and very mild disability than the other group. Of course, these are the very patients who are highly motivated to stay on such a diet, to prevent any disease progression, so they are better represented in the good dieters group. I am unimpressed with these criticisms. Despite the criticisms, the authors who made them argued that the dietary fat hypothesis is just as plausible as other, more fashionable hypotheses, and should be further explored. While scientists are exploring, I know what I'll be doing.

The damning editorial

After scratching my head for a long time over why Professor Swank's research has been ignored, I went back to *The Lancet* to see what sort of reaction the paper provoked amongst the readership. As a past editor of a medical journal, I am always intrigued to see the response of readers to major pieces of research. It is often difficult to predict what readers will find controversial and worth writing to the journal about. All journals have a Letters to the Editor section. Editors like to see these sections full of comments about the important papers we publish. Often, important points about the paper come to light when other doctors who read the paper compare the results to their own experience, or shed new insight on the topic from their research. What surprised me when I went back to the journal was that the paper, which I considered a major piece of research into MS, and certainly controversial, did not attract a single letter to the editor. Not one. Again I scratched my head. Then I flipped back a few pages and saw the answer.

Most journals have a policy of publishing comments on important papers in the same issue. As we have seen, these editorials are designed to give an expert view of where that research fits into the overall scheme of things. *The Lancet* is one of the premier medical journals in the world. *The Lancet*, along with the *British Medical Journal*, *Journal of the American Medical Association* and *New England Journal of Medicine*, constitute the 'Big Four' medical journals in the world. Their influence on medical thinking is profound. Their editorials are even more influential than the individual research papers, representing as they do elite medical opinion on the scientific value of the paper to which they refer.

The Lancet at the time had a policy, one which in general has been criticised by many other editors, of publishing anonymous editorials. Many journals, such as the *Medical Journal of Australia*, commission experts to write editorials on papers they publish, but tell the readership who these experts are. In that way they become accountable for the opinions they espouse, just as the authors of the original papers are. The policy of not identifying the authors of the editorials has been criticised as encouraging unbalanced editorials. One-upmanship is alive and well in medicine, and experts who can take a shot at other experts' work under the cover of secrecy are liable to do so. Incidentally, *The Lancet* has since changed its policy and now identifies the authors of such reviews, calling them commentaries rather than editorials.

The editorial in *The Lancet* on Professor Swank's paper was critical of the study.[11] The author, unnamed, correctly criticised the paper for not being randomised; that is, the patients were not randomly allocated to low and normal fat in the diet. Rightly the editorial author suggested that those patients who relapsed would be more likely not to follow the diet. However, in summing up, this unnamed author wrote 'the role of lipids in MS must remain not proven'. Carrying with it the impressive and prestigious stamp of *The Lancet*, this was a powerful message. I am sure many thousands of neurologists the world over looked at this and thought, well there goes the diet theory. It helps to explain why patients recently diagnosed with MS who question their neurologist about diet are told, as a friend of mine was recently, 'They've been looking at diet for years. If there was anything in it, they would have found it years ago.'

> Swank's work may have been discounted by some colleagues because of a critical anonymous editorial.

Must the evidence be absolutely conclusive though? Certainly if we are talking about a powerful drug with toxic side effects, we have a duty to be absolutely certain it works before offering it to our patients. But what about a therapy with positive side effects like reduced incidence of heart attack, high blood pressure, depression and so on, especially if the disease is incurable and the study results suggest a strong benefit? Even if the therapy didn't work for MS, surely as doctors we would be happy to see our patients' general health improving with better diet.

It is ironic to think that the great strength of Swank's study, that is its duration of 34 years, turned out to be its great weakness. It is rare to find any clinical trials in the medical literature of such duration. The interferon trials in MS, for example, have typically been of around one to two years' duration. When Swank started his study in 1949, the standard of proof in medicine was to test a new therapy out on patients and assess whether they got better or not. This must seem a sensible way to assess these things to the average person. Indeed, the 1934 Nobel Prize in Medicine, the first won by an American, went to Dr George Minot for his work on a chopped liver diet in pernicious anaemia. Minot gave his patients the chopped liver diet, followed them for about nine months, and found that they all did far better than any patients with the disease had previously. People who defaulted on the diet got sick again very quickly.

The parallels with Swank's work are obvious. But because of the duration of Swank's study, by the time it was published in 1990 the standard of proof in medicine had changed dramatically. Randomised controlled trials had become the accepted level of evidence. Ironically, this important piece of research potentially could have won Swank a Nobel Prize had it been published at the time he started it; by the time it was finished it was consigned to the 'unproven' basket and largely dismissed by a doubting medical profession. This is despite the fact that the disease was considered incurable, at the time had no other therapies which were effective, and the only side effects of treatment with Swank's diet were positive. Interestingly, the treatment for pernicious anaemia, that is vitamin B12 that is found in liver, has never been studied in an RCT. We accepted the work of Minot, yet we rejected the work of Swank. Curious.

It is important here to note that Swank was a highly respected, leading academic neurologist. He was born in 1909 in Washington, received a BS at the University of Washington in 1930 and an MD and PhD in 1935 from Northwestern University in Chicago. He founded the Swank MS Clinic in Oregon, taught at Harvard from 1945 to 1948 and the famous McGill University from 1948 to 1954, and was professor and head of the neurology division at the University of Oregon Medical School from 1954 to 1976. Swank published six books and 170 articles in his field and received numerous honours. He died in 2008 at the age of 99, just a few months short of his 100th birthday.

We sometimes become sceptical about things we read on the Internet with all its uncensored and unverified content, and can easily mistake quackery for real science. Professor Swank's work, though, clearly comes from the mainstream of academic neurology. The dismissal of his work is surprising considering he was seen by his colleagues as such a leader in MS management, teaching and research.

Could it have been an RCT?

Could performing a genuine RCT have removed the doubts? I don't think so. We would be left with the same problem. Many people, despite their best intentions, simply cannot stick to a diet. If we randomly allocated people to one group who had a low saturated-fat diet and others who ate a 'normal' diet, there would still be many who defaulted on the diet. Let's assume that this therapy really works. Those who stayed with the diet would have impressive results and stop relapsing. The group who was allocated to the normal diet would have bad results. The critics would then pinpoint the defaulters in the diet group, who would have a bad result and say, well they started relapsing and so gave up on the diet. We are left with those who stayed on the diet who would have done well anyway because they had a benign form of the disease. Whichever way the researchers went they would get the same criticism, and the case would still be considered 'not proven'.

Just as an aside, it is difficult to imagine that the 72 good dieters out of 144 patients in Swank's study all had benign disease, and that was the explanation for why they did so well. We have already seen that in most studies the benign group accounts for 6–20 per cent of cases, nowhere near 50 per cent. Incidentally, in his paper Swank is quite categorical that patients who defaulted on the diet, even many years after beginning it, soon relapsed. As the neurologist who was monitoring these patients carefully, he was the only one in a position to know whether defaulting on the diet came first, or the relapse came first. Again, as in interpreting all of the medical literature, we come down to a question of trust in the integrity of the researcher in reporting data, and Swank's reputation was one of the utmost integrity.

WHAT CONSTITUTES PROOF IN SCIENCE?

It is worth discussing the concept of proof in science here. Imagine the difference if Swank's paper had been presented to an audience of people with MS. While many would not have the scientific background to understand the difficulties in the methods he used, and the valid scientific criticisms of the paper, they could see for themselves what potential there was in this therapy. Better yet, imagine if it was presented to a group of patients and their doctors. The doctors would have to justify why they had written off a therapy with such amazing potential. This is a disease described as incurable. Do we need absolute proof? As Dr Bernie Siegel says, in the face of uncertainty there's nothing wrong with hope. It seems that the way in which this paper was presented to the medical world has effectively stopped it being offered to patients, except by a small group of 'believers' and presumably the original researchers. Let us not forget that these researchers were also eminent neurologists. While other experts did not agree about the validity of their findings, that is not unusual in medicine. The point at issue was how conclusive this evidence was.

We must remember that in medicine there is no such thing as proof. The editorial stating that this diet remained not proven was only stating the obvious; it was not the strength of the effect of the diet that was being questioned, but rather how much confidence the medical profession could have in prescribing it, how strong the evidence of the effect was. Because the study was not an RCT, the evidence was felt to be weaker than if it was. But even if it was an RCT, that does not constitute proof. For instance, if the p value was 0.05, then the difference between the groups still may have occurred by chance every twenty times the study was performed, even if there was no real difference between the two treatments at all.

In Swank's study the evidence may not have been as strong as if it was an RCT, but the size of the effect was stunning. Later we will see that interferon, which has been 'proven' in a properly constructed RCT, reduced the relapse rate by one-third in MS. Swank's diet in contrast reduced the relapse rate by three times this amount to nearly zero (one relapse every ten to twenty years). The magnitude of the effect was many times greater than for any other therapy tried in MS, despite the questions about the strength of the evidence. The relapse rate reduction once stable on the diet for those who could stick to it was of the order of 95 per cent. I am disappointed that more was not made of this extremely impressive research, and that some of my colleagues continue not to offer this therapy to newly diagnosed patients.

And again I would make the point that Swank's diet had a huge advantage over other tried therapies. It was not a therapy like interferon, in which patients passively receive treatment from a medical practitioner. It involved patients actively controlling their illness with a major lifestyle change. The power that such control gives patients should not be underestimated, and may have significant effects as well on their immune function and mental state. This issue will be explored in the chapter on the mind–body connection.

OTHER WORK ON LOW SATURATED-FAT DIETS

Since writing the first book, a number of other studies on low saturated-fat diets in MS have come to my attention. I am indebted to one of the members of the first MS Self-Help and Support Group we ran through the Gawler Foundation, who showed me the work of Dr Catherine Kousmine. Published in 1984, written in French, and translated into Italian, German and Spanish but not English, Dr Kousmine's book *La Sclerose en Plaques est Guerrissable* (Multiple Sclerosis is Curable) outlines 55 cases she treated over a period of nineteen to 26 years. She treated the patients with a diet very similar to Professor Swank's, supplemented with 1–2 tablespoons of cold pressed oil (sunflower, linseed or wheatgerm), and gave them a cream substitute made from linseed oil.

Like Swank's patients they did remarkably well, with most of them stabilising their condition and a number improving. Of the 55 patients, twenty had progressive forms of MS and the rest relapsing-remitting. Eight dropped out after stopping the diet, but of those who stayed in the study only one deteriorated due to MS, while four developed cancer and one scleroderma. In most cases response to the diet was very good. Again, it is unusual to find studies of such duration in medical research, and we would be unwise I think to ignore the findings, even though the study was not a randomised controlled trial. Dr Kousmine trained initially in science, then in medicine, and specialised in paediatrics.

She wrote another book entitled *Be and Stay Well Until 80 or More*, in which she outlined her views on the damage caused by typical high saturated-fat and processed food Western diets. Much of this is of course now accepted by the medical profession, but her views were strongly criticised at the time by her colleagues. Dr Kousmine herself lived to the age of 88. Just to show how much in medicine is old news being rediscovered, researchers from Norway have recently shown that a low saturated-fat diet plus omega-3 supplementation was helpful in a group of patients with MS, and suggested this area needs more formal study![12]

> Other studies of low saturated-fat diets support the work of Swank.

In 2005, the first RCT on dietary fat in MS was published.[13] This was unfortunately only a very small study of limited duration but is an important addition to the evidence base on dietary fats in MS. In a one-year study, 31 patients with relapsing-remitting MS were assigned to a low-fat diet (15% of calories) supplemented with fish oil or the standard American Heart Association heart diet in which fat made up 30 per cent of calories, supplemented with olive oil.

Immediately we can see problems with this study which might weaken the effects we have seen in Swank's study. Firstly it was a relatively short study: the maximal benefit of diet in Swank's study did not occur until at least the three-year mark. Secondly, the fat reduction was not specifically directed at saturated fat, and both groups lowered their fat intake. Thirdly, it was a small study: only 27 patients were available for analysis of the 31 enrolled. Lastly, olive oil is likely to have some benefit based on animal work in experimental MS, so should not have been used as a control treatment. Additionally, only around two-thirds of the participants were able to stick to their diets.

Despite these issues, the study showed that patients felt better according to standard MS quality of life questionnaires. But more importantly, their relapse rates fell quite significantly from pre-trial rates, more so for the fish oil group. In fact the fish oil group had a mean relapse rate of 1.14 relapses per year in the year prior to the trial, and dropped by 0.79, a reduction of 69 per cent, and the olive oil group had a pre-trial rate of 1.17 which dropped by 0.69, a 59 per cent reduction (personal communication, Bianca Weinstock-Guttman, 2008). These findings were statistically significant despite the small numbers of participants. Interestingly, the drop of 69 per cent for the low-fat plus fish oil group is remarkably similar to the relapse rate reduction in the first year of Swank's study (see Figure 1). This should really give us confidence that the findings in Swank's study were real.

The authors concluded that despite the study limitations, a low-fat diet supplemented with omega-3 fatty acids may complement the beneficial effects of concurrent disease-modifying therapies. They suggested this because virtually all patients were on disease-modifying drugs for the year prior and the year of the study. The 69 per cent relapse rate reduction associated with the diet compares very favourably with the reduction of about 30 per cent for these drugs in the major clinical trials, and would appear to be additive in benefit. The MS community is crying out for more well-designed research in the area, and researchers have speculated that with more research diet may well become standard treatment in the future.[14] It is interesting to note that I have been unable to find a single clinical study of a low-fat diet in MS that has not shown these strongly positive findings, regardless of methodology. Why, then, are such diets often dismissed by doctors?

SUPPORT FOR SWANK'S WORK FROM BASIC SCIENCE

In my research of fats in MS, I came across a number of old papers containing some very interesting findings. Scientists at the Hormel Institute and the Mayo Clinic in Minnesota looked at the fatty acid composition of plasma in fourteen patients with MS and compared this with 100 patients without MS. They published their findings in the *Proceedings of the National Academy of Science of the USA* in 1989.[15] Their findings were impressive. The cells of MS patients were comprised of significantly less polyunsaturated fatty acids than those of people without MS. More importantly, these fats had been replaced in the cells by saturated fatty acids.

This was replicated at around the same time in two other studies, both of which showed deficiencies in omega-3 fatty acids in cell membranes of people with MS.[16, 17] A 2007 review of the subject by British researchers published in the *British Journal of Nutrition* concluded that epidemiological, biochemical, animal model and clinical trial data strongly suggest that polyunsaturated fatty acids have a role in the development and treatment of MS.[18] The authors noted that disturbed essential fatty acid metabolism in MS causes a loss of long chain polyunsaturated fatty acids in cell membranes, causing problems with CNS structure and function. So here we have another possible explanation of why a diet rich in polyunsaturates and markedly restricted in saturated fats might improve the condition of people with MS.

In my work at the Gawler Foundation, I have been asked to look at the fatty acid profile of the cells of some people with MS. A similar finding has emerged. These people with MS, even those on the Swank diet, tend to preferentially take up saturated fats and incorporate them into their cells, even if they are only there in very small quantities in their diets. Hence the aim is to restrict saturated fats to almost zero in the diet. Again, it is somewhat surprising that little further research has been done in the area. But further work has been done in essential fatty acid supplementation.

ESSENTIAL FATTY ACID SUPPLEMENTS

This is where the story gets really interesting. Early work had shown that by adding polyunsaturated fats to the diet in the form of an omega-6 fatty acid, linoleic acid, there was a tendency towards slower progression of MS, but the results were a little inconclusive. These were three formal randomised controlled trials, but all of them were poorly set up.[19, 20, 21] For a start, none cut down the patients' intake of saturated fat. It is known that saturated fat competes with unsaturated fats for uptake into cell membranes and in biological pathways. Saturated fat is tough; it usually wins in these contests, and this seems to be especially so for people with MS. Secondly, the control groups did not really take an inactive substance. They were given oleic acid, or olive oil.

Olive oil has been shown to reduce the severity of experimental auto-immune encephalomyelitis.[22] We have also seen that countries like Italy, where the olive oil intake is high, have a low incidence of MS. Oleic acid gets taken up into cell membranes like the polyunsaturates, and is flexible and pliable, unlike saturated fatty acids. Finally, the numbers were too small in each individual study to get a statistically significant effect. So, a group of investigators pooled the results and looked at the overall effect, allowing for some differences between the studies.[23] They did show a statistically significant decrease in the rate of deterioration with linoleic acid supplementation, but only for those with minimal or no disability at entry to the study.

More recently, the UK National Health Service National Institute for Health and Clinical Excellence (NICE) produced guidelines for doctors managing multiple sclerosis. This set of consensus guidelines from experts in MS summarised all the available evidence on therapies in MS and made recommendations for doctors to follow. These guidelines make very interesting reading for people with MS and can be accessed easily on the Internet. I will refer to their recommendations elsewhere where relevant, but here it is important to note that they recommended that 'people with MS should be advised that linoleic acid 17–23g/day may reduce progression of disability'.[24] For people who are told by healthcare workers, as many people with MS I know have been, that diet has no role in the treatment of MS, it may be a good idea to refer them to these guidelines.

> Polyunsaturated fat supplementation has been shown to slow the progression of MS.

Another trial by Fitzgerald and co-workers in 1987 looked at the effects of nutritional counselling on outcome.[25] These investigators were working on behalf of a group called ARMS (Action for Research into Multiple Sclerosis). The group was formed by a number of patients with MS who were distressed about the lack of available therapies offered to them after diagnosis. Judy Graham, who wrote the excellent book *Multiple Sclerosis: A self-help guide to its management*,[26] was one of them. Much of the story of this group is reported here for those who are interested. They approached a group of researchers at the Central Middlesex Hospital in London, hoping to further research the disease and come up with some therapies. Their thrust was dietary. Professor Michael Crawford, Professor of Nutrition at Nottingham University, devised a diet which was high in essential fatty acids and provided a good intake of vitamins and minerals.

What made it hard for people on this diet was that the researchers asked patients to get these levels through normal diet and not by supplementation. While most people would find this extremely difficult, I discuss later the evidence that supplements of vitamins and antioxidants are not only not as good as getting these substances through diet, but positively harmful.

Two hundred people with MS entered the study. Predictably there was a high drop-out rate as the diet, testing and analyses were quite rigorous. Eighty-three remained in the study for 34 months. They were counselled to decrease saturated fat intake and increase polyunsaturated fats, as well as increasing antioxidants. This is where the fat part of the diet differed from Swank's. Unlike Swank, patients were able to eat saturated fats, but had to ensure the ratio of polyunsaturated to saturated fats remained high. For those who complied with the recommendations, as judged by rigorous dietary analysis, there was no significant deterioration in disability; for the poor dieters, the disability worsened significantly (p<0.022). One interesting aspect of the study was that the investigators were able to prove that the good dieters did modify their diet by monitoring levels of the fats in the blood.

For those more interested in the ARMS diet, Geraldine Fitzgerald and Fenella Briscoe, two of the nutritionists working with ARMS, in 1989 released a diet book entitled *Multiple Sclerosis. Healthy menus to help in the management of multiple sclerosis.*[27] They note here the recommended general dietary guidelines for the ARMS diet as follows:

1. Use polyunsaturated margarines and oils.
2. Eat at least 3 helpings of fish each week.
3. Eat 225g (½lb) liver each week.
4. Eat a large helping of dark green vegetables daily.
5. Eat some raw vegetables daily, as a salad.
6. Eat some linseeds daily.
7. Eat some fresh fruit daily.
8. Eat as much fresh food as possible in preference to processed food.
9. Choose lean cuts of meat, and trim all fat away before cooking.
10. Avoid hard animal fats like butter, lard, suet, dripping, and fatty foods such as cream, hard cheese, etc.
11. Eat wholegrain cereals and wholemeal bread rather than refined cereals.
12. Cut down on sugar and foods containing sugar.

The overriding guideline for the ARMS nutritionists was not so much the absolute amount of saturated fat in the diet, as the ratio of polyunsaturated fat to saturated fat. I find it hard to agree with the suggestion to eat liver and meat in this diet, as well as margarine, given what we now know about trans-fatty acids in margarine and the role of saturated fats in the causation of MS.

Omega-3 versus omega-6 fatty acids

With the increasing knowledge about fats today, the story gets even more interesting. The studies mentioned to date have looked at omega-6 supplementation. We now know that omega-3 fatty acids work to suppress immune system disorders and omega-6s seem to worsen them, although not nearly as much as saturated fats. Additionally, we have good evidence that MS is infrequent in places where fish (high in omega-3s) is eaten a lot. Japan for instance has a very low incidence. Perhaps omega-3 supplementation would be a better way to go than omega-6.

Some of the same investigators who had done the omega-6 work decided to do an RCT to test this.[28] Again, one of the difficulties was patient numbers, but also the investigators felt they couldn't ethically use a placebo inactive treatment as omega-6s had already been shown to work. So the control group took omega-6s. Once again there was no strict avoidance of animal fats; rather, the patients were 'given dietary advice to encourage a low intake of animal fat and a plentiful intake of omega-6 fatty acids'. So we have no record of how much animal fat patients in each group had, and the untreated group was actually receiving treatment with omega-6 fatty acids, which had previously been shown to work in MS. So was the group treated with the omega-3 fatty acids.

Not surprisingly the investigators failed to find a statistically significant difference. If omega-3s were better, one would expect both groups to get better but the omega-3 group to be ahead. This is what they found: the omega-3 group did better; 79 patients were unchanged or better and 66 were worse at two years. Of the omega-6 group, 65 were the same or better, and 82 were worse. The p value for this difference was 0.07, not quite making the usual 0.05 accepted significance level. Although the researchers were ethically right in not asking the control group patients to miss out on the benefits of dietary changes, this decision almost certainly cost them the chance to get a p value which would be regarded as 'proof' by doctors in general.

We now also have the work from the first RCT of diet in MS referred to previously which found a statistically significant improvement in the group which took fish oil.[13] A Dutch review in 2005 concluded that fish oil may be beneficial in MS both through its immune mechanism of action and through structural effects within the CN,[29] much as has been discussed in this chapter.

COMPARISON WITH ILLNESS PROGRESSION IN OTHER TRIALS

Good evidence of comparisons in illness progression is published in Swank's *Diet Book*. He compared the percentage of patients in his study who survived over the course of the study with four untreated groups of patients for which he could get data (Figure 3). These were from studies by Allison reported in the journal *Brain*,[30] Maclean and Berkson reported in the *Journal of the American Medical Association*,[31] Miller reported in *Acta Medica Scandinavica*,[32] and a study from the Veterans Administration MS Study Group reported in *Archives of Neurology*.[33] After fifteen years around a quarter of patients in these four groups had died, whereas only 6 per cent of Swank's patients had. At 30 years, 63 per cent of the untreated patients had died, compared with 18 per cent of those on the low saturated-fat diet. After 36 years, 70 per cent of untreated patients were dead, whereas only 21 per cent of Swank's patients were.

Figure 3: Percentage of patients surviving in each of five studies over time

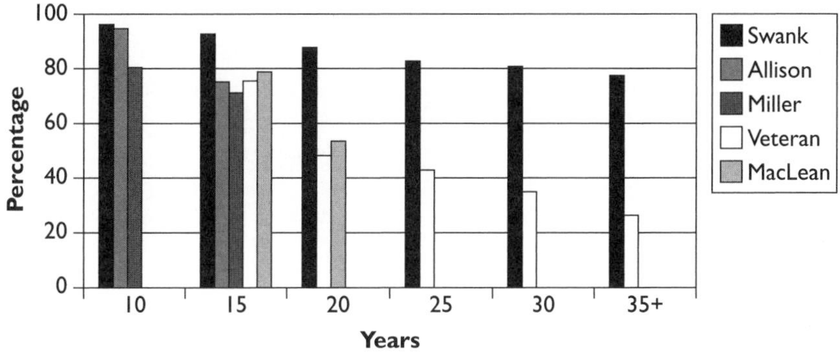

OVERVIEW

The evidence is extremely convincing. All the studies in MS where a low saturated-fat diet has been used as a therapy have had similar results; there are no studies with contradictory findings. Dietary fats play a major part in the development and progression of MS. Manipulating the intake of fats has a great effect on outcome. It seems clear that the most important part of this equation is to dramatically cut down saturated fats from all sources. Just adding polyunsaturated essential fatty acids to the diet slows disease progression. If the findings of Swank and others reported here are real, and we have every reason to believe that they are, it is much more effective, however, and seems to almost halt the disease altogether if saturated fats are cut out.

The fat story is likely to get even more interesting as knowledge increases. Evidence is starting to emerge that polyunsaturated fatty acids play an important protective role in the CNS,[34, 35] and some researchers in the field are starting to call for a re-appraisal of the role of fats in the development of MS.[36] In a few years, we may see a more complete acceptance of the role of fats in neurological disease just as we have in heart disease. Scientists are now beginning to propose that vegan diets with additional fish oil (plus vitamin D supplementation, about which I shall talk more later), through their immune system effects, can be used to prevent the onset of MS in susceptible people.[37]

7

DIETARY SUPPLEMENTS: EVIDENCE ABOUT MULTI-VITAMINS, ANTIOXIDANTS AND OTHERS

Why is it not possible to take a vitamin pill to obtain the same effect as a balanced diet?

Goran Bjelakovic

SUPPLEMENTS

In addition to diet, Swank placed all of the patients in his studies on a multivitamin a day. The area of vitamin supplements is one where there has historically been much conjecture, debate and opinion but little real evidence. And what evidence there is has until recently been contra-dictory. This is now changing. And it is important to consider, as with medications used in MS, the influence of powerful industries marketing their products, and this always muddies the waters.

While we have known for centuries that a diet rich in micronutrients, specifically vitamins, minerals and antioxidants, is helpful in preventing a range of diseases and slowing down the ageing process, it has not been clear whether extracting those nutrients, concentrating them and taking them in supplement form has any benefits. Like essential fatty acids, many of these compounds cannot be made in the body and must be

---

SUMMARISING THE EVIDENCE

- Antioxidants have been recommended for many inflammatory conditions including MS, although there has been little evidence to support any beneficial effect.
- Major meta-analyses of all RCTs on the health benefits of antioxidants and vitamin supplements compared to placebo have now been undertaken.
  - Beta-carotene, vitamin A and vitamin E supplements have been consistently shown to cause an increase in overall death rate in these studies, from about a 4 per cent increase for vitamin E alone to about 29 per cent for a combination.
  - Regular multivitamins have been associated with a one-third increase in risk of advanced prostate cancer, and nearly a doubling of risk of death from the disease.
- The B group vitamins are extremely important for normal brain function; they have not been shown to have the same risks.
  - Vitamin B12 is non-toxic and is frequently low in people with MS and those on a vegan diet.

EVIDENCE-BASED RECOMMENDATIONS

- Antioxidants and multivitamins are not recommended for people with MS.
- For people with MS wishing to take a vitamin supplement, a B group mixture is the best choice.
- It may be prudent to take vitamin B12 supplements if adhering to a plant-based diet.

---

ingested in the diet. A whole industry has grown up around extracting or synthesising these nutrients, and convincing us through clever marketing that taking these 'magic ingredients' in a tablet or capsule on a regular basis will keep us well or help us recover from disease. This is a bit like the modern pharmaceutical industry, which would have us believe that

we can live lifestyles known to accelerate ageing and contribute to countless illnesses and then reverse the effects with a single tablet—effectively
that we can have our cake and eat it too.

Intuitively this doesn't make sense. There is balance in all things.
A diet rich in fruit and vegetables is likely to have its great health-giving
benefits because of the combination of all the nutrients in the whole
package. Eating junk, and then supplementing with one, two or more of
the individual nutrients can't possibly replicate the value of the original
food. Yet for many people it is hard to resist the temptation of fast foods
with their strong, addictive flavours, feeling content in the knowledge
that they can be healthy despite this by taking vitamins.

ANTIOXIDANTS

Despite intensive research, it is unclear which particular constituents of
fruits and vegetables might be beneficial for health, but the antioxidant
vitamins and elements have been most studied. The focus has been on
antioxidants because it has been assumed that antioxidants may prevent
damage to cells from oxidation. We know that oxidation plays a role
in ageing and in many diseases, including cardiovascular diseases and
cancer.

Oxidation is a chemical process. This can best be visualised by imagining a piece of shiny silver left in the air for a few weeks. Gradually it
will lose its lustre and develop a grey coating. This happens because the
silver has combined with oxygen, in so doing giving up some of its electrons. The same thing happens with highly unsaturated oils. If a bottle of
linseed or walnut oil is left out in the air and heat it will quickly become
rancid, or oxidised.

The same thing is happening all the time in our bodies. Our bodies
are oxygen-rich environments. Oxygen is coursing through all our
tissues continually. While oxygen is necessary to keep us alive, it also
causes oxidation of our bodily tissues. In so doing, products of oxidation are released. Some of the names of these may be familiar. A lot has
been written now about free radicals. These are oxidation by-products
and are in themselves thought to be quite harmful. Additionally, in
these days of pollution, radiation, chemical pesticides and environmental contaminants, there are free radicals lurking all around us in
our external environment. If we smoke, we take in megadoses of free

radicals. These compounds are quite unstable and are looking to find an electron to stabilise themselves. These electrons come from our tissues, causing oxidation.

The balance existing between these by-products and the so-called antioxidant defences is thought to be a key factor in preventing the development of diseases such as cancer, heart disease and the auto-immune diseases including MS.[1] There is also accumulating evidence that these free radicals are responsible for much of the ageing process. There is now a large amount of literature describing the role of oxidation and lipid (fat) peroxidation in the development of MS. Many researchers have shown increases in the by-products of oxidation in people with MS compared to healthy volunteers,[2, 3] and in experimental MS in animals.[4] It has also been shown that during an attack of MS, these by-products overwhelm the antioxidant defence system. What hasn't yet been shown is whether improving the antioxidant status of patients with MS can influence the progression of disease, or how improving the antioxidant status using diet compares with the use of supplements.

Moving to a diet rich in vegetables, fruit, nuts, seeds and grains ensures a potent dietary mixture of vitamins, minerals and antioxidants. It also ensures that these substances are in their natural state, balanced with other food factors essential for their optimal function. Some foods seem to be powerhouses of antioxidants, for instance berries like blueberries, cruciferous vegetables like broccoli, grape seeds, red wine and tea.

THE RISKS ASSOCIATED WITH ANTIOXIDANT AND MULTIVITAMIN SUPPLEMENTS

The question then is could we take antioxidant supplements instead of or in addition to getting them through our food. When these compounds are taken as supplements, there has until recently been very little evidence, despite much interest and research in the area, that they make any difference at all to health. It was in fact assumed that, even if they had no benefit, at least they were doing no harm, and so could be taken almost as a form of insurance against an unhealthy lifestyle. Several major well-conducted studies published in the early 2000s have cast serious doubt over this assumption, raising the likelihood that taking antioxidant and vitamin supplements probably does very real harm.[5–11] These studies were systematic reviews or meta-analyses of all the published randomised controlled trials on multivitamins and antioxidant supplements in various diseases, and their effect on overall mortality. Meta-analysis is considered the most powerful form of medical evidence. Researchers analyse pooled data from all comparable trials. This means large patient numbers and greater likelihood of finding real effects rather than those caused by chance.

Vivekananthan's study from the Cleveland Clinic Foundation looked at seven RCTs of vitamin E and eight of beta-carotene supplementation versus placebo or no intervention in heart disease.[5] These studies involved around 220,000 patients. There was no effect from vitamin E supplementation, but beta-carotene supplementation resulted in a 7 per cent increase (p=0.003) in deaths overall, and a 10 per cent increase (p=0.003) in death from heart disease.

Bjelakovic's group from Copenhagen looked at various supplements in the prevention of cancers of the digestive system.[6, 7] They examined trials involving over 170,000 people, and found no benefit of beta-carotene, vitamin A or vitamin E in reducing the incidence of these cancers. However, again, they found an increase in the overall death rate of the people who took these supplements versus those taking placebo. For beta-carotene and vitamin A combination supplements there was a 29 per cent increase in mortality, and for beta-carotene together with vitamin E there was a 10 per cent increase.

Miller and colleagues from the Johns Hopkins School of Medicine examined nearly 136,000 people in nineteen clinical trials, taking either vitamin E alone or in combination with other supplements.[8] They found an alarming increase in the overall death rate of those taking high dose vitamin E (400IU or more per day), with a clear dose-response relationship, that is, the higher the dose the more likely that death was the outcome. The size of the increase in risk was alarming, with an extra 39 deaths per 10,000 people (p=0.035) taking the high-dose supplements compared with those not taking vitamin E.

Lawson from the National Cancer Institute, Bethesda looked at the relationship between multivitamin use and the five-year risk of prostate cancer in over 295,000 men in the National Institutes of Health Diet and Health Study who were cancer free at enrolment in 1995 and 1996.[10] They found a 32 per cent increased risk of advanced prostate cancer, and a massive 98 per cent increased risk of death in those men taking multivitamin supplements more than seven times a week. Because the study was very large, and was prospective, thus reducing bias from hindsight, the results were very likely to be accurate.

The risk of taking antioxidant vitamin supplements was characterised further by Bjelakovic's group from Copenhagen in 2007.[11] This major meta-analysis looked at the death rate from all causes for people taking antioxidant supplements versus no treatment in 68 trials with nearly a quarter of a million participants. They separated the trials into those of high and low quality. The high quality trials showed a clear increase in risk for those taking the supplements, with a 4 per cent increase in death rate for those taking vitamin E alone, 7 per cent increase for those taking beta-carotene, and 16 per cent increase for those taking vitamin A.

These results are of great concern, particularly as it has been shown by the 1987, 1992 and 2000 National Health Interview Surveys that in the United States, vitamin and mineral supplement use increased from just under a quarter of all adults in 1987 to over a third in 2000.[12] This is probably similar in most developed countries.

> Vitamins A (and its precursor beta-carotene) and E should not be taken as supplements; meta-analyses of clinical trials show they increase overall death rates.

Bjelakovic's editorial summed up the situation by asking: 'Why is it not possible to take a vitamin pill to obtain the same effect as a balanced diet?'[13] He stated that: 'Antioxidant supplements in pills are synthetic, factory processed, and may not be safe compared with their naturally occurring counterparts.' He hypothesised that one explanation for the increase in death rate due to antioxidant supplementation was that these supplements were given to people in middle- and high-income countries who already have diets with plenty of vitamins and trace elements.

Should we take antioxidant or multivitamin supplements?

Swank placed all of the patients in his landmark study on a low satu-rated-fat diet in MS on a multivitamin supplement. It was on this basis that I recommended in the first book that people with MS take a multi-vitamin daily. But that was before definitive evidence was available about their unexpected negative effects on health. The evidence now seems clear that taking multivitamins, particularly the antioxidants vitamin E and A (and its precursor beta-carotene), cannot be considered beneficial, or even safe, and should be avoided by people eating a healthy diet. On a diet like that recommended in this book, the intake of these and other essential vitamins should be quite high.

There have been many recommendations to supplement with quite large doses of vitamin E to guard against lipid peroxidation for people taking unsaturated oil supplements. Besides the above research about increasing death rates from vitamin E supplementation, research is now coming out on fish oil plus vitamin E supplementation for a range of diseases, but mainly in the area of heart disease. While the studies show a very beneficial effect for fish oil supplementation alone, they show no additional benefit from supplementing with vitamin E.[14]

BENEFICIAL INDIVIDUAL SUPPLEMENTS

So there is good evidence to suggest that people with MS should not take antioxidants or multivitamins. However, there are a number of individual supplemental vitamins which may be of value in MS according to available evidence.

Vitamin B12

Vitamin B12 is an extremely important nutrient. It is a B group vitamin found primarily in meat, especially liver, eggs and dairy products. No plant foods can be relied on as a definite source of vitamin B12. It is necessary for the maintenance of a healthy nervous system and plays a key role in the metabolism of fatty acids essential for the maintenance of myelin. Prolonged B12 deficiency can lead to nerve degeneration and irreversible neurological damage. Deficiency is more commonly caused by failure to absorb B12 from the intestine rather than a dietary deficiency.

People with low levels of acid in the stomach are susceptible to deficiency. Deficiency is well known to occur in vegans. As many people are taking drugs which lower stomach acid levels, like ranitidine or omeprazole, if they are also on a vegan diet there is a real risk of B12 deficiency. It can take many years for deficiency disease to develop after changing to diets low in B12. B12 deficiency is surprisingly common, even in people who are not on vegan diets or have low acid levels in their stomachs. One Australian study showed that about 23 per cent of people aged over 50 had low vitamin B12 levels.[15]

Fortunately vitamin B12 is completely non-toxic, so it is impossible to do any harm by taking supplements. People with MS on vegan diets like the one recommended in this book really should be taking regular vitamin B12 tablets, of the order of 250 to 1000 micrograms per week. It is quite effective by mouth and does not require injection,[16, 17, 18] contrary to popular belief, and is quite cheap.

MS and vitamin B12 deficiency are pretty similar diseases in terms of their inflammatory and neurodegenerative processes. It is actually hard to tell the difference between them sometimes, due to similarities in clinical features and MRI findings. In addition, decreased levels of vitamin B12 are fairly common in MS patients. In addition to its role in myelin formation discussed above, B12 has important immunomodulatory and neurotrophic effects, a bit like vitamin D. Researchers have raised the possibility of B12 causing MS, and suggested close monitoring of vitamin B12 levels in people with MS, as well as B12 supplementation.[19]

The B group vitamins in general are extremely important, particularly to normal brain function. They are involved in a multitude of chemical reactions within the body, including the metabolism of fats. They are quite cheap and readily absorbed. The dose may need to be increased if alcohol intake is high. The B group also includes folate. Folate deficiency has most recently been shown to be involved in causing Alzheimer's disease. Folate is intimately related to normal nerve cell development, as shown by the reduced incidence of spina bifida in babies born to mothers taking folate supplements.[20] It also reduces homocysteine levels.

Vitamin B3 (nicotinamide) has been shown in the animal model of MS to prevent degeneration of axons, and thereby to protect the animals against the usual progression of the disease if given before the disease is induced, and improve the disease once present.[21] There is great potential here for treatment of MS, but research is still required in humans to support these findings. This data supports the view that if any vitamin supplements are likely to be helpful in MS they are the B group vitamins.

Vitamin C

One of the major antioxidants is vitamin C. You can get large amounts of this vitamin from a vegan diet, particularly from fresh fruit and vegetables. I can find little evidence from the large scale clinical trials to show that supplementation has any benefit for a variety of different diseases. But a number of authorities report quite striking improvements in individual patients in conditions such as cancer, particularly when it is given intravenously, so I am loath to recommend against it. On the basis of the above meta-analyses, unlike the other antioxidants, vitamin C appears to be safe, even in large doses.

Flavonoids

The best known source of flavonoids is grapes, hence the well-documented health benefits of low to moderate consumption of red wine. Some of the most powerful of these compounds, though, occur in grape seeds. There are several commercial formulations of these compounds, and one might consider taking them despite the lack of any current evidence about their effectiveness or potential for harm. However, as with other antioxidants, they work best in their natural form, in combination with the other chemicals in their original state. So I don't recommend taking these supplements.

Ordinary tea also contains chemicals called polyphenols which are powerful antioxidants. Asian green tea has higher concentrations again. Studies of people drinking only two or more cups of tea a day have shown major reductions in heart disease, stroke, and other degenerative diseases.[22] Drinking too much, though, can cause problems because of the caffeine intake.

Iron

Many people are concerned that they will become iron deficient on a vegan plus seafood diet. This is really a theoretical risk, as a good vegan diet has a reasonable amount of iron in it. It is more of an issue for women, particularly those who have heavy periods. If this applies, it is possible to get iron levels checked periodically, or to take a small supplement. Excess iron is actually quite toxic and it is certainly better to be getting a small amount rather than a lot.

Indeed, US researchers have noted that abnormal iron accumulation is common in a variety of neurodegenerative diseases, including MS, and there is evidence that iron plays a role in promoting inflammation.[23] They showed that the common Th1 pro-inflammatory cytokines were more toxic to nerve cells if they were loaded with iron. An Egyptian study examining iron metabolism in twenty people with MS compared with ten healthy controls concluded that iron overload may play a part in the development and progression of MS.[24] So concerns about iron deficiency for people on the Recovery Program diet are probably unwarranted.

Glucosamine

Most of us have heard of the benefits, now clinically 'proven', of glucosamine in arthritis. Glucosamine is an extract from the shells of shellfish and is sold in capsule form from most health food shops. Recently it has been shown in experimental animals to produce a shift in the balance of the Th1/Th2 immune response towards a suppressive Th2 response, and to significantly suppress the animal form of MS, EAE, in the laboratory.[25] The authors suggested a potential use for glucosamine either alone or in combination with disease-modifying drugs to enhance their benefit and reduce their doses in MS and possibly other auto-immune disorders.

Alpha-lipoic acid

Alpha-lipoic acid (LA) is an antioxidant which has been shown to have favourable immune effects in the laboratory,[26] to suppress and treat the animal model of MS, EAE,[27] and to stabilise the blood-brain barrier in an animal model.[28] It has been further studied in humans.[29] In a fourteen-day placebo-controlled study, the investigators found that LA inhibited enzymes responsible for helping T cells get access to the CNS. They postulated that it may therefore prove useful in treating MS. They found that oral LA was generally well tolerated by patients. LA may ultimately be a useful treatment for MS.

OVERVIEW

There is no evidence that antioxidants or vitamin supplements improve the outcome from MS. The very influential Nurses Health Study in the United States, looking at the development of MS in over 176,000 US nurses, found no association between the intake of the antioxidant vitamins C or E, or dietary carotenoids (such as beta-carotene) and the development of MS, either taken as vitamin supplements or calculated from the foods they ate.[30] Recent evidence has raised serious concerns about taking multivitamins regularly on the basis that they increase overall death rates in controlled clinical trials. They are not recommended in MS, although individual vitamins may be necessary for people following a vegan plus seafood diet, including vitamin B12 and iron. B group vitamins in general are thought to be helpful for optimal brain function.

8

SUNLIGHT EXPOSURE AND VITAMIN D: EVIDENCE OF BENEFIT IN MS

There needs to be a better appreciation of the importance of vitamin D for overall health and wellbeing

M.F. Holick

Now we come to an extremely important part of the story. Despite all the public health messages we have had over the last decade or so about the harmful effects of sunlight, research is now clearly showing that regular sun exposure is essential for optimal health. Much of this research started with its benefits in MS. The evidence has gradually been mounting, to the point that there is now no doubt that inadequate exposure to sunlight, particularly in winter, increases the chances of susceptible people developing MS. Additionally, taking vitamin D, the hormone produced in the body by exposure to sunlight, has been clearly shown to reduce the risk.

I know personally that I avoided the sun over the fifteen years or so prior to my diagnosis of MS, particularly since having children. We hear so much about covering up our kids, about hats and sunscreen. Soon I was just as covered up and smothered in sunscreen as the kids; little did I know that it was doing me no good at all.

SUMMARISING THE EVIDENCE

- Adequate exposure to sunlight is essential for optimal human health.
- The health benefits of sunlight are mediated through at least vitamin D, formed in the skin from the action of ultraviolet B light.
- Sun avoidance due to fears of skin cancer is causing an epidemic of vitamin D deficiency in Western countries.
  - Vitamin D deficiency is implicated in osteoporosis, depression, high blood pressure, cardiovascular disease and autoimmune diseases like MS, rheumatoid arthritis and diabetes as well as certain cancers.
- Lack of sun exposure and subsequent vitamin D deficiency are implicated in causing MS; this is supported by epidemiological, laboratory, animal and human research.
  - Lack of winter sun in childhood raises the risk of developing MS in later life.
  - Low dose (>400IU per day) vitamin D supplementation reduces the risk of developing MS by 40 per cent; blood levels of vitamin D above 100nmol/L are associated with a two-thirds reduction in risk of developing MS.
  - There is seasonal variation in the activity of the disease process in MS, related to changing vitamin D levels.
- Currently recommended vitamin D supplementation doses are too low, and 'normal' blood levels are set too low; a blood level considerably higher than currently accepted normal levels may be optimal in MS.
- If vitamin D levels are adequate, there is no need for calcium supplementation.

EVIDENCE-BASED RECOMMENDATIONS

- People with MS should get fifteen minutes of sun on as much of the body as possible three to five times a week, with more in winter and less in summer.

- A vitamin D supplement of 5000IU should be taken daily in winter, or year round for people not getting sun exposure in summer.
- It is sensible for people with MS to keep blood levels of vitamin D around 150nmol/L, checked annually.

SUNLIGHT AND HEALTH

Since the first book, the journals have been full of scientific papers suggesting that we have overdone sun avoidance in Western society, and that sun avoidance may be even more harmful than overexposure.[1] A number of authorities are now pointing out that, due to sun avoidance, Americans are in the middle of an epidemic of vitamin D deficiency[2, 3] and that paradoxically vitamin D deficiency is emerging as a major public health issue in sunny Australia.[4] The problem is so great that it has been described as a pandemic.[5] It has been estimated that in 2004 sun avoidance cost the United States US$40–56 million in terms of the cost of its health consequences.[6]

> There is an epidemic of vitamin D deficiency due to sun avoidance in Western countries.

The risks of sun avoidance greatly outweigh the risks associated with sun exposure.[7]

Sun avoidance increases the risk of a whole range of diseases. The evidence is clear about vitamin D deficiency causing bone problems like osteoporosis and fractures, now in almost epidemic proportions in Western societies, but it also increases the risk of falling in the first place.[8] This is particularly true in winter when vitamin D levels are lower because of lack of sun exposure. In Geelong in south-eastern Australia, it has been shown that falls and fractures are more likely in winter when vitamin D levels are at their lowest.[9] One large study showed that supplementing people with vitamin D reduced the incidence of falls by around 50 per cent.[10]

But there is a much wider problem with sun avoidance and vitamin D deficiency. Muscle weakness, depression, high blood pressure,[11] cardiovascular disease,[12] and auto-immune diseases like rheumatoid arthritis and diabetes[13, 14, 15] are also linked to low vitamin D levels. Recent high quality epidemiological data and meta-analysis have shown that type 1 diabetes, an auto-immune disease similar to MS but attacking the pancreas, becomes considerably more common as ultraviolet light exposure from sunlight falls,[16] and can be reduced in incidence by about 30 per cent with vitamin D supplementation.[17]

Additionally, certain cancers, particularly the cancers of the reproductive system, seem to be associated with sun avoidance.[18] This effect appears to far outweigh the known effect of too much sun causing skin cancer. Overall, a 2007 meta-analysis of all the studies on vitamin D supplementation showed that people supplementing with even small doses of vitamin D had on average a 7 per cent reduction in death rates from all causes during the studies.[19] A 2008 paper looked at vitamin D levels in over 13,000 American adults in a nutrition survey, and their death rates.[20] People in the lowest quartile of vitamin D levels (under 44nmol/L in their study) had a 26 per cent higher death rate from all causes than those with the highest quartile of vitamin D levels, independent of other factors. It is clear that there are great health benefits from ensuring adequate levels of vitamin D.[21]

SUNLIGHT AND MS

Recently there has been growing interest in using sunlight and vitamin D in preventing and treating MS. While we still await results from a number of studies which have begun investigating this, there is now enough accumulating evidence to suggest this is an important part of the whole package of staying well for people with MS. Let's examine the evidence.

The geographical evidence

The paper I presented earlier about the epidemiology of MS is even more interesting in regard to latitude differences in MS incidence.[22] For a long time it has been known that there is a striking geographical disparity in the incidence of MS from country to country. While the study showed that this was in part related to saturated fat consumption, and the ratio of polyunsaturated fats to saturated fats, it also found another independent variable—latitude. At first sight, this appears relatively meaningless.

Why would there be virtually no MS at the equator, and the incidence
rise in direct proportion to how far we go towards the poles? Esparza and
co-workers list the countries studied in order of mortality rates from MS
and compare this with latitude, that is, distance from the equator. With
a few exceptions—the exceptions being where fish consumption is very
high—it is very nearly a direct correlation (see Table 8). This has also
been shown within countries[14, 23] and even north of the Arctic Circle.[24]
Why should this be so? It appears that the answer is sunlight. More and
more reports are now hypothesising that sunlight is one of the factors that
may prevent the development of MS[25, 26, 27] and there is a growing body of
experimental work to support this hypothesis. Many scientists now suggest
that sunlight plays a protective role in a number of auto-immune diseases
including MS, type 1 diabetes and rheumatoid arthritis.[13] The evidence
in respect to MS and diabetes from epidemiological studies is convincing,
and there has also been some quite stunning animal work showing that
the animal model of MS can be prevented by pretreatment with light, and
that disease progression is slowed with regular light therapy.

> MS is more common further from the equator due to lack of
> sunlight.

There are a number of possible ways in which sunlight might improve
MS. Professor Michel Dumas, of the Institut d'Epidémiologie et de Neurol-
ogie Tropicale in Limoges, France, feels that there may be five factors
involved, acting through suppression of the immune system by the ultraviolet light in sunlight.[28] These are decreased production of certain cells in
the skin involved in the immune response; reduction in certain proteins
on these cells which are necessary for activating immune cells; increased
production of interleukin–10, an anti-inflammatory cytokine; reduction
of interleukin–12, a cytokine responsible for immune cell activation;

Table 8: MS mortality rates (per million people) for men and women aged 45–74 by
latitude 1983–1989

	Mortality rates		
COUNTRY	WOMEN	MEN	LATITUDE (°)
Denmark	48.6	43.0	N55.7
United Kingdom	45.9	29.6	N51.2
Ireland	40.6	25.8	N53.4

Switzerland	39.7	29.6	N47.4
Poland	37.3	34.8	N52.5
Czechoslovakia	36.8	28.9	N50.1
Norway	32.8	29.7	N60.2
Hungary	30.4	21.4	N47.5
East Germany	30.3	21.9	N52.5
Netherlands	30.1	23.7	N52.1
West Germany	29.1	22.7	N52.5
Sweden	25.2	16.9	N59.4
Belgium	24.7	28.2	N49.6
New Zealand	24.5	14.6	S41.3
Austria	24.2	14.0	N48.3
Canada	22.6	16.9	N46.7
United States	19.6	13.5	N38.6
France	18.9	12.7	N49.0
Iceland	18.2	15.4	N64.1
Finland	15.6	17.7	N60.3
Romania	14.4	15.4	N44.5
Yugoslavia	14.3	11.8	N44.8
Australia	13.5	7.7	S33.9
Italy	13.2	9.8	N41.8
Bulgaria	11.1	11.0	N42.7
Greece	9.7	9.0	N38.0
Malta	9.3	12.0	N36.8
Argentina	8.4	9.1	S34.6
Cuba	8.0	3.8	N23.2
Portugal	7.8	11.5	N38.8
Spain	7.1	7.4	N40.4
Israel	7.0	5.4	N32.0
Japan	1.4	1.0	N35.7
South Korea	0.5	1.3	N37.5
Hong Kong	0.4	0.2	N22.3
Singapore	0.0	0.1	N1.4
Mean	20.0	16.0	43.9

(Modified from Esparza et al.[22], courtesy Oxford University Press.)

and lastly but probably most importantly, synthesis of vitamin D3. The hormone melatonin is likely to be involved as well.

The vitamin D theory

The vitamin D theory was first proposed by Goldberg in 1974.[29] He felt that getting insufficient sunlight to form vitamin D could be the trigger for MS in genetically susceptible people. He even went so far as to calculate, on the basis of amount of sunshine in areas with little MS and the rate at which vitamin D is formed in the body, that it would take 3800 international units of vitamin D daily to prevent the onset of MS. Incredibly, exactly this dose has recently been calculated to be the amount of vitamin D required to maintain a steady, reasonable vitamin D level.[30]

The theory has now been revisited and refined.[31] Vitamin D is formed in the body from the action of sunlight on the skin. Ultraviolet light consists of ultraviolet A, B and C wavelengths. UVB acts on one of the by-products of cholesterol metabolism in the skin to form chemicals which then become vitamin D. We all know about vitamin D from the stories of coal mining children who got rickets from inadequate sunlight. So vitamin D is intimately involved in the normal growth and development of bone, and in the absorption of calcium from our food and its deposition in bone.

What has become clear in more recent times is that vitamin D has profound effects on the immune system. This is well known to those of us who get cold sores. Every time I used to go out in the sun, I came out in a cold sore on my lip. This was because the herpes virus continues to live in our nerves once we have been infected, and when the immune system is suppressed the virus can cause its damage.

Vitamin D functions in the body by attaching to a specific receptor in cells. Receptors can be thought of as the locks into which a particular key, in this case vitamin D, fits. The exciting news from the standpoint of this theory was the discovery that these receptors are present on the white blood cells involved in the immune response in MS. So it was felt that vitamin D must play some part in regulating the immune system. As previously described, a number of animal experiments have shown that the animal model of MS is either stopped from developing or progressing by giving vitamin D supplements or by light therapy.[32, 33]

There is now a lot of evidence that vitamin D is intimately involved not only in immune system function, but also brain function.[34] It appears that vitamin D has protective effects and immunomodulatory effects (ability to affect/change immune system function) in the brain, and is useful in neurodegenerative and neuroimmune diseases, typified by MS. Researchers have concluded that its immunomodulatory potency is equivalent to other currently used immunosuppressants yet without their typical sometimes severe side effects.[35]

Goldberg's study on vitamin D supplementation

For a long time there was little human experimental work, but this is now changing. In 1986, Goldberg himself performed a study of vitamin D supplementation in MS patients.[36] Unfortunately, the numbers in this study were very small. Only sixteen patients were entered into the study. There was no control group, and Goldberg compared the patients' relapse rates after supplementation with those before. A number of confounding factors make this study difficult to interpret. Goldberg gave patients 5000 units of vitamin D per day. He did this by giving them 20g of cod liver oil a day. This meant he was also supplying substantial amounts of omega-3 fish oils. He also gave large doses of calcium and magnesium. The results showed that there were 2.7 times as many relapses per year before the supplements than after, with a p value of <0.005. Some previous studies had suggested that the relapse rate falls with time the longer patients have MS, so he corrected for that, but the result was still significantly better with supplementation.

A number of the patients dropped out of the study, and the numbers were small. Nonetheless, none of the patients who stayed on the supplements for the study period failed to have a lower rate of relapsing than before the supplements. Even in the group of six patients who dropped out, mostly because they didn't want to keep taking supplements, the relapse rate overall fell, with only two getting worse in terms of number of relapses per year. These two had been in the study only eight and four months respectively. It is a great pity that it has taken so long for this work to be followed up.

Embry's study on vitamin D levels

A paper from *Annals of Neurology* in 2000 confirmed that low levels of vitamin D correlate with the number of lesions seen on MRI.[37] Embry and colleagues compared monthly vitamin D blood levels in 415 patients from a particular area in Germany with the number of lesions detected on MRI scanning in MS patients from the same area. High levels of vitamin D correlated closely with low levels of disease activity and vice versa. This paper supports the previous data. The authors recommended that doctors may wish to treat their patients with year-round supplements of 3000–4000IU per day of vitamin D. Interestingly, an Australian study suggests that vitamin D supplementation may prevent some of the negative seasonal variation in mood which can occur during winter when vitamin D levels are known to be low.[38]

Other studies

A 2005 study from Finland added further support to the idea that low vitamin D levels may precipitate relapses.[39] Researchers measured vitamin D levels during relapses and compared these with levels during remission. They found the levels to be lower during a relapse and concluded that vitamin D may be involved in the regulation of disease activity in MS. They found that although levels were lower during relapses, they were mostly still in what would currently be considered to be the 'normal' range. Later I will discuss vitamin D levels in much more detail, but it seems likely that just having a normal vitamin D level may not be enough to significantly reduce the risk of relapses; a 'high' level may be more protective. A follow-up study in 2007 by the same group demonstrated that relapses were more common the lower the vitamin D level in people with MS.[40]

Argentine researchers publishing in the world's top neurology journal, *Brain*, in 2009 showed that vitamin D levels were significantly lower in people with MS than a control population of people without the illness; further, levels were again shown to be lower during relapses than when in remission.[41] A further study from Turkey showed that people with MS had significantly lower levels of vitamin D than people without MS.[42] The authors showed that 61 per cent of MS patients had low vitamin D levels, and that many had osteoporosis and muscle pain due to the low vitamin D levels. Similarly, a US study of MS patients in a long-term care facility showed high levels of osteoporosis, suggesting vitamin D deficiency.[43] So many authorities now recommend that people with MS get adequate vitamin D both to control the illness itself, but also to minimise the risk of complications like falls and fractures.[44] Additionally, research from the US Nurses Health Study looking at MS risk showed that vitamin D supplementation reduced the risk of developing MS by 40 per cent, and this was with very low dose supplementation.[45]

An important paper published in 2006 added further evidence that higher vitamin D levels protect against the possibility of getting MS. US researchers examined the stored blood of over 7 million army recruits from 1992–2004 and compared the vitamin D levels with their risk of developing MS.[46] They found 257 new cases of MS in the group. There was a significant decrease in risk with increasing vitamin D levels among Anglo Americans, but not African Americans or Hispanics, who had lower vitamin D levels than Anglo Americans. Interestingly, when looking at the actual levels of vitamin D, levels of around 100nmol/L or more seemed to be protective, with almost a two-thirds reduction in risk for those with these higher levels. Later I make the case that currently accepted 'normal' levels of vitamin D are actually too low, and that people with MS need to sustain a level of around 150nmol/L.

Epidemiological evidence about sun exposure and MS

An important piece of the evidence jigsaw was published in 2000 by Freedman and co-workers from the Radiation Epidemiology Branch of the National Cancer Institute in Maryland in the United States.[47] We have previously seen the value of case-control studies in evaluating the potential effects of different diets in MS. These workers looked at the effects of sunlight on MS using the death rate from MS in 24 US states as a measure. The study was substantial, with causes of death determined from all death certificates in these states over the period 1984–1995. MS patients were matched against control patients of the same age dying of other diseases, and results were analysed allowing for age, sex, race and socioeconomic status.

The results added great weight to the earlier epidemiological data. The researchers showed that the more sunlight people were exposed to in the course of their work, the less likely they were to die from MS. Further, people with high occupational exposure to sunlight who also had high exposure out of work had the lowest death rates by far, with an odds ratio of only 0.24, that is, they were only 24 per cent as likely to die from MS as those with low sun exposure. Swedish researchers provided further support in 2009, showing that those with high occupational exposure to sunlight had a 48 per cent chance of dying of MS, and those with intermediate exposure 88 per cent, compared with those with low exposure.[48]

Another study from Oxford University on a very large database of people in the United Kingdom found that people with MS were only half as likely to get skin cancer.[49] They had similar rates of all other cancers, so it seemed likely that sun was affording some protection against MS, in that people getting more skin cancer due to their sun exposure were much less likely to get MS.

This research was important evidence for the beneficial effects of sunlight in MS. What we now need is a well-constructed RCT with patients randomised to a reasonable amount of sunlight (or solarium UV light) or minimal sunlight daily, followed with MRI, similar to the large interferon and glatiramer studies. It would not surprise if the effect of sunlight was more marked than either of these drug therapies. Embry's paper seemed to suggest a roughly 50–70 per cent reduction in the number of MS lesions when UV exposure was at its maximum in summer compared to mid-winter, so we may see that sort of level of benefit for people getting regular sunlight. And this effect size may be even higher as maximal vitamin D levels were not particularly high in Embry's study.

Australian data

An interesting study from the Menzies Centre for Population Health Research in Tasmania, the Australian state furthest from the equator, looked at the rates of MS and malignant melanoma in each of the major cities of the states of Australia and compared them with the amount of sunlight in the area. We already accept without question the causative role of sunlight, specifically ultraviolet radiation, in the development of malignant melanoma, the most lethal of the skin cancers, and the reason behind much of the public health message about avoiding sun exposure. The scientists conducting this study showed that the correlation between low ultraviolet radiation and MS was considerably stronger than that between high UV and melanoma.[50]

> Adequate vitamin D, from sunlight or supplements, lowers the risk of developing MS.

Again, this is very strong evidence supporting the role of lack of sunlight in MS causation. Indeed, an editorial in the premier Australian medical journal, the *Medical Journal of Australia*, entitled 'Ultraviolet radiation and health: friend and foe', highlighted the beneficial effects of adequate UV exposure, and the possible role of lack of UV in MS.[51] There has since been good experimental work from Tasmania showing that adequate sun exposure, particularly in winter and between the ages of six to fifteen especially, reduced the risk of developing MS in later life by about two-thirds.[52] This has been strongly supported by an interesting US study in 79 pairs of identical twins, comparing their sun exposure in childhood with whether they developed MS in later life.[53] Each of the nine sun exposure-related activities during childhood they asked about conveyed strong protection against MS, ranging from 43 per cent to 75 per cent reduction in risk. They concluded that the benefits of sun exposure were independent of genetic susceptibility to the disease.

Further study of the Tasmanian population was undertaken by Canadian researchers from the University of British Columbia.[54] They studied 142 people with relapsing-remitting MS. The lowest relapse rate throughout the year of 0.5 per 1000 days occurred in February (mid to late summer); this compared with a rate of 1.1 per 1000 days (p=0.018) for the rest of the year, a 55 per cent reduction. This correlated with higher UV exposure and high vitamin D levels. Again, this supported the protective role of sun exposure against relapses.

Sunlight is by far the most efficient way of getting vitamin D. 'Contrary to popular belief, you cannot get enough vitamin D to meet your biological needs by ingesting fortified foods,' says professor Colleen Hayes, from the Department of Biochemistry, University of Wisconsin, Madison. 'Urged by the fear of skin cancer, individuals are avoiding sun exposure and using sunscreens. Somewhere, there is a balance between too much sun and melanoma risk or too little sun and auto-immune disease.' An interesting point to make here is that it has long been known that regular, moderate sun exposure, as opposed to getting sunburnt periodically, may protect against melanoma.[55] The fear of skin cancer with small, regular amounts of sunlight exposure may in fact be quite irrational.

MELATONIN

There is more to the sunlight story than vitamin D. UV light on the skin results in a suntan. A hormone, melatonin, which regulates skin colour, is normally released from the pineal gland. When UV light hits the skin, melatonin release is inhibited. The lack of melatonin then causes the pigment cells in the skin to increase the amount of pigment in the skin, resulting in a tan. What has been shown recently is that this hormone, melatonin, has powerful effects on the immune system, promoting inflammation. So with sunlight the melatonin level falls, and the immune system is suppressed. This is likely to be a second mechanism whereby sunlight suppresses immune function.[56]

IMPLICATIONS FOR PEOPLE WITH MS

No formal RCT of sunlight exposure in people with MS has yet been done, although early uncontrolled research on vitamin D supplementation is encouraging. While the scientific evidence is accumulating, what should those of us with MS do? My observation of people with MS over the years has been that very few have a suntan. This could be because the messages from authorities not only in general have been to avoid the sun, but neurologists have advised people with MS to avoid it as sunlight may precipitate relapses. This is one area where I disagree with Professor Swank. In his MS diet book, he advises strongly against going out in the sun for just this reason. He says that 'direct sunlight can quickly weaken most patients and can produce exacerbation of disease in many. This is to be avoided by all sensitive patients.' I disagree. I cannot find anything in the medical literature to support this contention.

Indeed, apart from the epidemiological evidence to the contrary, there have also been seasonal studies of relapses in populations of people with MS.[57, 58] The findings have generally been that relapses are more likely in the winter months. While some of this may be due to the effects of virus infections,[59] there certainly appears to be no increase in incidence in summer.

HOW MUCH SUN IS ENOUGH?

After reading a review of vitamin D production from sunlight,[60] I contacted the article's author, Dr Vieth, to ask how much sun I needed to get the recommended amount of vitamin D. It turns out that a person will probably get enough by getting all over sun (such as when swimming in a pair of bathers) for about ten to fifteen minutes on a day where the standard UV index is 7. Each point on the UV index scale is equivalent to 25mW of energy per square metre of exposed skin. So if the UV index is 14, you need half the time for the same amount of vitamin D. The UV index in Melbourne, Australia, is about maximum 12 in summer, and 1 in winter; in Perth it is about 14 in summer and 2 in winter. The UV index anywhere in Australia can be checked at www.bom.gov.au, the Bureau of Meteorology website, and there are similar websites for other countries. In the United Kingdom the website is www.metoffice.gov.uk and in the United States they tend to be state-based organisations.

What Dr Vieth recommended was getting the dose of UV light just short of getting some colour in the skin on each occasion. Over time, this tends to develop into a 'healthy' tan. Most daily weather reports recommend a safe amount of time in the sun; this is what to aim for. In addition, Dr Vieth suggested exposure three to five times a week is probably enough. It is important to note here that this amount of whole-body sun exposure will generate the maximum amount of vitamin D possible, that is, about 10,000 to 15,000 international units (IU). Staying longer in the sun doesn't cause any more vitamin D to be made, and is clearly a bad idea in that it raises the risk of other diseases, particularly skin cancer. Exposing a smaller area of the body for a longer period doesn't work either, as once all the vitamin D is made in a given area of skin (in the 15 minutes or so) no more is made until the chemical in the skin is formed again, roughly by the next day.

> Ten–15 minutes of sun three to five times a week promotes optimal health.

This amount of sun exposure is very safe, as evidenced by the report of the ANZ Bone and Mineral Society, Endocrine Society of Australia and Osteoporosis Australia which recommended six to eight minutes of sun in summer and 25 minutes of sun in winter to prevent osteoporosis.[61] Unfortunately their recommendation was just to get this exposure on the hands, face and arms. As noted previously, people who get this amount of exposure over the whole body get much, much more vitamin D, and the evidence suggests that more vitamin D is needed for MS than for osteoporosis prevention.

There are a few important points to clarify about UV radiation. As noted earlier, UV light is made up of UVA, UVB and UVC. UVB is the one that produces vitamin D when it hits the skin. All UV light gets through water without problems, so swimming doesn't reduce the amount of vitamin D produced. However, ordinary glass absorbs UVB while letting the UVA through, so it's impossible to get vitamin D by sitting inside and getting the sun through a glass window. You need to be outside. Most solariums have a mixture of UVA and UVB but it may be advisable to check with the solarium that this is the case before using a sun-bed to get adequate vitamin D on cloudy days.

For those worried about skin cancer and other damage from the UV radiation, there has been a substantial rethinking of this issue in recent times. A paper from the University of Bristol in the prestigious *British Medical Journal* in 1999 created a stir when the authors suggested that perhaps we have overdone the public health messages about sunlight, and that, in moderation, it may not be as harmful as was thought.[62] They further suggested that the benefit it may have for certain diseases may outweigh the harmful increase in skin cancer incidence.

Additional evidence has now emerged to support this. An epidemiological study of cancer rates in Europe showed that lack of adequate exposure to sunlight was likely to result in a large increase in the rates of cancers other than skin cancer. Indeed, the suggestion was that around 25 per cent of breast cancers are due to lack of sun exposure. The *Medical Journal of Australia* reported in 2002 that sun avoidance was now as or more dangerous than overexposure.[51] A paper from Boston published in the *Journal of Cell Biochemistry* in 2003 suggested that chronic vitamin D deficiency may have quite serious consequences for health, such as increased risk of high blood pressure, MS, cancers of the colon, prostate, breast and ovary, and type 1 diabetes.[63]

It is interesting to watch the medical pendulum swing in these matters; what is considered dogma in one generation is often rejected by the next. One just has to look at the duodenal ulcer story to see how medical dogma can change overnight. For generations the role of diet in causing duodenal ulcers was considered paramount, and people with ulcers were put on bland anti-ulcer diets. Then along came Australian researchers, who showed that an ordinary bacterium caused the problem and now people with duodenal ulcers are cured with antibiotics and the diet has been consigned to history. But to challenge a doctor about the diet in its heyday would have been considered mad. Indeed, the original researchers who discovered the bacterium were for some time thought to be just that. They are of course now Nobel Prize winners. Interesting.

But getting back to sunshine and MS, personally I find few things as enjoyable as sitting in the sun with my shirt off, reading a book, or walking along a beach in my bathers. If there is a better way to feel and stay well, I'd love to know what it is. I think the evidence is now very strong that this is the way to go.

VITAMIN D SUPPLEMENTS

I have studied this area in a great deal of detail since the first book. Much of the work in this area has been done by Reinhold Vieth, whom I contacted about vitamin D when first diagnosed. It seems clear that we in the medical profession have been overly concerned with the potential for toxicity from supplementing with vitamin D, and that we have under-estimated the doses required for optimal health quite significantly. Vitamin D levels in the body can be easily measured with a simple blood test. A level of less than 25nmol/L is considered currently to represent moderate to severe deficiency and a level of 25–50nmol/L mild deficiency.

There is quite a bit of evidence that we have set these levels too low and that optimal levels are really quite a bit higher.[64] Even at these levels, it has been shown that 80 per cent of women and 70 per cent of men living in hostels in the Australian states of Victoria, New South Wales and Western Australia are deficient.[8] In women in the city of Geelong, 30 per cent had deficiency in summer and 43 per cent in winter, and the rate of falls and fractures was higher in winter.[9, 65]

> People with MS should check their level of vitamin D annually and keep it around 150nmol/L.

The recommended daily allowance of vitamin D in Australia is 200IU. This amount of vitamin D is way too low. It is based on the amount required to prevent rickets, but is not nearly enough to prevent the diseases mentioned in this chapter. It is equivalent to the amount of vitamin D your skin would make in six seconds of all over sun in Perth on a summer's day. Vieth and others have shown that in sunny countries where these diseases are uncommon, the vitamin D levels are at least 100–140nmol/L, and more like 135–225nmol/L, and that a level of 200nmol/L may actually be optimal.[7] Others have suggested a level as high as 250nmol/L may be optimal.[66]

Laboratories are now changing their recommendations in this area. Many Australian laboratories are now reporting the range of 70–250nmol/L as being the therapeutic range. People with MS should aim for at least the middle of that range. To achieve a level of 100nmol/L requires a daily intake of about 4000IU of vitamin D for people who are not getting any sun. To get to 150nmol/L needs about 10,000IU a day in the absence of sunlight. It has been shown that average healthy men's bodies use about 3000 to 5000IU a day.[30]

It is important to note that it is not possible to get toxicity from vitamin D if it all comes from the sun. Only supplements can potentially produce toxic levels. The only published toxicity, however, is from supplements of 40,000IU a day.[60] Indeed, Vieth and colleagues reported via the Internet a groundbreaking dose escalation study of vitamin D3 in people with MS.[67] More recently this has been published in a major journal.[68] They gave increasing doses of the hormone to twelve people over 28 weeks, increasing the dose from 4000IU per day up to 40,000IU per day. Measured levels of vitamin D in the blood of these people were extraordinarily high, much higher than what we have previously regarded as toxic, with average levels increasing to around 400nmol/L and the highest measured level 800nmol/L.

Despite these apparently 'toxic' levels, no patient developed high calcium levels or any side effects. Although this study aimed to look at the safety of high dose vitamin D supplements and was not primarily designed to detect outcomes in the medical condition of these people with MS, it is interesting to note that the mean number of new MS lesions more than halved over the short period of the study from 1.75 to 0.83 (p=0.03). It is clear now that supplementation with vitamin D at quite high doses is very safe, and the way is now clear to use these larger doses in research situations to examine the effect on relapse rates and disease progression.

Further results from this study were presented at the annual meeting of the American Academy of Neurology in 2009. There was a dramatic difference between those people with MS who took high doses (averaging 14,000IU of vitamin D per day) versus the standard dose recommended by most doctors (averaging 1000IU per day). For those who took the higher dose, only 14 per cent had a relapse during the study, versus 40 per cent for those who took the lower dose. Measures of their immune system balance also showed a move away from an inflammatory profile. People with vitamin D levels above 100nmol/L did best.

In contrast, other investigators have trialled a synthetic form of the activated vitamin D3, calcitriol, in a pilot study in patients with MS.[69] They used a dose about ten times higher than its recommended dose in kidney disease, and found that a number of patients developed side effects and high calcium levels. They did find that the patients' condition improved, and that is an encouraging step in the continuing development of vitamin D as a treatment for MS.

The right form of vitamin D to take is vitamin D3 or cholecalciferol. This is the natural form that is made in the body in response to sunlight. In Australia, because it is such a sunny country, regulators have not in the past allowed vitamin D to be sold in high dose supplement form. Until recently, the only form available in Australia was vitamin D2 or ergocalciferol. This is synthetic, available on prescription only, and is not the optimal form to take. It is also expensive. Vitamin D3 on the other hand is cheap, and because it is naturally occurring cannot be patented by drug companies. The easiest way to obtain supplies at a reasonable strength is over the Internet. A 5000IU capsule is available quite cheaply at www.vitamin-D-max.com, a US company, or www.seeknatural.co.uk/product–1798.html, a UK company, and a 2400IU capsule from www.iherb.com. Both are fine for children as the capsules can be broken apart and the powder sprinkled on food such as morning cereal, and the softgel capsule in olive oil can be squeezed onto food or into drinks.

My recommendation is that when first diagnosed, people should ask to be tested for their vitamin D level immediately. It is very common for this first level to be low, and often this is why the attack happened. Australian researchers are now calling for 'active detection of vitamin D insufficiency among people with MS and intervention to restore vitamin D status to adequate levels . . . as part of the clinical management of MS'.[70] Many neurologists I know are now doing this routinely at diagnosis. If the level is very low, it can be brought up very quickly with a one-off megadose of vitamin D followed by regular capsules.[71]

For people with initial levels indicating severe deficiency (less than 12.5nmol/L), a one-off megadose of 600,000IU raised levels to an average of 73nmol/L.[71] This is still probably half the level which may be reasonable in MS, but it can be seen that even large doses of this vitamin are quite safe. My suggestion is to get a one-off dose like this if the initial level is low, and then take a regular supplement of around 5000IU a day in winter, or more if required, to get the level to around 150nmol/L. The level should be checked at the end of each winter of supplementation to make sure it is not being overdone. It may in fact be more important for men to keep their vitamin D levels high and check their levels frequently as it has been shown that women with MS have considerably higher levels than men with MS.[72] My own last two levels at the end of winter were 149 and 150nmol/L; these were achieved with frequent sunshine plus supplementation with around 5000IU a day on days when I didn't get any sun. Holick, a world authority on vitamin D, suggests annually checking one's vitamin D level as a routine.[3]

> A very low vitamin D level can be raised quickly and safely with a one-off megadose of vitamin D.

Supplementing with vitamin D at 5000IU per day is now thought to be very safe, although in the past many medical authorities have been concerned about the possibility of side effects with doses of this magnitude. Hathcock et al. have applied the risk assessment methodology used by the Food and Nutrition Board in the United States to derive a revised safe Tolerable Upper Intake Level (UL) for vitamin D3.[73] Their risk assessment based on relevant, well-designed human clinical trials of vitamin D3 concluded that the UL is 10,000IU vitamin D3 per day, that is, it is safe to take up to 10,000IU of vitamin D3 per day. Even with plenty of sun exposure, supplementing even up to this dose appears to be quite safe.

To illustrate the safety limits of supplementation, Kimball and Vieth reported in 2008 the cases of two men who had been supplementing with vitamin D.[74] One had been taking 8000IU per day for three years. This resulted in a blood level of 260nmol/L, and no changes in any measured parameters of calcium. The second, a 39-year-old man with MS, had been steadily increasing his self-prescribed dose of vitamin D over four years, from 8000IU per day to a whopping 88,000IU per day. This latter level would be expected to produce some toxic effects. In fact, the amount of calcium in his urine started to rise, and then blood calcium levels started to go up, with a vitamin D level in his blood of 1126nmol/L. He displayed no symptoms, though. At that point he stopped taking vitamin D, and within two months all his blood tests were normal, although vitamin D levels remained high at 656nmol/L. While not recommended, this at least shows that it takes very large doses of vitamin D to produce any increase in calcium levels and toxicity.

VITAMIN D AND BONE HEALTH

It is interesting to note that most Western societies have overdone their public health messages about sun avoidance, so much that a very large proportion of their populations are low in vitamin D or frankly deficient. As the main effect of vitamin D in the body is to extract calcium from the food we eat and incorporate it into bone, this has resulted in a virtual epidemic of osteoporosis in Western countries. Rather than modify the messages to promote modest sun exposure, which as we have seen has a range of health benefits, the response has been to recommend calcium supplementation. As a result, we have a huge food industry growing up around adding calcium to foods and encouraging substantial dairy consumption.

The evidence, however, is that this is not making an impact on osteoporosis and bone fractures. In fact, there is evidence that populations that eat mainly vegetarian or vegan diets have lower rates of osteoporosis and fractures. A study from Harvard in the late 1990s for instance showed that the incidence of forearm and hip fractures in men was no lower in those with high calcium intakes than those with low intakes.[75] Likewise, a very large prospective study from Boston of over 77,000 women showed there was no difference in fracture rates in women with high calcium intakes compared with those with low intakes.[76] Indeed, there was a trend to higher fracture rates in those with high calcium intakes. A detailed review of the literature shows that there is no evidence that increasing cow's milk consumption has any beneficial effect on children's bone health.[77] The Centre for Nutrition and Food Safety at the University of Surrey recommended that a 'fruit and vegetable' approach to osteoporosis may provide a very sensible alternative therapy for osteoporosis, and is likely to have many other health benefits.[78]

McCarty suggests that vegan diets in combination with vitamin D supplementation represent the best alternative to getting adequate sun exposure, in terms of achieving the wide-ranging health protection conferred by optimal sun exposure.[79] This seems to be related to the amount of phosphate in the diet; phosphate is low in vegan diets, whereas calcium supplements tend to raise the phosphate.

The problem with widespread calcium supplementation for populations of people with low vitamin D levels is that most of the calcium that is added to food is not absorbed into the body because of the low vitamin D. It has been shown, for example, that people with a blood level of vitamin D of 86.5nmol/L absorb two-thirds more calcium than those with blood levels of 50nmol/L, yet both levels have been until recently considered normal.[80] For people with osteoporosis, the best thing to do is get out in the sun regularly as per the guidelines in this book, not eat more calcium. And, of course, it's easier to exercise more when outside, further strengthening bones. MS and osteoporosis often go hand in hand, especially for people with advanced disease, because they don't exercise much and don't get outside much. People with MS must get out in the sun.

The risks associated with calcium supplementation

As we have discussed, the main job of vitamin D in the body is to absorb calcium from the diet and lay it down in bone, thus forming normally strong, healthy bones.

Unfortunately, given the evidence that we are in the midst of an epidemic of vitamin D deficiency and that vitamin D levels are falling in the community, and hence not enough calcium is being absorbed, osteoporosis has become widespread, resulting in a large number of fractures of long bones and the hip, particularly in our elderly.

Instead of treating the cause of this problem—that is, getting people out in the sun more often or, failing that, supplementing with adequate doses of vitamin D—a whole industry of calcium supplementation has appeared. As consumers, we now face constant advertisements about whether we are getting enough calcium, designed to get us to take calcium supplements. The dairy industry has seen an opening here to market its products as high in calcium and therefore healthy, obscuring the very real health risks associated with dairy products, particularly for people with multiple sclerosis.

It has actually taken a long time for researchers to begin to investigate whether this widespread calcium supplementation is doing any good or, more particularly, whether it is possibly doing harm. After all, many of our elderly are on drugs called calcium channel blockers, particularly those with heart and vascular disease, and intuitively it seems problematic to be giving them the very mineral whose effects we are trying to block in the body.

Recently, a number of well designed trials and meta-analyses have raised serious doubts about the safety of calcium supplementation. A major randomised controlled trial from the University of Auckland, published in 2008 in the *British Medical Journal*, examined 1471 postmenopausal women.[81] Of these, 732 were randomised to calcium supplementation and 739 to placebo. Heart attacks were more common in the calcium group than in the placebo group (45 versus 19, p=0.01). The investigators also looked at the combined end point of heart attack, stroke or sudden death, and found that this was also more common in the calcium group (101 versus 54, p=0.008). It should probably come as no surprise that calcium supplementation in these elderly women was associated with increases in serious cardiovascular event rates.

This increased risk might even be considered acceptable by some if the benefits of calcium supplementation were very marked. But there are serious doubts about whether there is really any benefit in terms of bone health from supplementing with calcium. Interestingly, researchers from the same institution showed that calcium supplementation actually increased hip fracture risk by 50 per cent.[82] A 2007 meta-analysis from the Harvard School of Public Health reported that pooled randomised controlled trials showed no reduction in hip fracture risk with calcium supplementation, and that an increased risk was possible.[83] For other fractures, there was a neutral effect.

It really is time for a re-appraisal of the whole calcium–vitamin D issue in health. Clearly, vitamin D is very important for a variety of reasons, not least its helpful effects on mood, muscle strength, cancer, vascular and auto-immune disease. A real problem is that when we do supplement with vitamin D, we generally use too low a dose. We need to raise the level to a minimum of 75nmol/L to get any benefit at all for bone health,[84] and it probably needs to be twice that to really get the full health benefits for other conditions. We know, for example, that a level of 100nmol/L or so is the threshold level above which there is a great protective effect against developing MS.[46]

As for calcium, like many other heavily marketed supplements, now that the evidence is coming in we can see that it pays to be very, very selective about what supplements to take. Supplements need to be taken for a good reason, with a therapeutic aim in mind, and utilising the best available evidence to support their use. For people with adequate vitamin D levels (and for people in most geographic regions this means supplementation with relatively large doses of vitamin D in winter), calcium supplementation is completely unnecessary. For those who avoid the sun or cannot get much sun in winter, and those with osteoporosis, supplementation with around 5000IU of vitamin D daily is recommended, rather than with calcium. Calcium supplementation, on the basis of current evidence, poses too great a risk to human health and is not recommended.

OVERVIEW

Many experts, on the basis of epidemiological data showing less MS where there is more sun, animal work on improving experimental auto-immune encephalomyelitis with light therapy, reduced risk of MS with adequate sunlight or vitamin D supplementation and limited human studies, now believe that sunlight improves MS. I find the evidence convincing. There is an urgent need for more RCTs on this simple, safe therapy. In the meantime, people with MS can feel comfortable that sunlight is likely to improve their outcome from the disease, and protect them from many others in addition. Provided the amount of UV radiation is not excessive, this is a very safe therapy, with the bonus of being very pleasurable. In winter, in most places in the world, a vitamin D supplement is necessary to keep vitamin D levels optimal at around 150nmol/L. This is rapidly becoming accepted medical practice in the treatment of MS.

9

OTHER LIFESTYLE ISSUES:
EVIDENCE ABOUT EXERCISE, STRESS, DEPRESSION AND SMOKING

Living a healthy lifestyle will only deprive you of poor health, lethargy, and fat

Jill Johnson

EXERCISE

As long ago as 1974, Professor Ritchie Russell, Professor of Clinical Neurology in Oxford, published a book entitled *Multiple Sclerosis: Control of the disease* in which he detailed a specific exercise program he felt arrested disease progression in MS.[1] It was called the Rest-Exercise Program (REP). The program involved people with MS doing short bursts of vigorous exercise, preferably in the lying position, such as press-ups or weight-lifting exercises, followed by periods of rest. Russell thought this would help by protecting the blood-brain barrier which we know is intimately involved in the development of MS. He reports in his book details of 21 patients of various ages and the good results they achieved with this therapy.

Since then there has been an accumulation of evidence about the beneficial effects of exercise on many Western diseases. Regular,

SUMMARISING THE EVIDENCE

- Exercise improves fitness and function in MS.
  - Exercise improves mood, wellbeing and quality of life in people with MS.
  - Laboratory research shows that exercise releases certain proteins that protect brain cells.
- Stressful life events are associated with an increased risk of relapse in MS.
- Depression is very common in people with MS; at least 50 per cent of people with MS experience it at some time.
  - The presence or absence of depression may be the most important factor in determining quality of life for people with MS.
  - Getting depressed can make the disease worse through shifting the immune system towards a Th1 response.
- Smoking (active and passive) increases the risk of developing MS, and of it becoming progressive.

EVIDENCE-BASED RECOMMENDATIONS

- People with MS should undertake regular, vigorous exercise if possible.
  - There are options for those with more severe disability, including personalised gym programs and hydrotherapy.
- Management of stress is important; this may involve keeping a diary, counselling, meditation or more specific strategies.
- Preventing depression is important; a range of strategies is useful including omega-3 supplements, adequate sunlight and vitamin D, exercise, counselling and meditation.
- People with MS should quit smoking, as should family members who are at higher risk of developing MS.

vigorous exercise for instance has been shown to be associated with a 50 per cent reduction in the risk of death from established breast cancer.[2] More recently the same sort of benefit has been seen with bowel cancer.

It is likely that exercise has an anti-inflammatory effect, and we have seen the importance of shifting the balance in MS away from inflammation.[3] In the 1970s, there was quite a strong prevailing medical opinion that people with MS should avoid exercise, that it could somehow be detrimental. There is now good evidence that exercise improves fitness and function in mild MS and maintains function for people with moderate to severe disability.[4] RCTs have also shown that moderate aerobic exercise does not worsen symptoms of MS.[5] There is strong evidence that exercise therapy, including aerobic exercise and resistance training, improves muscle power function, exercise tolerance functions and mobility-related activities such as walking in people with significant disability.[6-12] Exercise also improves mood, general well-being,[8, 13, 14] fatigue[15, 16] and quality of life.[17] Walking distance has been shown to be increased with regular treadmill training.[18] Interestingly, some of the benefit of exercise in MS seems to be more pronounced in women.[19] Exercise has been shown to be superior to neurological rehabilitation in improving exercise tolerance and walking ability in people with mild to moderate MS.[20]

Regular exercise is safe for people with MS and improves function, mood and quality of life.

There is growing indirect evidence that excercise may be helpful too. Two proteins, brain-derived neurotrophic factor (BDNF) and nerve growth factor (NGF), have been shown to have some protective effects for neurons in MS, helping them repair. Gold and colleagues have shown that exercise significantly increases the levels of these proteins in people with MS.[21] German researchers have also shown increased levels of neurotrophic factors in people with MS who undergo exercise training.[22] Further, they summarise literature on exercise also playing a role in preventing cognitive decline. Here again I have to speak from experience in saying that twenty to 30 minutes of vigorous exercise a day makes me feel much better, both physically and mentally.

There is good work already showing that regular exercise significantly reduces the chances of depression, and improves the quality of life for people with MS.[13] A 2008 review of the literature concluded that 'evidence exists for recommending participation in endurance training at low to moderate intensity, as the existing literature demonstrates that MS patients can both tolerate and benefit from this training modality. Also, resistance training of moderate intensity seems to be well tolerated and to have beneficial effects on MS patients.'[23] It seems there is a complex interplay between lack of exercise causing depression and fatigue, and fatigue causing depression.[24] Aerobic exercise is very helpful in breaking this cycle, but needs to be regular to maintain the benefits.[25]

Unfortunately, recent studies have shown that people with MS do less exercise than those in the general population.[26, 27] Again, it is important to consider the benefits of this lifestyle change, not only for general health, but specifically for MS. It is important to say here that not only does exercise improve symptoms in MS and prevent depression, it has been suggested that it may also modify the course of the illness through a neuroprotective effect.[28] Other researchers have suggested that regular exercise could reduce long-term disability by promoting neuroprotection, neuroregeneration and neuroplasticity through the production of nerve growth factors,[29] and by inducing immune modulation through alteration in cytokines and stress hormones.[30]

So it appears likely that exercise, like diet, is effective against both the major ways in which MS causes its damage, immune activation and degeneration. My feeling is that this is very likely, just as it has benefits in modifying the progression of many other immune-mediated and degenerative diseases. A US study of 611 people with MS provided some confirmation, showing that exercise had a positive impact on the progression of disability as well as quality of life.[31]

STRESS

There has long been a view that stressful events may precipitate relapses in MS. It is well known that major life events like marriage breakdown, moving house, losing or changing jobs, losing close friends or loved ones and so on may have a profound effect on our general wellbeing. While people have felt that such events may trigger relapses in MS, there has been little good science on the subject until recently. A number of papers published in reputable journals have now looked closely at the subject from several angles. It appears clear that major life events, or more particularly our reaction to them, can often trigger MS attacks. This is where meditation can be so valuable, in minimising the harmful effects of these stresses.

There is no doubt that stress precipitates relapses in MS.

Scientists at UCLA have summarised basic molecular and animal experimental research, as well as human clinical and epidemiological studies, showing that stress can precipitate relapses and worsening disability through a variety of mechanisms including an 'overshooting' of the inflammatory response, and through worsening degeneration.[32] I have previously described the immune system balance of Th1 versus Th2 cytokines which is intimately involved in the development of relapses in people with MS. Swiss researchers conducted a prospective study in fourteen healthy medical students to see whether a psychologically stressful event, in this case the students' final examination, could modify one of the known Th1 cytokines, tumour necrosis factor alpha (TNF-alpha) levels. They showed a significant increase of TNF-alpha starting the next day, suggesting the possibility that stress can precipitate relapses by its effect on the immune system.[33]

Ackerman and colleagues from the Department of Psychiatry at the University of Pittsburgh studied 50 women with MS, following on a weekly basis the occurrence of major life events such as those listed above, and their MS disease activity.[34] I was surprised to see that nearly half of all major life events were followed within six weeks by a relapse. Relapses were, however, more common in those people who were more clearly affected by the events, as demonstrated by a higher resting heart rate and blood pressure. Meditation has been shown to reduce these and is likely to therefore have a very positive effect on minimising the risks of relapse after major life events for those of us who regularly meditate. I should note here that in an eighteen-month period some years ago every single one of the stressful events I list above happened to me, yet I remain well. I have given my health regime a pretty good 'road test', and derive considerable confidence from that.

US researchers have studied the development of new MRI lesions in 36 people with MS and correlated these with stressful life events. After major life stresses, people were roughly 1.6 times more likely to develop a new lesion in the next eight weeks.[35] It should be noted that the p value in this study was 0.0008, clearly indicating that the findings did not occur by chance. This study also noted that those with coping mechanisms could reduce this risk.[36] Again this lends support to the potentially beneficial effects of meditation in MS. In 2006, the same research group summarised the effects of stress on MS, noting that 'a growing literature reports that stressful life events are associated with exacerbation and the subsequent development of brain lesions in patients with multiple sclerosis'.[37] It has further been suggested that acute short-term stressors generally cause no problems. In contrast, stressors such as interpersonal conflicts, loss and complicated bereavement, poor social support, anxiety and depression are risk factors for MS exacerbations.[38]

A Dutch study examined 73 patients with relapsing-remitting MS at an MS clinic.[39] During the study period, 70 had major stressful events. Stress resulted in a more than doubling of the exacerbation rate (relative risk 2.2, p=0.014) during the following four weeks. The researchers also noted a threefold increase in relapses following infections during the study, but this was independent of the stress associated with the infection.

A unique study from Israel looked at the development of relapses in people with MS who were exposed to rocket attacks on civilian centres in northern Israel during the 2006 war between Hezbollah and Israel.[40] The researchers clearly showed that there was a major increase in the number of relapses for these people during the 33 days of the war compared with the periods both before and after.

A 2008 Greek study looked at 26 women with MS for an average of over a year, noting the number and type of stressful life events they had and their subsequent risk of relapses.[41] Experiencing three or more of these stresses during a four-week period caused a fivefold increase in MS relapse rate (p=0.003). Having at least one stressful event associated with psychological effects lasting over two weeks was associated with three times (p<0.05) the rate of MS relapses during the following four weeks. This study is strong evidence of the association between stress and relapses in MS because it was studied prospectively.

Overall, the evidence is quite congruent and clear. Stress plays a major role in MS relapses and strategies need to be developed to minimise the effects of stressful life events.

DEPRESSION

One of the potential consequences of stress is the development of depression. Depression is very common in people with MS, being diagnosed in over 50 per cent of people with MS at some time during the course of the disease.[42] One Italian study found that 46 per cent of patients in their study had major depressive disorder[43] and a Norwegian study revealed that 59 per cent of patients assessed had depression.[44] An Australian study found higher rates, with 67 per cent of surveyed people with MS being depressed.[45] Further, it has also been found in quite a large study that one in four people with MS has unrecognised and undiagnosed symptoms of depression.[46] It has been shown that people with MS who experience depression mostly do not seek medical help or treatment,[47] although in a large Canadian study, 40 per cent of people with MS had been treated with antidepressants during the study period.[48] Researchers have shown that the single most important factor in determining the quality of life of people with MS is not disability or fatigue or work, but the presence or absence of depression.[49]

This has been supported by a US study showing that depression was the best predictor of quality of life for people with MS, and that cognitive function was the best predictor of ability to work.[50] A major US consensus statement on depression in MS reported that depression was common in MS, had a major negative impact on quality of life, and was under-recognised and under-treated.[51] US researchers have suggested that the key issues promoting depression in MS are social support, coping ability, how people feel about themselves and the illness, and stress.[52]

> Depression is very common in people with MS and probably worsens the physical disease.

An important point to note about depression in MS is that the development of depression almost certainly worsens the physical disease by shifting the immune balance towards a predominantly Th1 response.[53] Further, it has been shown that treatment of depression corrects this immune disturbance[53, 54, 55] and so probably slows disease progression. Depression, along with fatigue, not only worsens the psychological but also the physical impact of the disease on people with MS.[56]

Researchers have looked at depression in MS and compared it with the incidence of depression in other chronic diseases.[57] They found that depression is a specific feature of MS. That is, while having MS can cause one to get depressed, as can non-specific factors in having a chronic disease in general, there is something very specific about the disease process in MS which makes people with MS much more likely to get depressed. Further, it is not only the physical progression of the illness that increases the distress of people with MS about their health. In fact, the 'invisible' features of MS such as pain and depression are much more likely to precipitate health distress than the more visible features.[58]

So, avoiding depression takes on a much more important role in the management of this illness than is generally recognised by most treating doctors. Hope and positivity are important factors in avoiding depression, but it is worth pointing out that there is now a lot of evidence to show that physical factors are important as well. The omega-3 fatty acids have a key role here. We have seen how effective these are in ensuring optimal cell membrane function, and improving the immune system. What is also becoming clear now is that a diet rich in omega-3s prevents depression.[59, 60, 61] This is probably also due to a membrane effect on the nerve cells in the brain.

Both animal and human work has now shown that fish oil supplementation improves learning. But there is also evidence that low eicosapentanoic acid (found in fish/fish oil) levels correlate with depression.[62] There are also data from large population studies which show that countries where fish forms a major part of the diet have much lower rates of depression than those where fish is not eaten much. Japan and Taiwan, for example, where fish consumption is the highest in the world, report rates of depression below 1 per cent of the population. West Germany, Canada and New Zealand, where fish consumption is very low, report rates of 5 per cent or over. There is also evidence from small uncontrolled studies that omega-3 supplements can improve depression. And there is now RCT evidence that omega-3 supplements improve depression in people with Parkinson's disease.[63] So another benefit from changing to the diet I have suggested is that there is less likelihood of depression.

As previously discussed, there is also good evidence that regular exercise prevents depression.[13] Given its other health benefits, exercise should form part of the health program of everybody who is able to do it. There is also longstanding evidence that low vitamin D levels are likely to precipitate or exacerbate depression and poor cognitive function.[64-7] This is a further reason to ensure that people with MS get adequate sun exposure, or take vitamin D supplements if that is not possible.

SMOKING

Smoking is a major lifestyle issue for those who seek optimal health, but we now have evidence of its specific detrimental effects in MS. There has been quite a bit of experimental data on the effect of smoking on the development of MS. It has suggested strongly what we would naturally suspect to be true, that smoking, with all its harmful effects on the body, has a role in MS development. An important point to emerge from a large study on nurses' health was the very clear association between cigarette smoking and MS.[68] The Nurses Health Study found that, compared with women who had never smoked, the risk of getting MS was 1.6 times greater for current smokers, and 1.2 times greater for past smokers. There was also a clear relationship between the duration of smoking and risk of MS. The risk was highest (1.7 times) for those who had smoked for over 25 years. This was supported by a Norwegian study which showed a very similar risk, with smokers 1.8 times more likely to develop MS than non-smokers.[69] A 2007 meta-analysis of all studies on smoking showed a significantly elevated risk of MS with smoking.[70] The author felt that the most likely reason for the association was unhealthy lifestyle behaviours of the smoking group, but I suspect the more likely cause is deliberately taking into the body the very potent cocktail of poisons involved in cigarette smoke.

Now there are enough reasons for anybody to give up smoking even without this data. With all the serious health problems smoking causes, from heart disease and lung cancer through to a range of other cancers, the single biggest positive health decision any smoker can make is to quit the habit. But for people with MS, or if MS runs in the family, there are even more compelling reasons to give up. This study didn't look at whether smoking worsens existing MS, just at whether it is associated with its initial development, but more recent studies examine the issue of how smoking influences MS progression.

Researchers at Harvard School of Public Health conducted a well designed case-control study on smokers with MS.[71] People with MS who had ever smoked were three to four times more likely to develop secondary progressive MS than those who had never smoked. A Swedish study in 2008 confirmed, in a group of 122 people with MS for a mean duration of six years, that smokers were significantly more likely to have progressive disease and to progress at an earlier age.[72]

A French case-control study showed that children were more than twice as likely to get MS if their parents smoked, and the longer they were exposed the more likely MS was to develop.[73] So passive smoking is harmful in MS as well. Another study from Austrian researchers published in 2008 showed that for people who had had an initial attack suggestive of MS, smokers were nearly twice as likely to go on and develop definite MS and to develop it earlier than non-smokers.[74] This has important implications for relatives of people with MS. Both passive smoking in the household and active smoking by as yet unaffected relatives make the development of MS more likely. A 2009 report from Johns Hopkins University to the AAN meeting in Seattle noted that those who started smoking earlier, in their study before the age of 17, were considerably more likely to develop MS.

> Cigarette smoking, both active and passive, increases the risk of developing MS, and of it becoming progressive.

Unfortunately, studies have shown that more people with MS smoke than in the general population.[26] Additionally, seeing a change in the sex distribution of MS, with proportionately more women getting the disease than men, scientists have suggested that this may be linked to the increasing rates of cigarette smoking in women.[75]

Smoking is an important potential modifier of the progression of MS. For people with MS who still smoke, this strong evidence means that making a positive choice about giving up smoking for better health in general is likely to favourably affect the course of MS as well. It is a reasonably simple lifestyle choice which can make a great difference to disease progression.

COGNITIVE FUNCTION

The term cognitive function describes higher mental functions such as awareness, perception, reasoning, judgment, ability to learn and remember details, and so on. There is growing evidence that cognitive function is progressively impaired in people with MS. The amount of impairment seems to relate quite closely to the loss of nerve cells which has been shown to accompany MS progression. This can be detected on MRI by a gradual shrinkage of the brain. An Italian study of 503 people with MS showed that 56 per cent had some degree of impairment of cognitive function.[76] Cognitive impairment was worse with longer duration of disease, increasing disability and with certain genetic background, although recent research has shown that it is present even very early in the disease and has an effect on quality of life.[77]

A US paper suggests that up to 70 per cent of people with MS have cognitive problems at some stage during the disease.[78] The cognitive problems are directly related to the amount of damage to the CNS, although it has been shown that specific cognitive disturbances are present even early in the disease.[79] Even people who have only an isolated episode of optic neuritis and otherwise appear to stay well have been shown to have significant cognitive decline 24 to 31 years later.[80] This adds weight to my view that the lifestyle changes I outline in this book should be started as early as possible after diagnosis.

German researchers have suggested that people with MS be tested for any decline in cognitive function as this is the most sensitive index of disease progression.[81] They suggest that subtle changes in cognitive function can be a useful way of determining whether disease-modifying therapies are working or not. Researchers have shown that, in addition to the more usual measures of cognitive function, decision making capacity is also affected in MS.[82] This can have a significant impact on daily life for people with MS, and contribute to disability.

OVERVIEW

Evidence is mounting that regular exercise has various benefits for people with MS. Not only does it make people feel better, improve quality of life and reduce the potential for depression, there is every likelihood that it positively affects the disease process itself. In contrast, stress and depression play a significant negative role. Efforts to minimise the impact of stress, manage it better, and lower the risk of depression are likely to reduce disease activity. Smoking has a negative health effect in general, but the evidence is now clear that it has a specific negative effect on people with MS. It is becoming more apparent that, like many other Western degenerative diseases, MS responds positively to healthy lifestyle choices.

10

OTHER FACTORS: EVIDENCE ABOUT GLUTEN, DENTAL AMALGAM, VACCINATIONS, HYPERBARIC OXYGEN AND OTHERS

Every really new idea looks crazy at first

Alfred North Whitehead

Since being diagnosed with MS, I have become very much more open-minded about many unconventional therapies people try for a whole host of diseases. Everyone is different. It is likely that different things trigger MS in different people. So it follows that we should not be too dogmatic about what might and might not work in any particular case. In the RCTs on MS, we see the results of what has happened to a group of people with MS. But in all the trials, some people got better, some stayed the same and some got worse. Interferon may slow the disease for one person, while another deteriorates. That person may find that glatiramer slows the disease for them. Alternatively, some other less conventional therapy may work.

Whatever works works. Each of us is not a clinical trial. If we find something that stops the disease for us, then that speaks for itself. Many people with MS have used the following therapies, and say they have worked. Below I present some evidence on which to base recommendations about them, but there are caveats regarding that evidence. Who

SUMMARISING THE EVIDENCE

- There is no real evidence of an association between gluten and MS.
- There is no proven link between dental amalgam and MS; the risk of developing MS for people with amalgam fillings is not significantly higher than for those without.
- There is conjecture about the role of hepatitis B vaccination in MS; some studies suggest a link.
- There is currently no evidence of any benefit from hyperbaric oxygen therapy in MS, although trials have been poorly designed.
- Bee-sting therapy does not seem to be of any benefit in MS.

EVIDENCE-BASED RECOMMENDATIONS

- Gluten-free diets are not necessary for most people with MS, unless there is a proven allergy for an individual.
- Taking amalgam fillings out is hazardous and the risk may outweigh the possible benefit in MS.
- People with MS may wish to carefully consider the risks of vaccinating their children against hepatitis B.
- Hyperbaric oxygen and bee-sting therapy are not recommended.

knows what research will find in the future about things we discount at present? Just as people with MS were being told in the past to stay out of the sun and avoid exercise, and we now know that this was having a negative impact on the disease and on their quality of life, so some of the more contentious strategies and therapies I discuss below may in time come to be used commonly.

GLUTEN

In her book *Multiple Sclerosis: A self-help guide to its management*, Judy Graham outlines the cases of two spectacular improvements after people radically changed their diet to eradicate substances to which they felt allergic.[1] These people were Roger MacDougall and Alan Greer. Roger gave away gluten initially, then sugar and all dairy produce. Alan excluded meat initially, then all other saturated fats, then a host of foods including gluten-containing foods. Both made stunning recoveries from advanced MS. Why this may have worked I don't know. Any one of the things, or some combination of them, which these people gave up might have been triggering their disease. The saturated fats were very likely to be implicated, from the evidence I have previously presented.

There is also a growing number of researchers who contend that, in an evolutionary sense, legumes and gluten in cereals are relatively recent additions to the human diet. These protein-rich foods may be implicated in a host of auto-immune diseases including MS. I have not seen enough evidence to convince myself that these foods should be avoided by people with MS, but some find the arguments convincing.

The most severe form of gluten intolerance is coeliac disease. Here, people develop serious digestive system disorders due to an immune response to the gluten in wheat. One might expect, if gluten was a key ingredient in the diet to avoid in MS, that people with MS might have a higher than usual incidence of coeliac disease or, vice versa, that people with coeliac disease might have a higher than expected incidence of MS. A major population study published in 2007 examined 14,000 people in Sweden with coeliac disease and compared them with 70,000 other people without the disease acting as controls.[2] One would have expected a higher rate of MS (or other CNS degenerative disease) in those people with coeliac disease than controls if gluten was involved in causing these diseases. In fact the researchers found no statistically significant association between coeliac disease and subsequent multiple sclerosis, Parkinson's disease, Alzheimer's disease, hereditary ataxia, the symptom ataxia, Huntington's disease, myasthenia gravis or spinal muscular atrophy. This is very strong evidence that there is no link with gluten.

If there was indeed a link, one should at least expect to find in people with MS antibodies to gluten which indicate intolerance. In fact, Italian researchers looking at 95 patients with MS found not a single patient with elevated antibody levels.[3] UK researchers tested 49 patients with MS for their antibody levels and found 12 per cent had raised levels; however, this compared with 13 per cent of unselected blood donors, so it was unlikely that people with MS had any special sensitivity to gluten.[4] Iranian researchers tested 166 people with MS for antibodies and compared them to people without MS.[5] They found no difference in antibody levels. Italian researchers in 2008 found no cases that had coeliac disease-related antibodies among 217 people with MS, but one case in the controls.[6] This patient was shown to have coeliac disease.

Italian researchers used an alternative approach to investigate this problem. They fed a gluten-free diet to animals with the experimental form of MS, EAE. Not only did the animals not improve, but they initially had a more severe disease course.[7] Interestingly, they later seemed to have less disability than the other animals, but given their initial deterioration it is difficult to be definite about any effect either way. In all, these papers add further evidence for the lack of any definite link between gluten intolerance and MS. In total, I have found this lack of hard evidence for any detrimental effect of gluten enough to not change my own diet to exclude wheat products, but would certainly change if evidence did emerge.

There is more information about gluten in MS at www.direct-ms.org, a website run by Direct-MS, a registered charity investigating the nutritional basis of MS. Those responsible for this site, however, have strong views that gluten is involved in MS despite the lack of clear evidence. In other respects, the site is excellent. Judy Graham's book also gives an excellent account of the possible role of allergy, in its broadest sense, in the management of MS. It is well worth reading, particularly for people having difficulty controlling MS with conventional means. I hope there is enough information on lifestyle change and medical therapies presented in this book to give most people a way of slowing the disease. But if not, and the disease still progresses, this sort of radical step may be an option.

My advice would not be to give up on other tried and true therapies. For people still relapsing despite a low saturated-fat/high omega-3 diet, and perhaps some drug therapy, it is probably best to stay on these if they are causing no problems, and perhaps investigate other medications. But, in addition, it may be helpful to be tested for gluten intolerance, and if that suggests a link then cut out wheat products and see how things go. Alternatively, some people may want to try it in any event. I can't see this doing any harm, and it might just hit the right trigger for a particular case of MS, although it is important to note that this is not based on any available evidence. It would be unwise, though, to put all your eggs in one basket, so to speak, and give up on the other therapies while doing this. I feel it is important to try to get as many things working in my favour as I can in controlling this illness.

A case-control study from the Harvard School of Public Health in 2006 showed that a history of allergies was not related to the risk of getting MS.[8] However, interestingly the researchers showed that taking regular antihistamines in the three years prior to diagnosis reduced the risk of getting MS by about 80 per cent, so there is probably more to the story.

DENTAL AMALGAM

Interest in this area stemmed from an early observation about the geographical distribution of MS. Ingalls, a doctor from the renowned Framingham Epidemiology Study Center in Massachusetts noted that the incidence of MS seemed to follow the incidence of dental caries.[9] Knowing that mercury (which forms part of dental amalgam in fillings) has been implicated in neurological disease, the theory was formed that perhaps the amalgam in fillings was causing MS. Ingalls, who himself was diagnosed with MS, felt that other heavy metals including lead may also play a causative role in MS. He published another paper a few years later describing an outbreak of a cluster of 30 to 40 cases of MS and other neurological syndromes in Ohio.[10] He found some evidence that this was related to heavy metal contamination of local water, particularly with chromium and cadmium.

One of the difficulties with this theory is that the incidence of dental caries may just be a marker for some other factor which is really contributing to the development of MS. An interesting case-control study from Leicester found that people with MS had more dental caries than those without.[11] It also found that people with more mercury amalgam fillings had higher mercury levels in their bodies, but it found no higher incidence of MS in those with fillings. So the association of dental caries with MS may just be a reflection of some other variable which is also related to dental caries, and not dental amalgam.

For instance, dental caries is most common in more affluent societies. If we look at the incidence of MS in the world, it is most common in affluent countries. Saturated fat consumption is also highest in affluent countries. Perhaps the observation of MS following the incidence of dental caries had more to do with this than with dental amalgam. This is supported by other case-control studies.[12, 13] Although the issue remains contentious, a major 2001 review concluded there was no significant health risk from dental amalgam.[14] A subsequent review in 2005 concluded that there was no evidence of any association of amalgam with neurodegenerative diseases or auto-immune diseases, but that more research is needed with regard to MS.[15] A further systematic review in 2007 reported that there was a slight increase in the risk of developing MS for people with amalgam fillings which was consistent across studies but was not statistically significant.[16]

Although many people with MS have had their fillings removed as a result, there is as yet no evidence of any sort that I can find to indicate that this might be helpful. Critics of the technique will point out that MS has developed in many, many people who have no fillings or have dentures. Mum, for example, had dentures as a very young woman. She once told me it was fashionable in those days in Europe to get all your teeth taken out, so they wouldn't cause you any problems later. It was many years until she developed MS.

On the other hand, many people approach their recovery from serious illness in a very holistic way, and feel that removing all possible toxic substances from their bodies and environment is essential. Removing their dental fillings may be part of this process. It certainly seems that people with many amalgam fillings have higher levels of mercury in their bodies. Personally, I think that if someone feels this is an important issue then they should go ahead and do it, although it is not based on any available evidence. But I wouldn't advise people getting all their fillings replaced as a trial to see if it will help, if they are doing all the other things recommended in this book. Like asbestos roofs in houses, the hazardous material is probably safer left alone, where it will release much less of its toxicity than if drilled and removed. A reasonable approach would be to leave current amalgam fillings in place, but if any new ones are needed to get them made from a different material.

HEPATITIS B IMMUNISATION AND MS RISK

There has been a lot of conjecture about whether getting immunised against hepatitis B increases the risk of getting MS. Hepatitis B vaccine is genetically engineered and has been available since the 1980s. It is considered to be well tolerated by people, although there have been many reports of increased risk of MS associated with the immunisation. A large case-control study from the United States tested whether this was by chance, and found an alarming increase in the risk for several major auto-immune diseases, including MS. People getting hepatitis B vaccination were 5.2 times more likely to be diagnosed with MS than controls who were not vaccinated.[17] This is supported by a US case-control study which showed that people with MS were 3.1 times more likely to have been vaccinated in the three years prior to onset of symptoms than controls who did not have MS.[18] To confirm that this was a real effect specific to hepatitis vaccination, they checked whether tetanus or influenza vaccination resulted in any similar effect, and found none.

It seems likely that MS is not the only auto-immune disease which may be precipitated by hepatitis B vaccination. US researchers found significant numbers of people with other auto-immune disease after hepatitis B vaccination in a Vaccine Adverse Event Reporting System and the general medical literature.[19] They concluded that it should be considered there is a causal relationship between hepatitis B vaccination and serious auto-immune disorders among certain susceptible people.

For people already vaccinated for hepatitis B there is nothing that can be done about it. But it may be worth considering this information if the question comes up of having close family members or children vaccinated for hepatitis B, given that they already have a much higher risk of developing MS than the general community. A French group suggested in 2005 that this increased risk of MS with hepatitis B vaccination was due to a contaminant in the manufacturing process,[20] although UK researchers have found a highly significant degree of cross-reactivity between the hepatitis B vaccine and myelin oligodendrocyte glycoprotein, thought to be one of the targets for CNS auto-immunity in MS.[21]

HYPERBARIC OXYGEN THERAPY

One potential therapy which should be discussed in a little more detail is hyperbaric oxygen. This form of therapy has its supporters for the treatment of MS, as it does for many other diseases. I am fortunate to have been trained in hyperbaric medicine and to have worked in a Hyperbaric Medicine Unit. This gives me a little background in the area and helps my interpretation of the conflicting claims.

Hyperbaric chambers are the recompression facilities used to treat divers with 'the bends'. They are being increasingly used by elite sportspeople as a way of healing rapidly after injury, although there is little evidence to support this practice. Cross-referencing 'MS' with 'hyperbaric' in a Medline search produces a little under 100 references. A good summary of the available evidence was published in 1995 by two Dutch epidemiologists.[22] They found fourteen clinical trials in the literature on hyperbaric therapy for MS. Of these, eight were of sufficient quality to include in an overall analysis. Only one showed a result in favour of hyperbaric oxygen. Given what we know of statistics in these trials, there is a reasonable likelihood that this was the one chance positive result that might be expected. The respected Cochrane Collaboration published a systematic review of the available literature in 2004.[23] They concluded there was no consistent evidence of any benefit of hyperbaric oxygen in MS.

One of the difficulties of these trials is that most were for people with chronic progressive or chronic stable MS. This seems like just the wrong group of patients to treat. Hyperbaric oxygen therapy involves supplying oxygen, effectively at very high doses. This means that areas of inflammation, like MS lesions, would have better oxygenation of the damaged tissue and less swelling. In my view, this therapy should be trialled in MS patients who are having a relapse. This could quite possibly show a benefit.

The biggest of the studies, from Milwaukee in the United States, registered the results of over 300 patients treated with hyperbaric oxygen.[24] They were unable to show any benefit of treatment. I think this is how we must view hyperbaric therapy. For those few patients who get significant benefit from this therapy, there is no reason to abandon it. It is very safe, with only minor side effects, and it is not terribly difficult for patients. You just need a good book to while away the time in the chamber. But for most people it is likely to be ineffective.

OTHER THERAPIES

Many people have tried a range of other therapies for MS. These include homeopathy, naturopathy, osteopathy, ayurvedic medicine, massage, acupuncture and so on. Personally I find the occasional massage extremely relaxing and energising. Anything that promotes a feeling of wellbeing is likely to have beneficial effects on the immune system, and that can only do good. Gradually more and more of these therapies are being scrutinised in carefully performed RCTs and we can assess their true benefit or otherwise.

In 2005, Austrian researchers investigated an interesting new treatment modality for people with significant disability in MS, aimed at improving their function.[25] They applied a low frequency whole body vibration for quite short periods and compared this with a placebo. People receiving the vibration therapy improved in postural control and mobility. This therapy deserves wider testing although the effect may be indirect, such as through relaxation.

Bee-sting therapy

Another therapy which has had its proponents over the years has been bee-sting therapy. There has been little in the medical literature on which to base recommendations about this, with most of the reports of its benefits coming from anecdotes. A 2005 study of 26 patients used live bees stinging patients with relapsing-remitting MS three times a week.[26] The researchers found no reduction in disease activity, disability or fatigue and no improvement in quality of life, so this therapy is difficult to recommend. Others have tried immunising people with MS with bee venom extract. In a small study of nine patients, researchers found it to be safe but it did not seem to produce any benefit.[27]

OVERVIEW

I have described a few of the possible alternatives beyond mainstream approaches to good health using the diet and lifestyle changes previously discussed and conventional medicine. Most are unsupported by currently available evidence, however, they may be worth trying in individual cases.

11

THE MIND-BODY CONNECTION: EVIDENCE ABOUT THE ROLE OF THE MIND AND EMOTIONS IN HEALING

It's not what happens to us, but how we respond that ultimately matters

Jean Shinoda Bolen

This is one of the most interesting but least understood areas in medicine. In six years of medical school I learnt all about disease, micro-organisms and treatments we as doctors could give to patients to help them get better. To a much lesser extent, I learnt about how patient factors could predispose them to illness, and how various lifestyles and behaviours put people at risk of acquiring certain diseases. What was conspicuously absent was any discussion or study of the complex interplay between people's emotions, personalities and lives and the diseases to which they are predisposed, and what patients can do about disease in a holistic sense once they have developed it. There was discussion about cures, but little about healing.

Yet for most of the history of medicine, this has not been so. For previous generations of doctors, who had few effective resources with which to treat disease, there was strong emphasis on patient factors in disease. Great medical minds of prior times were convinced that patients held the key to their recovery from illness. But today's doctors, surrounded by a vast array of technological wonders and marvellous drug

SUMMARISING THE EVIDENCE

- There is little evidence about the role of the mind and emotions in healing, yet most of us intuitively understand the clear association.
- Survivors of serious illness share similar characteristics; they see the illness as a challenge, actively seek solutions, and engage wholeheartedly in the healing process.
- Repressed emotions and unresolved grief and conflict can trigger or worsen serious illness.
- Faith and hope are important companions in the healing process; it is important to replace fear with faith.
- An RCT has shown that writing down difficult feelings produced a 30 per cent improvement in people with chronic inflammatory diseases.
- Meditation has numerous health benefits and has been shown to be of value in auto-immune conditions.

EVIDENCE-BASED RECOMMENDATIONS

- Find avenues to express grief and difficult emotions.
- Consider keeping a diary, seeing a counsellor, or attending an MS group.
- Engage with the practice of meditation; even 20 minutes a day brings significant health benefits.

therapies, have lost sight of just how important the patient is in determining recovery from illness.

THE PATIENT'S INFLUENCE ON ILLNESS

For most of my career, since the influence of Ian Hislop as an intern, I have needed no convincing that emotions play a very significant role in the development of illness. Ian wrote two important books studying his long exploration of this area of medicine, entitled *Stress, Distress and Illness* and *The Feeling Being* which I can recommend to readers. While they are both written for the practising primary care physician, there is much in these books for the lay public if they have some background in medical terminology. It was only much more recently, though, when challenged by my own serious illness, that I started to explore the much more contentious area of patients influencing their actual recovery from illness.

I must thank Dr Joanne Samer here. Joanne is a general practitioner who practises in Perth. Not long after I was diagnosed with MS a number of important people entered my life, providing guidance when I most needed it. Joanne was one of them. Joanne was diagnosed with MS in 1994. Like me, she was galvanised into action by the diagnosis and began to look everywhere for things she could do to recover from the illness. Not for her the passive patient role. She began experimenting with nutritional supplements and emotional healing in its broadest sense. Unlike me, she did not go to the traditional medical literature for answers, because she did not trust it. When I first spoke to her, she knew nothing about Professor Swank's work.

I owe Joanne a great debt. Among other things, she introduced me to Bernie Siegel. It's worth noting before I talk about Bernie that Joanne was to develop thyroid cancer two years after being diagnosed with MS. As I write this, she has not only recovered from both illnesses and is practising medicine, but is lecturing others on the benefits of nutrition in illness. She is truly an inspirational woman, and has used the serious illnesses she had to positively change the course of her life.

BERNIE SIEGEL'S MESSAGE

But about Bernie. Bernie Siegel is a surgeon who works in New Haven, Connecticut. After years of trying to keep a detached, impersonal relationship with his surgical patients, he realised this was doing neither the patients nor himself any good. He now runs ECaP, a group for exceptional cancer patients. Unlike 'traditional' cancer surgeons, he actively encourages his patients to look everywhere for ways to heal, to explore every possibility, to become 'active' participants in their healing.

It was through reading Bernie's books that I realised the response I had to my illness was typical of survivors. In his book, *Love, Medicine and Miracles*, which every doctor should read, he describes what it is that sets apart these people who recover from serious illness.[1] In general they find the illness a challenge and an opportunity for personal growth. They tackle the illness actively, rather than being passive recipients of doctors' treatments. They go to every source for information, are open-minded about unconventional therapies, try everything. They feel empowered by the discoveries they make to take control of their illnesses and, indeed, their lives.

> The way people respond to illness profoundly affects outcome.

These are difficult ways for a conventionally trained doctor to respond to illness. To illustrate this, as Bernie says, imagine the different responses to the situation I am about to describe. A woman comes into a lecture theatre full of medical students. She describes how she was diagnosed with terminal cancer with secondaries everywhere just a few months ago, but that the latest scans show she is cured, that there are no more lesions. The students will be filled with awe, and ask how the patient did it, what she tried and so on. Imagine the room is full of doctors, particularly those who have been qualified for some time. The responses will be very different. They will suggest that the original pathology reports must have been mixed up with someone else's, that the scans must have been switched, that the tumour must have been benign. They will do almost anything rather than remain open to the possibility that this illness has been healed. What makes us become so closed-minded? Where do we lose our openness to such ideas?

I have had discussions with many of my colleagues along these lines, with colleagues who in other respects seem very open-minded and understanding. But they cannot bring themselves to make the leap to believe that these things are possible. They cannot accept that the mind is so powerful that not only can it create illness, but it can take it away. But why should that surprise us? Humans understand so little of the workings of the universe. Our perception is so limited by the particular physical make-up we have. Worse, with modern technology and media, we have become so convinced that we can control nature and our lives we forget that we are part of nature, and part of the energy that moves through all things. Every now and then something reminds us of our frailty and how interwoven we are into the fabric of life. Often it is serious illness. But mostly we live with the comfortable illusion that we have control over our environment and everything that happens to us.

There is a movement in medicine away from the conventional paternalistic view of impersonal doctors treating passive recipients of their care, patients who don't argue or say what they want and who are therefore not empowered to tackle the changes they must make to overcome disease. Visionary physicians like Deepak Chopra and Bernie Siegel lead this revolution. They understand what potential we have within us for modifying the course of disease, if only we choose to, and are allowed to use it. And of course we can learn much from individuals, such as Ian Gawler, who have themselves recovered from 'terminal' cancer. The messages from all of these people are surprisingly similar.

ILLNESS AS A CHALLENGE

It is from these doctors and others that I have got the message that serious illness is a challenge. Many patients come to regard it as a gift. Like other challenges in life, out of the kernel of the problem may come wonderful insights and answers that transform our lives. This has certainly been true for me. The list of what I have got from having MS outweighs the things I have lost many times over. I am sure this is so for many other people and many other illnesses.

For those of us with MS, and cancer, and many other serious diseases, it is worth remembering that the illness is part of us. I don't like to think of tackling my illness as a fight. It doesn't make sense to fight yourself—it just empowers the illness. It's just that some of the cells of our bodies are not behaving in the way we want them to behave. We have extraordinary power over how our bodies' cells behave. If we get anxious and our blood pressure rises, we lower our heart rate to compensate. We don't have to do it consciously, indeed we can't do it consciously. If we get too cold, we start our muscles shivering to generate heat. Similarly if we get infected with a virus, we mobilise our immune system to fight the invader and almost always win. When we break a bone, we don't have to tell our body how to heal itself. Built into the DNA in every cell in our bodies is the blueprint for fixing itself when things go wrong, for developing into an adult, for producing children.

But in MS and cancer, something goes wrong with the message. If we can do all these other things, why can't we control our bodies' cells and stop the process going wrong when it does? Well, the truth is that some people can. Countless case reports exist of patients terminally ill with cancer who go home and make a complete recovery. If they can do it we all can, if we can work out how. It only has to happen once to make it possible. The body has a tremendously effective ability to heal when it is in balance. The difficulty is in quietening the mind long enough to allow the body to return to this natural state of balance. This is where meditation comes in.

Some individuals who spend a lot of time getting in tune and harmony with their minds and bodies can do extraordinary things with them. Certain spiritual leaders in eastern religions who meditate regularly or use other techniques such as yoga have shown sceptics that they can raise their pulse rates to almost the exact number of beats per minute they wish to, and lower them again at will. Bernie Siegel tells of patients who are instructed under anaesthetic to lower their pulse rates, or slow down their rate of bleeding, and are able to do so. Before dismissing this, there is much scientific literature showing that some people, despite deep general anaesthesia, can recall under hypnosis exactly the conversations that went on in the operating theatre. Patients who have been told that they will be well and feel little pain after an operation have been shown to require less pain relief.

It is not much of a leap from here to understand that people can heal almost any illness. From my reading, what is important here is that, before people can heal illness, they must heal themselves. What opened my eyes to this was the marvellous work of Carolyn Myss, author of the best-selling *Anatomy of the Spirit*. This was the book that Ian Hislop suggested I start with when I first saw him. This book, along with *Quantum Healing* by Deepak Chopra, helped me understand the concept of the underlying energy that runs through all of us, the energy that we need to heal and the energy we are often wasting in our day-to-day lives.

Carolyn Myss and many other authors have shown that different personalities tend to predispose to different types of illness. The heart disease personality is well known. The hard driving executive with the type A personality, who eats poorly and often smokes and drops dead one day just before an important board meeting. What has been shown equally is that there is a cancer personality, or type C personality as Ian Gawler calls it. Cancer happens more often to people who have difficulty expressing anger, who keep their feelings in rather than letting them out, who would rather not bother anybody with their wants and desires. Indeed, Bernie Siegel cites interesting work showing that the personalities of a group of medical students could predict their disease patterns later in life at least as well as any other predictor.

Since beginning the MS retreats I run with Ian Gawler, we have noticed that there may be an MS personality as well. Certainly my sense is that MS people are strong-willed, fiercely independent and prefer not to accept help from anybody. I have seen a pattern, too, where this is often in reaction to having had difficult conflicting emotions in childhood, often resulting in suppressing anger about loved ones who have caused some injury or been unjust, and turning that anger inward instead. The metaphor of the body turning on itself is pretty apt.

TIME IS AN ILLUSION

An interesting follow on from this is the concept of freeing up the very powerful subconscious mind to enable us to deal with disease by working through unresolved conflicts and suppressed anger and grief. The key to understanding this is realising that the conscious mind does not have the power to heal us.

I like Wayne Dyer's view that the conscious mind is actually insane, because it believes in something it is not.[2] It believes it is the body, the accomplishments of a person, the history of a person. The conscious mind deals in thoughts. Every minute of every day we have a never-ending stream of thoughts passing through our minds. If we are focused on a particular problem, the thoughts may be centred around finding a solution, perhaps working through alternatives. More often than not, if we stop to actively listen to the thoughts, they are nonsense. There may be a strain of some song we have recently heard, playing along in front of an imaginary conversation with someone we have seen earlier or are about to see later. These constant thoughts rob us of the energy we need for healing. We waste that energy dealing in the abstract with countless unimportant matters we think about over and over again. Serious illness demands that we focus our available energy in the present, on healing ourselves. Most of what is happening in the conscious mind distracts us from actually being present in the now, in the present moment. Being centred in the present moment actually requires some effort and some commitment. It is all about being mindful of the distractions which constantly pull us away from the moment.

The present moment is all we have. Many people are locked into a lifetime of thoughts and inner wrestling about things that have long since passed, or will never happen. Yet those thoughts would have no existence, except for the fact that they are being thought by the thinker. If the thinker wasn't present right now, none of that would exist. This is very powerful stuff to consider for those people who feel that the past controls their lives. Many people feel that they would be better people, or far better able to cope or would be less anxious, if only certain things in the past hadn't happened. For instance, some blame their parents for not loving them sufficiently, or for always criticising them. This is often still the case many years after the parents are gone. But the only reason the parents' actions still exist in any sense is because of the thoughts that person is thinking *in the present moment.*

Again, I like Wayne Dyer's metaphor. See yourself as a ship on the ocean, looking down from above. Behind the boat stretches the wake. Is it possible for the wake to be driving the ship? No, it is just the history being left behind. The power to drive the ship lies within the ship itself.

On reflection, time is an illusion. Over the years, humans have become more and more sophisticated at measuring time exactly. The concept of what a person would be doing at 3 p.m. on a given day next week would have meant absolutely nothing to Stone Age people. Now, with superannuation, and booking ahead for holidays, and diaries full of appointments, we have come to believe in time as a very real thing. So much so that we spend much of the present moment either in the future or the past, or both, planning or worrying about what is going to happen or analysing or trying to work out what we should have done in situations that have already happened. We have precious little time left to be experiencing now. But in reality, now is all we ever will have. Right until the moment we lie on our deathbeds preparing to depart this life, we will still be in the present moment. How much of it will we have wasted before then by not being centred and present in the moment as we live? Excessive thinking in effect gradually removes us from the present moment by dulling our senses to what is really going on in our lives. The antidote to excessive thinking is to concentrate on feeling and sensing our physical bodies again in the present moment. This is where the technique of progressive muscle relaxation (PMR) as taught by Ian Gawler in his meditation workshops is of great benefit. As an introduction to meditation it is really good for relaxation, but more importantly, because the focus of concentration is on how the physical body is feeling, it helps to centre us again in our bodies, and hence helps us to live in the present moment. It has been shown to be of value in people with MS in a UK study.[3]

Very early on after being diagnosed with MS, as I was battling mentally to come to terms with it, I started focusing on where I wanted to get to with all the changes I was making. Diet, meditation, exercise, sunlight, visualisation. What was the aim of all of these things? The aim, I realised, was to keep myself the same as I am now. That is, my endpoint was identical to the process I was going through every day. What I was aiming at was not some distant future goal. I had my aim already. I was already fit, active and had essentially no disability. My aim, then, had to be to enjoy every day as I maintained that state. That was the very outcome I was after. I was already there.

This was a revelation in many respects. The whole trick was to ensure that I was living life to the full every day and enjoying the present moment, not concentrating on some far distant goal. If I did things right, that would take care of itself. I realised that every day is an end in itself. The process is the outcome. These two messages now hang on my study wall, 'Every day is an end in itself' and 'The process is the outcome'. They remind me, when I forget as we all do, to stay centred in the present moment.

Sometimes the continuous mind babble that we all have keeps returning to a theme. It might be how we have been harshly treated by a friend, or how we were hurt in a particular relationship. This indicates that at a deeper level, in the subconscious, we have not resolved an important issue in our lives. Our subconscious mind is very powerful. Until we satisfactorily resolve such issues, it will keep returning to the problem. This may not happen consciously, although it often does, but may take the form of dreams around a certain theme. Worse, it may take the form of illness. To have the necessary energy to heal the illness, we have to heal the underlying problem in our subconscious. To marshal all our energies to deal with the illness, we have to resolve those underlying issues so that the energy is ours again to deal with the illness.

Carolyn Myss shows in *Anatomy of the Spirit* how these destructive patterns develop, and how we can resolve some of these issues. Just by being aware of these mechanisms, we may liberate enough energy to begin dealing with the problems. Mainstream researchers are starting to explore this area too. A major review of the brain–immune connection in MS noted that psychological factors like mood and cognition exert a modulating effect on the immune system in MS.[4]

THE CONSCIOUS VERSUS SUBCONSCIOUS MIND

I was lucky enough to have a very good guide when I first got sick. I regard it as no coincidence that the right people keep popping up just when you most need them. To use Bernie Siegel's idea, coincidence is God's way of remaining anonymous. Ian Hislop started me off on the process of understanding the importance of unresolved issues years earlier. Then when I was diagnosed with MS, he helped me to start tackling issues that I had left unresolved. The first part of the process is to quiet the conscious mind enough to start to get in touch with the subconscious. This is the value of meditation. Some prefer other methods of quieting the mind: yoga, tai chi, playing music, gardening—all may be equally good, depending on personal preferences. Until the mind slows down though, and leaves enough gaps in the constant stream of mental chatter, the issues bubbling up from our subconscious remain elusive. While music or gardening may be helpful in quietening the mind, they are only really capable of slowing the mind a little. Meditation is the most helpful way of slowing the mind.

RESOLVING UNFINISHED BUSINESS

An early insight I had when Ian Hislop visited me after my diagnosis was to trust my instincts and feelings. Immediately on talking to him, I realised I had to attend to some important unfinished business. I suggest that it is important to listen carefully to the immediate gut-level reactions that occur when first hit with the shock of serious illness. Later, when things have settled down, it may be much easier and more comfortable not to confront the things that you instinctively felt needed sorting out. But they need to be confronted.

I had remained estranged from a work colleague for some years after a perceived injustice, and determined I would remedy that immediately. I had also consumed a lot of energy over the years ruminating over a past relationship in which I felt I had been betrayed. I resolved as well that I would go and have lunch with the person, in order to confront some of my own feelings and liberate my wasted energy. I did these things because I could see that I needed all my energy if I was to heal myself physically. But also, it was clear to me that all of us could benefit from liberating the energy we had tied up in these past events.

A useful way of looking at difficult issues that arise is to see them as lessons. Many spiritual teachers believe that life is a series of lessons to be learnt while we are here on Earth. By looking through major issues and conflicts to see what lessons we can learn, the damaging impact of those conflicts can be much reduced. It has been said that in life there are no friends or enemies, just teachers.

This is particularly important when we perceive ourselves to be the loser. Almost always something can be learned from the situation. This can put an end to dwelling on the issue and wasting energy which is so necessary to assist healing. It can turn a situation from a negative to a positive one, and assist our own personal growth and help us to learn much about ourselves and the way we handle difficult issues.

SYMBOLS AND DREAMS

Another important insight I gained from Bernie Siegel helped me to understand why Carolyn Myss keeps asking us to think about our lives symbolically. Bernie stresses the power of dreams. For the first time, I realised why dreams are so important. Humans have not always had the power of language. That skill developed with evolution, presumably with parallels in the physical development of certain parts of our brains. Before words, how did humans think? We must assume they thought in images. How do we dream? Most of us do so in images. When I think of my dreams they are usually visual, with few words. Dreaming represents the released expression of more basic and primitive parts of our minds, presumably the subconscious. When thoughts stop interrupting and getting in the way of our subconscious mind expressing itself, as in when we sleep or when we meditate, issues that are really important to us begin to emerge.

Hence Bernie exhorts us to pay attention to our dreams. He says that the more open we are to this, and the more we pay attention to our dreams, the more we will see the signposts and messages our subconscious minds have for us. This was illustrated to me very graphically. The very first night after I read this, I was determined to pay more attention to my dreams. Sure enough, I woke at about 3 a.m. I had been trying hard to find a way of visualising the MS disease process in my body. I had read that many cancer patients were able to effectively influence their disease by visualisation techniques, such as seeing their white cells as armed warriors shooting the cancer cells. I didn't find this a helpful image with MS, but I couldn't find any other that seemed to fit.

That night I dreamt I was walking with some friends up the road where I lived as a child. Parked on the side, encroaching on the road, were several large earthmoving machines. The machines were yellow with many little legs, which went up and down in progression when they were working, like a millipede. My friends crossed over the road, but I tried to get over a little further up, just as a big burly fellow in blue overalls climbed up on the biggest machine and started it up. The gap between it and the next machine was narrowing as I tried to get through, and my right little finger was caught between two of them. It wasn't badly damaged, but I could clearly feel it being squeezed between the two machines.

I woke in a cold sweat. Had I not been thinking about it, I would have gone back to sleep and not taken any notice. But I immediately saw the significance of it. It was just so obvious. The roads of my childhood were my nerve cells; what better symbols are there? Traffic passing up and down them all the time, connecting things together, and so on. The machines were the white cells of the immune system, and they were responsible for the continual process of tidying up the edges of the nerve cells. But they had encroached on the road and were actually damaging the pathways themselves. The burly driver indicated that something other than me was in control of them. The fact that he was so big and strong was a reflection of how powerful I perceived the illness to be. Amazingly, the little finger on my right hand had become caught between two of the machines. For a couple of days I had been getting odd sensations in just that finger. I had been worried that it might be a relapse. As Bernie said, once you start looking for it, it happens.

Now I had the ammunition I needed for my visualisations. Bernie had said that some people with MS liked to think of their white cells as the seven dwarfs. I simply could not buy that one; it just wasn't for me. But my subconscious, once I had given it free rein to come up with something, had provided exactly what I needed. For a long while, I visualised the machines every time I began meditating. I saw myself at the controls as the machines moved along the edges of the roads, but not onto them, tidying up the debris on the edge.

FAITH

It's extraordinary, I think, that in the many, many books written on spiritual matters there is such agreement between the authors on so many things. This really struck me as I started catching up on a part of my life I had ignored. Carolyn Myss' *Anatomy of the Spirit* led me to her other book *Why People Don't Heal and How They Can*.

On walking through a small bookshop in Perth called Wisdom Books, I came across a book whose cover I liked. A quote on the cover said something like 'A story not to be missed'. The picture on the cover was of an old man reclining, with a young man talking to him. I just thought, this looks interesting, bought it and took it home without knowing what it was about. I read it in one sitting. Incredibly, the book was about a university professor who develops an incurable neurological disease resulting in increasing paralysis, and about how one of his former students learns lessons about what is important in life by visiting him every Tuesday. The book is called *Tuesdays with Morrie*, and while it is a little painful to read early after the diagnosis of MS, it is uplifting and full of joy. It has since become a bestseller. See what I mean about coincidences? In the same bookshop I found a nice little parable about life by Dan Millman called *The Laws of Spirit* which is also really helpful. I soon began reading much of Deepak Chopra, and Joanne Samer introduced me to Bernie Siegel. People started buying me books about self-help and positivity. Things like Richard Carlson's *Don't Sweat the Small Stuff*, and others, are full of useful little insights to help us get in touch with ourselves a bit better. *Handbook for the Soul*, edited by Richard Carlson and Benjamin Shield, put together the ideas of many of these great late twentieth-century spiritual leaders. If your spirit is ever in need of a real lift, just read any one of these short pieces.

For me, the surprising thing was how closely they all thought about the spirit. For my whole life I had struggled with the concept of faith. I could not get involved with organised religion. It had no relevance for me. It seemed that many of the religious people I knew were less in tune with themselves than many who were not religious. I knew the history of organised religion and the heartaches and tragedies it had caused. I also had difficulty trying to believe in a god. Every different religion had a different god or gods. They couldn't all be right. But which one if any was?

> Faith involves living as if the outcome you want is the outcome that will happen.

I forget where I got the insight. Perhaps it was Dan Millman. Imagine there is some greater plan for everything in the universe. Imagine things aren't happening by accident. Imagine there is an intelligent energy running through all things, guiding them. Faith doesn't necessarily mean believing this. Faith is living life as if this were true. Belief isn't necessary to have faith. At first I found this hard to follow. Surely I had to believe it to have faith. But as I started putting my trust in this notion, it became easy. I started to live as if this was true, and it started to seem true. Things weren't happening by accident. I became aware of the most amazing courage which I hadn't been able to see before. I was still the same person with the same friends, yet suddenly there seemed to be another door open for me, and I could see so many things I had only glimpsed before. Conversations I had with people I had known for years suddenly seemed to have so much more substance, had a ring of truth and depth to them that I had only occasionally felt before. Now it seemed to be happening regularly.

I now feel that faith and belief form part of a continuum. My friend Siegfried Gutbrodt, formerly of the Gawler Foundation, specialises in laughter therapy. Siegfried always tells his audience about the positive effect of laughter on our bodies, about the good chemicals that are released during laughter. But, importantly, he points out that it can be faked. That even if you are not feeling too good but make the effort and have a big laugh, the same chemicals are released. It works too. Try it yourself if you don't believe it. It's amazing how much better you feel after a good laugh, even if you fake it. I use that analogy a little for the concept of faith becoming belief. Faith is a little bit like faking it, living life as if something is true but not necessarily believing it to be true. But if you live that way long enough you gradually start to believe it, and it gradually starts to happen.

When I started this regime of diet, sunlight, meditation and so on to take control of MS, even though I had seen all the evidence and collated it carefully I still had to convince myself to have faith and live as if it was going to work. The sceptical approach of some medical authorities can be very powerful, especially for a traditionally trained doctor. But as the years of good health have gone on, faith has given way to a growing belief. And more and more my belief is reinforced as I see evidence of other people with MS who show faith in their ability to overcome this illness.

Letting go

In the beginning, I realised that part of the trick as far as faith is concerned was to let go and just go with what was happening and what I was feeling and trust that things would work out. In the words of Bill Harris of Centerpoint Technology, 'Let whatever's happening be okay'. I had for some time felt professionally that to achieve things I needed to push hard. In most of the things in my life, I felt a sense that I was directing them which, I began to realise, was an illusion. Strangely, I began to thank MS for allowing me to feel like this, and for giving me these insights. I began to stop avoiding certain situations that I thought would be difficult or unpleasant and, surprisingly, I started finding new things in them. I started enjoying the company of people I hadn't previously really liked much, partly because I could see things in them that I hadn't seen before. I soon realised these were reflections of myself. I was allowing things to touch me that I hadn't allowed before. Many times I had the realisation that I had needed something to knock me onto this track. I could dimly see that if it hadn't been something as major as MS, I might have ignored it and continued unaware.

COMPASSION VERSUS BEING JUDGMENTAL

One of the great lessons I learnt came from Carolyn Myss' first book. I had for years regarded myself as a compassionate doctor. With many of the attitudes I had learnt from Ian Hislop, I felt that I had good empathy with patients and with their families. What I soon realised was that in some senses, I was using all my compassion at work and seemingly had very little left in the rest of my life. This was a hard lesson. Carolyn Myss points out that being compassionate is the opposite of being judgmental. This was hard to reconcile, because I felt I was a compassionate person, yet I also knew that I was very judgmental. When I realised that the two were essentially opposites, I knew that I had to change from being judgmental if I was to really become compassionate. Part of ceasing to be judgmental involved learning to forgive.

Forgiveness is an interesting virtue. While at face value it may seem that the act of forgiving has a lot of benefit in it for the person being forgiven, the forgiver may benefit greatly from forgiving. In many respects both parties can be winners. Forgiveness may not just be about working out grievances from the past and working actively to seek reconciliation, but rather it is something to be practised as a daily exercise. Just as we get back energy from forgiving those against whom we harbour negative feelings from the past, so we lose energy beginning the process anew every day. I began to try to actively deal with some of these issues on a day-to-day basis, as well as with people from my past.

Being judgmental is very easy. People are so different. It is tempting to criticise people for doing things differently from the way we are used to doing them. But what that does is close us to new possibilities, to understanding why people do things we are not used to, to appreciating the differences in people, and to being open to new ideas. It costs us dearly being critical and judgmental. Above all, it stops us being compassionate.

POSITIVITY

One of the things people say all the time when first diagnosed with serious illness is that it is important to be positive. I can see that this is true, but it is not as easy as it sounds. It is certainly no simple mental exercise to focus on the positives. I think the positives can come when you take the illness as a challenge to change your life. If the illness becomes a means to grow, then I feel that the positives start to flow from the process of change which accompanies that growth. For instance, in trying to become less judgmental and more compassionate, I have become more aware of the great courage and spirit shown by people with diseases so much worse than mine.

The day after I was diagnosed with MS, I went down to our local heated pool where I swim regularly. I swam the twenty laps almost in tears, feeling devastated about my future. When I got out, I sat down in the cafe upstairs. On the table in front of me was a magazine, which I vaguely started to read. It was the program for the wheelchair sports games held at the same venue recently. Inside was the story of a champion ten-year-old who had been born paralysed from the waist down, but had risen to the top of her chosen sport through years of often painful training and dedication. My illness looked so insignificant. Here was I, 45 years old, having lived a life that some would look on as so fortunate. I had had 45 years of perfect health and unlimited activity and, although the future was uncertain, I had every reason to feel that I would get many more years of life, and probably a fair amount of that time still being active.

Why did I sit down at that table with that magazine on it? I could just as easily ask why I became an academic physician who edited a journal for fifteen years and knows how to interpret medical evidence, and not a lawyer or an engineer. I was going to get MS anyway, whatever career I had. But without that background, I would have struggled to devise a way of dealing with the physical aspects of this disease. And I would not have been able to undertake this book, the culmination of many years of training. As a result, many people with MS may have lived very different lives.

More and more as I looked around me, I could see others worse off than myself. Once I started my search, I felt even luckier. When the Medline search turned up around 19,000 papers on MS, I didn't realise how lucky I was. A few weeks later a good friend found she was able to tell me she had post-polio syndrome after suffering polio as a child. This is well described in medical textbooks, yet no one seems to know what causes it. It occurs decades after polio and is characterised by worsening weakness. It was extraordinary that I had been blind to her symptoms, when it was so obvious that she walked with a pronounced limp. Eagerly, I told her I would look it up on the Internet and get back to her about what possible therapies there were. To my great surprise, only two papers came up when I typed in post-polio. And I had 19,000. Again I counted my lucky stars. Today there are twice that number on MS.

Being positive is not something you can will yourself to be. It came to me when I started taking an active role in the illness, and making changes to my life. It is now emerging that being positive and happy has a profound effect on the immune system. The term psychoneuro-immunology has been coined to reflect the study of the effect of mind and emotions on immune function. Allowing yourself to become depressed by the illness can literally make you sicker.

Fear versus faith

One of the ways in which this important energy we need for healing can be wasted is when we are consumed with fear. In many respects, fear is the opposite of faith. The earlier discussion about living in the present moment is relevant here too. MS is a frightening disease, particularly when first diagnosed. Most of us want to live a long, healthy life. So often we hear people say 'I hope I drop dead with a heart attack' or 'I hope I die in my sleep after a healthy life'. The fear of incapacity and a long, drawn out demise is distressing for most people. Yet that is precisely what comes to mind when given a diagnosis of MS. Suddenly the wheelchair comes into view, and being fed, and catheters and so on. But most people, when told, are comparatively well. It makes no sense to spend some of the precious time we have now, when we are well, consumed with worry about what might be when we are not well. Worse, using that energy worrying robs us of the energy we need to heal ourselves.

> Fear of the future is destructive; replace fear with faith.

Once again, Ian Hislop captured it perfectly when he sent me a short note early on. He said: 'The principle is straightforward. You have to replace fear with faith. Faith in yourself, your future, and perhaps in something which transcends both.' It is interesting how often people facing serious illness or death come to similar conclusions. Lance Armstrong, the famous Tour de France winning US cyclist who recovered from widespread testicular cancer, says in his great book about his recovery 'Hope . . . is the only antidote to fear' and 'I refused to let the fear completely blot out my optimism'.[5]

Hope

This leads to the associated concept of hope. For most of my medical career I have felt that it is important to be very honest with patients and their relatives. In emergency situations, where it is clear someone is going to die, I have always felt that I shouldn't try to play down the seriousness of the situation, or give the family 'false hope'. I feel that people should be allowed to prepare themselves for the worst, if this is the likely outcome. Bernie Siegel has convinced me, however, that there is no such thing as false hope. There is only 'false no hope'. While this does not apply quite so easily to the emergency situations in which I find myself, its relevance is more obvious with conditions such as cancer and multiple sclerosis.

While statistics help us describe the outcome for a particular group of patients, they are quite useless for any individual patient. There are always those who do better and those who do worse than the statistics. There are always extraordinary survivors, no matter how bleak the outcome or how advanced the disease. We can always have real hope that we will have a similar course. This is especially true for MS, which is such a variable disease. We know that there is a group of people who do very well, those with so-called benign MS. At the very least, why shouldn't we hope that we will be one of these people? How much better is it for someone to live positively in hope than negatively in depression, when there is a real possibility that they won't deteriorate. Researchers have shown one of the principal reasons for chronic sorrow in people with MS is their loss of hope.[6]

The problem with telling someone that she has six months to live, or will be disabled within two years, is that it may become a self-fulfilling prophecy. The doctor's relationship with the patient is charged with such authority, and patients usually do their best to please their doctors, so much so that patients will often live out exactly the script they have been given. By giving patients this 'false no hope' we weaken their resolve; we literally take away some of their power to heal the illness. This doesn't mean I now don't tell my patients the truth. But there are ways of being honest yet still preserving people's hope. Even the energy and hope of relatives surrounding a seriously ill person can buoy the patient. It defeats the human spirit to take this away from people.

> There is no such thing as 'false hope'; there is only 'false no hope'.

COUNSELLING

An important part of dealing with any serious illness is through counselling. One of Ian Hislop's suggestions for me early on was to get some professional help from a psychologist. I knew how important mental state and positivity were to successfully tackling the disease. With the background I had of living through Mum's illness and watching every step of her gradual decline, I knew I could have been set up for a bad outcome mentally. My initial reactions to the illness all involved seeing my outcome through the screen of what happened to Mum. It became very important to undo some of these preconceptions.

Ian had picked this up very early as we sat outside that first afternoon. Every time I mentioned Mum my voice began to tremble. There was obviously a significant amount of energy tied up in issues around Mum that I needed to resolve if that energy was to be available to me to tackle the illness. I rang a couple of clinical psychologists Ian had suggested. No one could fit me in. I started to realise that there is no such thing as a psychological emergency as far as some of these therapists are concerned. To me this was the closest thing to an emergency I could think of. I just felt I couldn't get on with dealing with MS without first resolving some of the issues surrounding Mum. If I didn't, I felt that I would be dealing with her illness, not my own.

Angrily, I had the insight that psychologists, who are well aware of the effect of added work pressures on their mental state, and interruptions, and working late, had structured their work lives to minimise these disruptive events. The net result was that I couldn't find anyone who could see me before three weeks. This just seemed too long. I wanted to start straightaway. Ian had given me some directions, and I felt I had to start the journey, but without the added weight of a whole lot of unresolved issues about Mum.

I got back in touch with Ian. Fortunately he was able to find me someone else and, of course, she was perfect. She was happy to see me the next week. It's hard to describe how frail a doctor in my position feels coming in to a clinical psychologist's office. I didn't feel any stigma about needing some counselling; I regarded it as a helpful service from someone professional and distant from the relationships I had been in. But I was a senior physician, suddenly being required to take on the role of a patient, feeling weak and vulnerable, as if my whole future had been plucked out of my life in front of my eyes.

Nada is a woman of my own age, with a laconic wit and a shining intelligence. She is not the bored, cynical psychologist who has heard it all before. She welcomed me with a touch on the shoulder, and within minutes I had a feeling of great rapport with her. She had the great knack of making me feel she was genuinely interested in me; I still feel she really was. The first session was just about who I was, how I thought, who my family was, how this was affecting me. I told her about Ian, and about all the things I had resolved to do, to confront some of my past conflicts. She was great. At the end she simply said, 'You don't have to do it all today.'

Why don't you do five things tomorrow that you know make you happy. That'll be a good start.' That helped me to realise that my usual modus operandi as an emergency physician faced with a major problem was to go and fix it. MS wasn't going to be like that.

In the second session, we concentrated on Mum. I told her all about Mum, MS and me, the relationship we had, how her illness had affected me. As I spoke I started to realise that I actually had quite a realistic view of Mum. I hadn't placed her on a false pedestal because of her illness, but had seen her many faults and accepted them without diminishing our relationship. The session was something of a revelation to me. I realised that I did not have much unfinished business with Mum. She and I had always been close and were quite frank with each other. A great weight came off my shoulders. There wasn't much to be done here. What I really needed to do, though, was to stop assuming I would be the same as Mum. By now I had started my search for answers, and this was getting easier. We had one more session, just on what practical things I could do to stop getting too entangled in my work commitments, but that was all.

I recommend everyone newly diagnosed with any major illness consider some psychological counselling. We need every bit of our energy to tackle the illness. If we are wasting any energy dealing with things we don't need, or if we are tackling things in unproductive ways, it is usually easy for trained professionals to spot. Of course ongoing counselling may also be important. I have found that the journey which MS started me on has become extremely difficult at times, and led me to explore issues I never imagined I would in my adult life. It is worth 'shopping around' a bit to find someone who really suits. Having done that in my case, I find that an ongoing professional relationship with someone who really knows me, and who I know I can trust, is enormously helpful when the inevitable difficulties crop up in my life.

HOW WE VIEW OURSELVES AND THE ILLNESS

Whenever I refer to MS, and people with it, I do so in a certain way. I never use the phrase 'MS sufferer' and I try to use the phrase 'MS patient' sparingly, and only in the context of medical studies. I do the same in my day-to-day life. The way we feel about the illness and refer to it has a big bearing on our outcome in my view. Again these are things I cannot prove. To use Carolyn Myss' terminology, 'biography becomes biology'. Like many others, she has seen that if people don't express their grief they end up radiating grief. They get depressed. If people can't say what they want, repress their real wants and desires and feel powerless, then something like cancer may literally start eating them away. If people see themselves as 'suffering' with MS, they will probably end up suffering and get more attacks.

Now I know a lot of people with advanced MS are suffering. I feel this very acutely. I saw and lived through Mum's suffering. But I am hoping that people who take a positive approach to this illness, take an active stance and make the necessary lifestyle changes, will do much better than if they allow it to dominate them. And people with advanced MS who are reading this may also get something out of reconsidering the attitude they have towards the illness.

I also don't refer to MS as 'my illness'. Once I get on too-cosy terms with this illness, I may just end up adopting it and needing it to get on with the rest of my life. I don't want the illness to become a central part of my life around which the rest revolves. By thinking of it as an illness about which I am actively doing something, but which I expect won't be there in an active form for most of the time, it allows me to focus on other, more important and productive areas of my life. I don't talk about 'fighting' MS. MS is a manifestation of an imbalance in my body. It is not some outside invader like malaria or a virus. All the cells involved in MS are my cells and part of me. It makes no sense for me to fight myself. It empowers the illness.

> The words and thoughts we use to describe illness are important; they can become a self-fulfilling prophecy.

What I am trying to do is tip the balance back to a more favourable one, where my immune system is not overactive and my nerves are in harmony with it. I feel I can do that with diet, meditation, sunlight and my attitude. It is not about fighting, it is about healing. Healing is multi-faceted. It is not just physical healing. Indeed, it is becoming clear that being sick spiritually impairs physical healing. Many of the ancient tribal healers knew this, but we are only now rediscovering it in a 'scientific' sense.

Feeling in control of the illness

There is considerable literature on the positive effects of people having a feeling of control over illness. Bernie Siegel's books are rich with anecdotes about people he has seen who have transformed themselves, and overcome serious illness, because they were active, positive participants in the process. Bernie describes the survivors of serious illness as people who, on learning of the diagnosis, actively seek out information, look for people to talk to who have overcome such illness, question their doctors about alternatives and generally become what doctors think of as 'difficult' patients.

This is one of the reasons I am so keen on what many people call 'complementary' or 'alternative' therapies, but many are just really healthy and healing lifestyle choices. These are generally things people actively do to change the course of an illness, such as dietary changes, exercise, meditation, getting adequate sunlight and so on. Why they should be called complementary or alternative is beyond me. In what way is improving nutrition and actively calming the mind alternative? Surely developing a toxic chemical in a laboratory and then injecting it into people, knowing that it will cause damage to their bone marrow, hair, gut and sense of wellbeing, is more alternative?

Fortunately we are seeing a move back towards more holistic medicine in many Western countries. Our eastern neighbours have known about these other therapies for centuries. Deepak Chopra has recently written about his rediscovery of ayurveda, the long time Indian traditional healing method. Many mainstream medical scientists are now using good scientific methods to prove these things about which we have known for centuries.

Researchers have investigated how people with MS respond to practitioners of so-called alternative medicine compared with conventional doctors.[7] They found that although MS patients got significant benefit from drug therapies and medical providers, practitioners of alternative medicine were rated significantly higher in listening skills, care and concern, and patient empowerment. The authors concluded that more study should be done on the benefits of emotional support gained from medical and alternative practitioners to quality of life in MS.

Writing down feelings

In April 1999, Smyth and co-workers from the Department of Psychiatry at the State University of New York published the results of a simple study in the *Journal of the American Medical Association* (*JAMA*).[8] They performed a well-constructed RCT, using 112 patients with chronic asthma or rheumatoid arthritis (RA). Like MS, RA is an auto-immune disease, but the target of the immune system is the joints rather than the nervous system. Asthma is also a disease mediated by the immune system. The 'treatment' group was asked to write on just one occasion about the most stressful event of their lives. The 'control' group was asked to write about a neutral topic.

With this simple intervention, that is, getting people to express feelings that may not have been completely released before, the 'treated' patients got better and the others did not. This should not surprise us, but to a sceptical medical community this scientific 'proof' was something of a shock. The p values were 0.001, so the result was unlikely to have occurred by chance. Further, the magnitude of the effect was stunning. The RA patients had a 28 per cent reduction in disease severity (this is about the same benefit as derived from interferon and glatiramer in MS), and the asthma patients a 19 per cent improvement in lung function. And this effect persisted for four months after the 'treatment'. Effects of this size and duration are difficult to achieve with drug therapies without producing side effects. Yet all this was achieved with only one session. Imagine if these people had regularly expressed their feelings.

JAMA carried a powerful editorial commenting on the article, by David Spiegel, a psychiatrist from Stanford University.[9] We have already seen how influential an editorial in a prestigious journal can be. This one is well worth reading. Perhaps the most surprising thing about the editorial is that he sounds surprised. Yet there is abundant scientific evidence of the effects of the mind and spirit on illness. Most of us know these things to be so resonant with truth that they require no proof. But the medical community has become sceptical in these days of miraculous drug therapy. This is despite evidence that people are more likely to die after than before their birthdays and holidays,[10] for example. Or evidence that patients with psoriasis (a chronic skin condition) heal faster with meditation training tapes played during treatment than without.[11] Or the abundant literature showing that patients who express their negative feelings[12] or develop a fighting spirit[13] do better in recovery from cancer. These things have been known for a long time. Spiegel concludes with an interesting point, which I quote in full:

> *Were the authors to have provided similar outcome evidence about a*
> *new drug, it is likely that it would be in widespread use within a short*

time. Why? We would think we understood the mechanism (whether we did or we did not) and there would be a mediating industry to promote its use. Manufacturers of paper and pencils are not likely to push journaling as a treatment addition for the management of asthma and rheumatoid arthritis.

I find these comments also extremely pertinent in relation to the previous discussion about Swank's work on saturated fats. Now, if Swank had tried a new margarine that did the same thing, the whole story would have been different. Firstly, it would have been much easier to perform a bona fide RCT, as patients would be taking something, not omitting something, in their diet. Once margarine therapy was 'proven', the marketing arm of the margarine company would have swung into action and people everywhere would be buying and eating it. And it would have been even more impressive if it had been a drug. The resources of some of the major pharmaceutical companies are enormous.

But this is to overlook the very important point about Swank's work. Not only does the dietary change physically alter the course of the illness, so does the mental change that comes with the feeling of control over the illness. Let us not discount the effect of the mind and spirit here. Spiegel finishes his editorial by saying: 'In this, and a growing number of studies, it is not simply mind over matter, but it is clear that mind matters.'

Bernie Siegel recommends, not only to people with serious disease but to everyone, that they start keeping a journal or diary. On the three-month 'anniversary' of being diagnosed with MS, I started mine. We were just coming back from holiday in the south-west of Western Australia, around the well-known Margaret River winery area. I chose the day to start because of the special significance I attached to three months without a relapse. I picked out a nice diary from our favourite general store in Dunsborough. It was purple and had a huge opening sunflower on the cover. A good symbol, I thought. For some time, I made it a daily ritual to sit down in the evening and write my thoughts about the day. I now do it when I get the feeling that something is going wrong or nagging at me. It gets me more in tune with how I am feeling.

Keeping a diary can be very helpful in the expression of difficult emotions.

There are many things I have done to which I can ascribe the sense of wellbeing I now have. The diary is certainly one of them. I am just so glad that mainstream medical researchers find this important enough to study and publish. It is about as far removed from giving injections of toxic chemicals to people as I can imagine, yet no less powerful. And the beauty is that the patient has control over it.

The diary has been really helpful to me. I can look back from time to time and see how I was feeling at certain times, see what things helped me stay positive and so on. Recently I re-read an entry I made about eight months after the diagnosis of MS. I had only just begun regular injections of medication, having made the decision that I should use every avenue open to me to control the illness even though I was not keen on injections. Within weeks of commencing, I started to feel really low. It is clear now on looking back through the entries I made at the time, that once I started injecting I began feeling like 'a sick patient'. To that point I had been so positive and full of faith and confidence, but paradoxically, the addition of injections to my regime was a powerful psychological blow to my confidence and made me see myself as sick.

The diary really helped, though. I sat down to write one night, and resolved as I was writing that I would let myself get no lower. I drew a little signpost with the date on it, and a message that this day marked the lowest point of my mood and that from here I would recover. And sure enough that is what happened.

MEDITATION

Another of my regular daily rituals is meditation, and I believe this is a key part of the overall package. There are many types of meditation. It is important to choose one that suits, and this may involve a bit of trial and error. My meditation started in 1975 when I took a year off medicine after getting perilously close to failing third year. Life at university had provided such attractions and alternatives to study that I was in a deep downward spiral. Straight As in first year had gone to straight Cs. Fortunately I had the sense to pull out. Equally fortunately, the faculty of medicine was generous enough to allow me a year to sort things out. I took off to Europe for a year as many young Australians do. Backpack on my back. Nowhere organised to stay. Just to experience it. Throwing my fate to the winds.

I was lucky enough, as the currents and eddies moved me around, to be drawn to a teacher of transcendental meditation (TM) when I was in Switzerland. Unbeknown to me, this older lady was apparently very senior in the organisation of TM. She taught me to meditate in her unit, and then invited me to stay on her farm with her. TM is a very useful meditation technique. Like many others it is based on a mantra, that is, a word or sound repeated over and over mentally. There is quite a science around the beneficial physical effects of meditation as well as the mental benefits. Much of this can be found in the mainstream medical literature. Regular meditators have lower blood pressure, less heart disease and so on. There are now over 1500 papers in the medical literature on the health benefits of meditation.

I used TM for several years, and then let it lapse after I qualified in medicine, just when I probably needed it the most. A few years later, when the long hours and being woken from sleep over and over again started to get to me, I learnt a different technique. This was part of a 'better sleep' program that I decided to attend. The meditation is called so-hum medi-tation and is based on an ancient Eastern technique. Essentially, while it also uses a mantra ('so-hum'), it uses it in combination, and in time with, focusing on the breathing. There are teachers around who can instruct in this method, but in essence one focuses on the in-breath, imagining it coming up from the stomach to the back of the throat through an imagi-nary passage, at the same time saying 'so' mentally. On the out-breath, going the other way, one says 'hum'. I find it extremely relaxing. It is best not to get hung up about any particular technique; whatever works for you is best. A really good description of meditation from Tibetan monk and well-known meditation teacher Sogyal Rinpoche can be found at www.buddhanet.net/e-learning/advicemed.htm.

Many people get more involved with meditation. I have become increasingly convinced that meditation should form a key part of healing from any disease. My work with Ian and Ruth Gawler at the Gawler Foun-dation has shown me the profound benefits of this simple technique. Ian's teaching has been that the body is capable of healing any illness. To heal, though, the body needs to be in a state of balance to allow its natural healing mechanisms to operate. Meditation can help achieve that balance. I now have a repertoire of meditation techniques, including the progres-sive muscle relaxation technique and breath awareness methods. Ian's book *Meditation Pure and Simple* is a must for anybody wishing to deepen their meditation. It helped me enormously and I recommend it strongly.

Meditation is very helpful in any chronic disease.

Slowing the mind is the correct physiological term for what actually happens in meditation. Normal brainwave recordings show many waves of a frequency of greater than 12 cycles per second with a fairly small amplitude (height), looking a bit like a saw tooth pattern, termed beta waves, together with waves of 8–12 cycles per second, termed alpha waves. As meditation proceeds, or as we get into reflective states while listening to music or gardening, the frequency slows. This is the state we get into early in meditation or when we are in that focused attention state, like when watching a movie, and other things are blocked out. For most people, this is where most meditation happens. In deeper alpha states we reach a twilight state like just drifting off to sleep, and the frequency drops further. This state is good for learning, and people feel very relaxed.

As meditation deepens the brainwave frequency slows further, to between 4–8 cycles per second, becoming theta waves. This is the brainwave pattern associated with dreaming during rapid eye movement sleep. It is also associated with visionary experiences, enhanced creativity and sudden breakthroughs. Some experienced meditators can get down to this level without difficulty.

As the brain quiets even further, the wave pattern continues to slow and grow in amplitude until we are experiencing waves which are large, but below 4 cycles per second. This is the delta wave pattern, and represents the subconscious mind. The brainwaves by now are very large and slow. This is the state of deep dreamless sleep, but if it is experienced with awareness, as during meditation, there is an intense feeling of oneness and connection with the underlying energy of life. Mystics and very experienced meditators describe this state in detail and clearly have experienced it. Getting into this awareness of the subconscious mind can throw up all sorts of emotional difficulties, as long-buried issues surface into awareness. But as a result it has the potential to be very healing too.

I meditate every day, almost always in the same spot. It helps to find a comfortable chair but not one that is so reclining or comfortable as to induce sleep. That is not the aim, although it is no major problem. I tend to meditate shortly after getting home from work, before dinner. It helps me separate my work life and pressures from my home life. By the time I emerge, I am usually relaxed and feeling a bit slow. It certainly helped to feel like that around mealtime in a house when there were small children running around and chores to be done before dinner.

A lot of people ask how I can find the time in a busy job with a full home life to fit in meditation, getting some sun and exercise, as well as all the other things I have to do each day. One of the answers is that I don't watch much TV. A long time ago I realised that our spirits reflect what we put into ourselves, what we think and what we are exposed to. If we put trash into our spirits, we will have trashy spirits. If we sit in front of TV and are constantly exposed to the violence and disasters that pass for news, and superficial sitcoms, our spirits reflect that. The difference between half an hour of meditation and half an hour watching the news is simply enormous. It is a study in opposites. I regard it as a priority to make time for myself each day, and meditation is one of those times. Others find alternatives to meditation that may be just as effective. Researchers have shown, for instance, that music therapy improves acceptance and reduces anxiety and depression in people with MS.[14]

ANALYSING ENERGY

Another thing I try to do each day, preferably a few times each day when I remember, is to analyse where I am at in an energy sense. Carolyn Myss describes this beautifully in *Anatomy of the Spirit*. It is easy to be consumed with internal poring over issues that have come up during the day. Or going over past difficulties that still haven't been resolved. Or ruminating about some perceived injustice that may have occurred some time ago. By taking time to stop occasionally and analyse where my energy is at, at that particular time, I can catch myself draining energy with such preoccupations. All of that energy is needed to tackle serious illness, and to centre myself in the present moment. Stopping, and catching myself doing these things, can lead to conscious decisions not to waste that energy, to put off the internal debate until later, or to make a decision to confront some issue rather than ruminating about it. I find this technique really helpful.

OVERVIEW

It is possible to heal all illness. Even if unable to heal an illness, how illness affects people is profoundly dependent on their reaction to it and their emotional state. But we need resources to tackle illness. It is important to get a sense of some control over the process. Conventional medicine, with its emphasis on patients behaving as expected and being passive recipients of care, serves us poorly in this regard. It is important for patients to be 'difficult', to be actively involved in their management. Equally, as doctors we need to not only learn to be tolerant of this 'difficult' behaviour, but respect it for what it is: the expression of a patient's ability to contribute to healing.

12

STEROIDS

It is preferable to prescribe oral rather than intravenous steroids for acute relapses in MS

D. Barnes

Now for drug therapies. I have deliberately placed them in the book to follow lifestyle changes to reflect the importance of diet, sunlight and the mind–body connection. But medical therapies for treating MS effectively are finally being developed and tested. In the next few chapters I examine them in detail.

While most of the advances in the medical management of MS have occurred in the last ten to fifteen years, the role of steroids in managing relapses has been accepted for many years. Most neurologists now prescribe steroids for acute relapses for people with relapsing-remitting MS. The evidence seems clear that they shorten recovery time from individual relapses. This contrasts with any of the other agents currently available, none of which appears to have any effect on improving the recovery from an acute relapse. For instance, natali-zumab, which potently affects the relapse rate in MS and which is discussed later, has no effect on recovery from an acute relapse.[1] What is not so clear about steroids is whether the actual amount of recovery is

SUMMARISING THE EVIDENCE

- A short course of steroids clearly improves the rate and extent of recovery of MS relapses.
  - There appears to be no difference between routes of administration; oral is as good as intravenous, and much less unpleasant.
  - Side effects are generally mild if the course is short.
  - There is no need to taper the dosage if the course is short.
- Long-term therapy with steroids in MS is not beneficial and has many side effects.
- Preliminary evidence suggests that intermittent, pulsed doses of steroids may be helpful in slowing disease progression.

EVIDENCE-BASED RECOMMENDATIONS

- For any relapse that is distressing oral steroids are recommended, as prednisone or prednisolone 500–1000mg daily for three to five days.
- Short courses of steroids should not be used more than three times a year.

improved, or what are the optimal doses; appropriate routes of administration, or benefits long term, if any.

'Steroids' is the accepted shortening of the term corticosteroids. Steroids in general are found naturally in plants and animals, but corticosteroids are those particular steroids secreted into the bloodstream by the adrenal gland. Many are now also synthesised in the laboratory. Typically the synthetic corticosteroids are many, many times more potent than those which occur naturally. Some will be familiar with the term anabolic steroids. These are the steroids used as performance-enhancing drugs by many sportspeople. Although the steroids used to treat MS are related to these drugs and share some of their properties, they are different drugs. I will use the term steroids here to denote corticosteroids.

HOW STEROIDS WORK

Steroids have widespread effects in the human body, but the effects for which they are used in MS are those related to suppression of the immune system and changing the balance of the immune system chemicals, the cytokines. As the relapses in MS are caused by inflammatory demyelinating lesions due to inappropriate immune system activation, this dampening effect on the immune system by steroids is a logical therapy. Many other therapies aimed at suppressing the immune system have been tried in MS, and this is probably at least partly how interferon works. I will discuss these further in the chapters to come in this section.

Some will be familiar with the use of steroid creams and lotions in inflammatory conditions of the skin such as dermatitis. Steroids are also administered by mouth or injection for inflammatory conditions such as rheumatoid arthritis, asthma and systemic lupus erythematosus, and for certain lymph tissue and other cancers. Here again, they work through immune suppression.

Studies of people with MS relapses who are being treated with steroids show that the steroids work by decreasing the levels of the 'bad' cytokines and eicosanoids and by making the cell membranes of the white cells more pliable and less sticky.[2] It is interesting to note how similar this is to the mechanism in which diet and essential fatty acid supplements work, but without side effects. Other evidence suggests that there is also an effect on the way the brain interprets the messages coming to it from the body's nerves.[3] MRI studies also show us that steroids significantly decrease the amount of swelling around individual MS lesions, causing better nerve transmission through these affected areas. These effects are seen on MRI within hours of taking the first dose.

Side effects of steroids

Fortunately steroids are relatively safe when used in short bursts of five to seven days or less. A few rare cases of bone problems have been reported, as well as pancreatitis, but these are exceedingly unlikely. When used continually long term they can cause weight gain, fluid retention, increased risk of infection, risk of stomach ulcers, muscle weakness, changes in behaviour including depression or psychosis, cataracts and osteoporosis. Long-term use is not a good idea in any condition, unless there is no real alternative. But used as a short, sharp burst for an acute relapse, these drugs are very safe and there should be no hesitation in using them.

RCTS OF STEROIDS IN MS

Studies over many years have shown a beneficial effect in recovery from acute relapses in MS when the relapses are treated with intravenous steroids. The most influential and well-conducted study initially was from Wales in 1987. Milligan and colleagues randomised 50 patients to receive either methylprednisolone (MP) 500mg intravenously (IV) for five days or an inactive placebo.[4] Assessments were carried out at one and four weeks after the treatment by a 'blinded' neurologist; 73 per cent of MP-treated patients improved compared with 29 per cent of those on placebo. The p value was 0.001. The treated group contained patients with classic relapsing-remitting MS but also patients with chronic progressive MS, and both categories benefited from MP. This study caused most neurologists around the world to subsequently offer patients IV MP for relapses.

Although most inflammatory diseases for which steroids have been used have shown similar benefit for IV and oral routes of administration, most neurologists have used steroids for MS only by the IV route. This seems to have stemmed from the results of a study by Beck and co-workers in the early 1990s.[5] They studied the use of steroids in the condition optic neuritis, discussed earlier. This is where the nerves to the eyes become inflamed, causing visual disturbance. It has long been known that the majority of people who develop this condition eventually go on to get MS. Beck and colleagues showed that IV MP seemed to delay the development of MS in these patients for longer than oral MP. While this may have just been a quirk in the way the results fell in that particular study, it was very influential in its effect on the prescribing habits of neurologists. Most tended to give only IV steroids after the results of that study were published, even for people who had typical MS relapses and not optic neuritis.

This was first challenged by the results of a small study of 35 patients which showed equivalent benefit for oral and IV steroids.[6] Because of the size of the study, most doctors did not change their prescribing practice to favour oral steroids, despite the advantages of this route. A more recent study further clarified this question. Workers from London showed in a well-constructed RCT comparing oral prednisolone versus intravenous MP that oral was just as good as intravenous. Barnes and co-workers compared oral versus IV steroids in 80 patients.[7] There was no difference between the groups in terms of degree of neurological improvement at one, four, twelve or 24 weeks after therapy. Indeed, there was a slight trend to better results for the orally treated group.

Both of these studies could be criticised for using the Kurtzke scale to measure disease progression rather than, say, the number of new lesions on MRI. I disagree. The clinically significant end-point in MS studies needs to be whether people get better or worse from a disability point of view, not whether their scans look better or worse. Personally, I see the use of the disability scale as a strength, not a weakness of these studies.

The most recent of these studies was from Copenhagen. Sellebjerg and co-workers randomised 51 patients with an acute relapse of MS lasting less than four weeks to receive either placebo orally or oral prednisolone 500mg per day for five days, then a tapering-off dose.[8] After one, three and eight weeks, 4 per cent, 24 per cent and 32 per cent in the placebo group and 31 per cent, 54 per cent and 65 per cent in the prednisolone group improved 1 point on the Kurtzke Scale score (all $p<0.05$). Patients also rated their symptoms as having improved much more with the steroids at three weeks ($p=0.005$) and eight weeks ($p=0.0007$). No significant side effects were noted.

Dose and route of administration

This study really confirmed the very significant improvements people can get by using steroids when they have a relapse. Most doctors will now offer this therapy for a relapse. But if only IV steroids are offered, it is worth mentioning the evidence that oral steroids are just as good. There is nothing like quoting the original study to assist your case. From the patient's point of view, oral is really much better. For a start, no special expertise is needed to administer the drug, which means no day hospitals and inconvenience. Secondly, there is no discomfort, bruising and so on. It's worth pressing this issue.

Oral and intravenous steroids are probably equivalent in effect.

There is still, however, considerable debate about the optimal dosage of steroids and the duration of the course. Indeed, there are still neurologists who will never prescribe steroids, believing that they confer no benefit despite the evidence. In the United Kingdom, this is about 5 per cent of neurologists. Most use them for selected relapses but not all, and about 50 per cent use them for all relapses. Similarly there is a lot of variation in whether oral or IV steroids are usually used. UK neurologists overwhelmingly favour IV, despite the evidence presented above that oral is likely to be just as effective. Over 90 per cent use IV steroids, and only about 5 per cent routinely use oral steroids.[9]

The commonest dosage schedules for steroids in acute relapses are oral prednisone or prednisolone 500mg a day for five days, or IV methylprednisolone 500mg or 1000mg a day for three days. The UK National Institute for Health and Clinical Excellence (NICE) guidelines recommend either 500mg–1g of IV methylprednisolone for three to five days, or 500mg–2g oral prednisolone for three to five days. The oral and intravenous doses have been shown to be roughly equivalent in terms of biological availability.[10] Further, the NICE guidelines suggest that steroids shouldn't be used more than three times a year, or for more than three weeks at a time in any given episode. It is also important to note that tapering doses after the initial course are not needed, despite being commonly prescribed. A study from Detroit showed that there was no difference in outcome with or without a tapering dose,[11] and the shorter the course the safer the drug is.

Another intriguing possibility raised recently is that the course of steroids may be more effective if it is given at night.[12] Because there is a natural rhythm of steroid secretion in the body, varying between day and night, Israeli researchers compared outcomes and side effects of steroid therapy for relapses between one group of people with MS given the treatment during the day and the other at night.[12] The outcome was better for those receiving the treatment at night, side effects were fewer and patients expressed a clear preference for night-time treatment.

Most neurologists treat only some relapses. They argue that only attacks which are severe and likely to leave some disability should be treated. I disagree to some extent, and so do the NICE guidelines. From the point of view of a patient, all relapses can leave lasting symptoms which can be quite distressing, even if just disturbances in sensation, and some of these sensory lesions may result in quite a bit of pain in the long run. Therefore I favour treating most relapses unless they are very frequent, in which case a maintenance immunosuppressant medication might be best considered. The NICE guidelines recommend treating 'an acute episode sufficient to cause distressing symptoms or an increased limitation on activities'.[13] So what constitutes 'distressing' is clearly up to the patient.

A short course of steroids is safe and effective for treating relapses.

I think it is a good idea to discuss with the neurologist the possibility of keeping a dose of steroids at home in case of a relapse, and what sort of symptoms might warrant starting the course. Sometimes it can take quite a while to get an appointment with a neurologist, and the earlier these drugs are started in a relapse the more effective they are likely to be. Many patients and their neurologists will be comfortable with this sort of approach, although clearly it is not for everyone. Not everyone feels confident enough about what exactly constitutes a relapse.

LONG-TERM THERAPY WITH STEROIDS

If steroids are so effective when given in short, sharp courses for relapses, surely they would be of benefit in preventing relapses if given longer term. We know, for instance, that when steroids are given for a first attack, there is a longer delay to the second than if they are not given. Perhaps, if they are used continually, there would be fewer attacks. The trouble here is the side effects of long-term use of steroids. In short intermittent courses steroids are remarkably well tolerated, considering what powerful drugs they are. In long-term use, however, they have the very unpleasant side effects I have presented, some of which are probably more unpleasant than the disease they are being used to treat. That is especially so when we can't yet tell which patients are going to fall into the benign group. If you are not going to ever have more than one or two attacks, it is certainly not worth taking powerful drugs with side effects.

Long-term continual treatment of MS with steroids was shown over 40 years ago to be unhelpful.[14] However, there still remains the possibility that intermittent so-called 'pulses' of steroids, which have minimal side effects, will be beneficial in slowing the rate of progression to disability.

A 2006 German study looked at monthly IV doses of methylprednisolone 500mg in a group of nine MS patients who were getting monthly MRIs.[15] After six months on treatment, there was a 44 per cent reduction in number of new lesions compared with the baseline six months on no therapy (p=0.013). This warrants further study.

Additionally, a study from Los Angeles compared two different dosages of MP given every other month for two years to patients with secondary progressive MS.[16] The investigators studied 108 patients and found that the group with higher dose MP took longer to go into a sustained progression of disability than those with the lower dose. This suggests there may be significant benefit from intermittent pulsed steroid therapy in progressive forms of MS. Another interesting piece of research from Germany has studied a novel way of giving the steroids. After repeatedly administering a long-acting steroid directly into the spinal fluid, essentially by the same technique as lumbar puncture, patients with progressive MS experienced substantial improvements in walking distance and speed.[17, 18] Larger studies may help determine whether this has a place in the management of people with progressive MS.

OVERVIEW

There is convincing evidence that steroids are useful in improving the recovery after a relapse of MS. It is probable that steroids delay the onset of the next episode as well. The oral route seems to be as effective as the IV route. There is also likely to be a role for long-term intermittent high dose steroids, but more work is needed before this will be clear. For the time being, for most relapses, there should be no delay in starting a short course of steroids. In some cases, it may be worth speaking to your doctor about keeping some steroids at home in case of a relapse so that they can be started early.

13

INTERFERONS

If neurologists agree that these compounds have a moderate effect, but that the effect needs to be confirmed in long-term trials, patients and their doctors deserve an explanation . . .

Clanet and Cucheratt

Interferons have now been used to treat MS for over a decade. The interferons and glatiramer acetate which I will discuss more in the next chapter are collectively described as 'disease-modifying agents'. Their action is such that they are intended to modify the course of the disease rather than make a difference to current symptoms. Some of the newer agents just being released onto the market will fall into that category as well. Interferons belong to a class of chemical messengers in the body. In the chapter on MS and the immune system, it was noted that essential fatty acids are converted in the body into chemicals called eicosanoids and cytokines. These messenger chemicals have a role in regulating the function of the immune system. Some of these messengers promote inflammation and some suppress it. Interferons belong to the cytokine class of chemicals.

SUMMARISING THE EVIDENCE

- Interferons are only modestly effective (30%) in reducing relapse rate in MS.
- The evidence of benefit in reducing rate of progression to disability is less convincing.
- It is unclear how long the interferons remain effective with continued use; it may be as short as twelve months.
- Neutralising antibodies which reduce the drug's effectiveness may be formed.
- There are many problems with the clinical trials, including drug company sponsorship, issues with unblinding and failure to account for drop-outs from the studies, weakening the findings.
- Side effects of the interferons, some of them serious, are often a problem.

EVIDENCE-BASED RECOMMENDATIONS

- For people with MS who don't experience or can tolerate side effects interferons may be a suitable treatment option, but the effect is at best modest.

WHAT IS INTERFERON?

Interferon was first described in 1957. It was found to be secreted by cells exposed to viruses and interfered with replication of the virus, hence the name. Subsequently, three main species of interferon have been described in humans: alpha and beta interferon, belonging to type I; and gamma interferon, belonging to type II. The type I interferons tend to suppress the immune system and have been studied in the treatment of MS, and the type II interferons tend to promote inflammation. More sub-types have been discovered in other animals, and probably will continue to be. The interferons arise from genes which are quite ancient in an evolutionary sense, through most animal species.

Interferon alpha and beta are produced by most cells in response to infection with viruses. Most viruses are sensitive to these anti-viral actions. Interferon gamma is produced only by certain white cells in response to some immune stimuli.

The interferons in general have anti-viral actions, effects on the immune system, and inhibit the growth of tumours. It is not certain which action is responsible for their therapeutic effect in MS. Interestingly, as long ago as 1979, decreased interferon production was demonstrated from the white cells of patients with MS.[1] The interferons have also been used in treating hepatitis C, malignant melanoma and granulomatous disease. In these diseases, there is usually considerable discussion with the patient before embarking on treatment with interferons because of the serious side effects they can cause.

THE INTERFERON TRIALS

There has now been a large number of RCTs studying the effects on MS of interferon therapy, although all to my knowledge have been drug company-sponsored trials. We know that the results of drug company-sponsored trials are not as robust as those of independently funded trials, and are more often favourable to the drug being studied. Despite this, many observers now feel that, because of the interferons (and glatiramer), MS is a treatable disease. Most of the work has been on interferon beta-1b (IFN-b1b) and interferon beta-1a (IFN-b1a), although interferon alpha-2a (IFN-a2a) has also been studied. It is worth going over the most important of these trials in a little detail to get a sound understanding of the pros and cons of this form of treatment for MS.

Small studies in the early 1980s showed that interferons given directly into the spinal fluid[2] and then by injection[3] reduced the number of relapses in people with MS. The first large-scale study was by the IFNB Multiple Sclerosis Study Group, published in *Neurology* in 1993.[4] This was a study of 372 patients in eleven centres. Patients were randomly assigned to receive placebo (inactive injection), IFN-b1b 1.6 million units, or IFN-b1b 8 million units, given by subcutaneous injection every second day for two to three years. The results were interesting. The relapse rate for the placebo (untreated) group was quite high at 1.27 relapses per year. With the lower dose of interferon the relapse rate was reduced about 8 per cent to 1.17 relapses a year, and with the bigger dose was reduced by about 34 per cent to 0.84 relapses a year. Because the number of patients in the study was quite large the differences were significant, with p values of 0.01 and 0.009 respectively, so the differences were unlikely to have occurred by chance. The severity of relapses was also shown to be reduced significantly.

Two years later, the same investigators presented further follow-up of these patients.[5] It was hoped that by following them for longer, a reduction in progression of disability could be demonstrated. Patients were now studied for up to five years. Interferon continued to reduce the relapse rate, by about a third in the higher dose group, and the MRI evidence supported this, with untreated patients developing many more new lesions. In contrast, treated patients did not suffer significantly more lesions. However, differences were not significant at the p<.05 level after the second year, and only five patients completed the five years of the study. Importantly, the five-year study failed to show any significant decrease in progression of disability.

One of the difficulties in this trial was the size of the placebo response. This is something that is not often mentioned in discussions about the interferon or other drug studies, but there is every reason to suspect that the placebo response will be quite large in MS. In addition, the natural history of the disease is that the number of annual relapses falls over time. This makes it hard to assess whether a drug is making any difference to what would have normally happened. In this study, taking data directly from the reported results, from the end of the first year to the fifth year in the study the placebo group went from an annual relapse rate of 1.44 to 0.81, a 44 per cent reduction. The high-dose interferon group went from 0.96 after the first year to 0.57 in the fifth, a 41 per cent reduction. The authors responded to this by stating that: 'This phenomenon diminishes the statistical power to demonstrate a significant treatment effect in the later years of this and other relapse-prevention trials.' There are other interpretations of this data. One could argue that placebo had a greater effect after the first year of study than the drug.

Interferons are only modestly effective in reducing the number of relapses in MS; there is doubt about whether they have much effect on disease progression.

Despite the apparent reduction in number of relapses overall in the treated groups and MRI evidence that there were significantly fewer new MS lesions, the investigators were unable to detect any difference in the progression of disability between the treated and untreated groups in either the two-year or the five-year study. This is of great concern for people with MS. An editorial on both studies in the prestigious *British Medical Journal* in 1996 commented on the fact that the drug had been hurriedly licensed for use in the United Kingdom on the basis of these studies.[6] It concluded that its licensing was a very 'high risk strategy' and: 'We remain in total ignorance of the long term benefits and side effects of interferon beta in patients with multiple sclerosis.'

These findings have largely been reproduced in subsequent interferon studies, with minor differences. One of the difficulties in interpreting the findings of these studies has been that, although there is clear evidence of a decrease in relapse rate, the effects on the progression of disability in general have been disappointing. Only one trial, the European interferon b1b trial (this trial being in secondary progressive MS rather than relapsing-remitting MS), showed an effect on progression to disability.[7] The delay in progression achieved with three years of interferon treatment was of the order of nine to twelve months, with a drop in the percentage of patients becoming wheelchair bound from 25 per cent for the placebo group to 17 per cent for the interferon group.

There is now some indirect evidence that the disease-modifying drugs, including the interferons which are the most widely prescribed of them, do slow illness progression. Data were presented at the 21st Congress of the European Committee for Treatment and Research in Multiple Sclerosis (ECTRIMS) in Greece in October 2005. Researchers at the University of Alberta in Canada looked at 1752 people with MS at the Dalhousie MS Research Unit between 1979 and 2004. They used Kurtzke's EDSS scale to compare progression of MS before and after these disease-modifying treatments became available for MS. Before these therapies, the median time from diagnosis to walking with a cane was 14.5 years, and 18.1 years (25% slower) after they became available. They were able to compare people who had declined these treatments, and these people continued to deteriorate at the same rate as before the treatments became available.

Neutralising antibodies and blood tests

A large number of treated patients developed antibodies against the inter-ferons (neutralising antibodies or NABs), which reduced the effectiveness of the treatment, mostly making it equivalent to no treatment at all. There is a lot of discussion and controversy about whether this is significant or not, and whether it makes any difference to the treatment effect long term. A study of 101 patients taking interferons from the National Neurology Hospital in London published in 2003 reported that over a 26 month period, 38 per cent of Rebif (IFN-b1a) treated patients and 44 per cent of Betaferon (IFN-b1b) treated patients developed neutralising antibod-ies.[8] None of the Avonex (IFN-b1a) treated patients did. The down side, however, for patients taking Avonex in this study was that none of them remained relapse-free for the period of study, whereas 19 per cent of the Betaferon treated patients did, along with 27 per cent of the Rebif treated patients. Overall, the authors were disappointed to report that nearly half of the patients treated with interferons had continuing evidence of disease activity, either with disabling relapses or insidious progression of the illness, over the relatively short period of study.

More recently, a Swiss study over four years showed that neutral-ising antibodies to Avonex also reduced the effectiveness of therapy,[9] and another Swiss study over two years also showed that neutralising antibodies during Rebif therapy were common and reduced treatment effectiveness.[10] Italian researchers concluded that the development of neutralising antibodies significantly influenced the effectiveness of inter-feron beta.[11] A 2007 Expert Panel report concluded that 'neutralising antibody testing is a critical component of care for MS patients because it provides information on one of the most important factors determining clinical responsiveness to IFNbeta therapy'.[12] People taking interferon should ask their neurologist about this. Many neurologists now use a different test, the molecular genetic test of interferon bioactivity.

In all the interferon studies, many patients have had side effects and subsequently pulled out of treatment. This means regular blood testing to detect any abnormalities caused by the drug. Because the studies have gone for up to five years at a maximum, we don't know how long these benefits will be sustained. Finally, and most important of all, the benefit is relatively small.

Later I will discuss whether these trials really 'prove' the benefit of type I interferons, but even if we accept that they do the benefit is quite small, at around a one-third reduction in the number of relapses. Nevertheless, many authorities are recommending interferon as first-line treatment for people with MS on the basis of these studies. Further, a number of groups are calling for all newly diagnosed patients to be offered either interferon or other recently 'proven' agents such as glatiramer. The MS Society of Canada for instance has suggested this practice to all its members.

More recent research suggests that interferon alpha given by mouth rather than injection may also be effective.[13] If this is confirmed, it offers a much more acceptable treatment option than treatment by injection. Another promising avenue currently being researched is of a nasal spray. This has been shown to be a useful way of delivering the drug in monkeys[14] and may soon be trialled in humans.

SIDE EFFECTS OF INTERFERON THERAPY

To put this part of the picture into perspective, it is worth setting out here in full the adverse reactions listed in the prescribing information for medical practitioners that comes with one of the commercial preparations of IFN-b1b:

> ADVERSE REACTIONS: Inj. Site reactions; flu-like symptoms; CNS disturbances incl. depression and suicidal ideation; leucopenia; elevated hepatic enzymes; severe hypersensitivity reactions.
>
> Also listed are contraindications and precautions, that is conditions in which the drug should either not be prescribed, or should be prescribed with care:
>
> CONTRAINDICATIONS: Pregnancy; history of severe depressive disorders, suicide ideation; decompensated hepatic disease; refractory epilepsy.
>
> PRECAUTIONS: Depression; seizures; cardiac disease; myelosuppression; renal impairment (monitor); lactation.

This makes fairly depressing reading for anyone contemplating starting interferon therapy. Most patients of course do not get most of these effects. Flu-like illness, however, is very, very common. So is headache.[15] Most people find that they feel ill on the day of injection, with an acute flu-like syndrome consisting of fever, chills, headache, muscle pains, joint pains, nausea and perhaps vomiting and diarrhoea. These effects can be to some extent minimised with other drugs again. However, most people are loath to take another drug to offset the side effects of the first drug. These drugs, such as ibuprofen, of course have their own side effects.

Indeed, a friend of mine who has MS required surgery after perforating a stomach ulcer after a few months on ibuprofen therapy to minimise the flu-like effects of interferon. Most people, however, find that they gradually become tolerant of the flu-like side effects. Rather more serious are the other side effects referred to above, and the fact the interferon can impair fertility and should not be used during pregnancy.

Much has been written about the potential for increased risk of depression with the interferons. This is particularly important given how common depression is in MS, and how it can worsen the physical disease. Depression is a well known side effect of interferon alpha treatment; its occurrence with the interferon betas used in MS is less well established, but the risk appears real.[16]

> Side effects of interferon therapy are very common, and can be serious.

One side effect about which little is written is loss of hair. Over a third of patients had hair loss in the studies in which this was reported.[17, 18] Indeed in one of the studies, over half the patients had this distressing symptom in the first six months of treatment. Importantly, few of the interferon studies have reported the side effects of these drugs after two years, so we have little knowledge about the long-term side effects of taking these drugs.

One of the few to do so was a large Canadian study.[19] This followed up 844 patients on all the interferons over six years in British Columbia. Distressingly, they found that over a third (36.9%) of patients on the interferons developed liver disease as measured by elevations in liver enzymes. This was a considerably higher rate than reported in the clinical trials of the agents. It raises serious questions about the real side effect profile of these agents in actual practice as opposed to the clinical trial setting.

Several other side effects have been reported and are potentially very serious, but are often not mentioned when these drugs are prescribed. It appears that thyroid disease is very common in people taking the interferons. In one large long-term follow-up study, 24 per cent of patients taking the interferons for MS developed thyroid dysfunction, mostly under-activity of the thyroid, and 23 per cent developed thyroid auto-immunity.[20] Most (two-thirds) developed this within the first year of treatment.

This is a serious issue, and under-activity of the thyroid can be hard to diagnose and is easily mistaken for fatigue or depression, both common in MS. But thyroid under-activity may need urgent treatment, although it often settles without treatment when caused by interferon therapy, although this may not be so in long-term treatment.[21] So patients on the interferons should have their thyroid function monitored closely while on therapy, particularly in the first year.[21] Other serious potential side effects are pancreatitis,[22] skin problems[23] and peripheral neuropathy which can produce neurological effects difficult to distinguish from MS.[24]

It seems that the side effects of interferon are more common in younger patients and those with smaller body size. Side effects seem to be the commonest reason for stopping the drug in the first year or two of therapy. In one Irish study of 394 patients taking interferons for MS, 28 per cent of people stopped taking the drug within five years of starting therapy.[25] Those stopping due to side effects did so relatively early, at a median time of one year, whereas those stopping due to failure of the treatment to be effective stopped at three years. Significantly, more people with secondary progressive disease stopped because of treatment failure than people with relapsing-remitting MS.

It should also be noted that interferons should be stopped by women with MS who are taking them if they try to get pregnant. One large study showed very significant increases in the rate of stillbirths and low birth weight babies to women taking interferons.[26] There were also significant fetal malformations. Other serious concerns have been raised about the potential for the occurrence of cancers in long-term users of interferons. Although not statistically significant, one study showed a trend to more cancers in people with MS who were on interferons.[27]

CONCERNS ABOUT THE INTERFERON STUDIES

One major concern with the methodology of all the interferon studies is that, because the side effects of the interferons are so prominent, many if not most patients receiving interferon as opposed to inactive placebo guess correctly that they are taking the active drug. This is of great concern in studies which are supposed to be blinded, that is, the participants are not meant to know whether they are getting the active drug or placebo, nor are their doctors.

As we have seen, the placebo effect in general is the term applied to the benefit that patients get when they expect to get better if they think they are receiving an active treatment. This effect can often be quite large, as it has been in a number of clinical trials in MS including the original interferon B trial.[4] The placebo effect may result in substantial improvements in the course of a disease, and when a study is effectively 'unblinded' because people know that they are getting the active drug it raises the distinct possibility that the beneficial effects seen in the study may be partly or even completely due to the placebo effect. That is, the drug itself may not be particularly effective in treating the disease at all, and the benefits are being caused by patients expecting to get better. If patients know they are getting the active treatment it is also very likely that this information will be transmitted to the treating doctors, introducing bias into their assessments. Indeed, an early trial of cyclophosphamide in MS quite elegantly showed that if the treating neurologists were unblinded and knew which treatment the patients were getting they assessed the drug as improving the patients' condition, whereas in reality it had not.[28]

> Problems with the methodology of the interferon studies weaken the evidence that they are of benefit.

In the IFNB five year study for example,[5] 80 per cent of patients in the high-dose interferon group correctly guessed their treatment. This seriously weakens the conclusion that interferon was effective in that study, as the placebo effect may have played a major role in producing this apparent benefit. We have already seen how much the relapse rate fell for the patients in the placebo group in that study. Another major weakness of the study was the high rate of patient drop out, with 20 per cent of those in the high-dose group opting to drop out of the study or be unavailable for follow-up and subsequent analysis. A real possibility when the drop-out rate is so high is that the patients who continued to deteriorate despite treatment gave up and left the study. This would have the effect of artificially making the treatment look better than it really was by leaving those who did well in the study available for final analysis.

This was in fact the only one of the interferon studies to report what happened to patients who dropped out and, sure enough, they had a higher relapse rate, more active disease and became more disabled than those who remained in the study. This is the very criticism that has been levelled at Swank's study, but goes seemingly ignored in the RCTs on interferon.

An Italian group of neuroepidemiologists led by Filippini formally reviewed all the interferon studies to assess their adequacy, and reached some perhaps surprising conclusions.[29] They found that the evidence from the studies was not strong enough to draw any conclusions about the benefit of interferons beyond the first year of treatment, and that even in the first year the interferons could only be said to slightly reduce the number of patients who had relapses. They showed, for instance, in assessing all the studies, that the available evidence did not indicate that the interferons had any effect on the number of hospital admissions the treated patients had, or their need for steroids for relapses. If interferons were truly effective, one might have expected some improvement in both these measures in line with the drop in the number of relapses.

They noted that the commonest problem with the studies was the high rate of patient drop out, leaving only three-quarters of those patients enrolled in the studies they reviewed available for final analysis. They also found that the evidence the interferons delayed or prevented disease progression was inconclusive. This is supported by more recent evidence looking at the experience of 1173 patients in Italy with the three common formulations of interferon, Betaferon, Rebif and Avonex.[30] These researchers showed that at four years, despite falls in relapse rates, there was still on average a significant increase in disability. They showed that approximately 1 in 5 of the patients on Betaferon pulled out of therapy because of side effects, this being approximately three times the number of patients pulling out who were on the other drugs.

Another Italian study in 2005 reported that, in a large group of people treated with interferons, there was a substantial (59%) reduction in relapse rate over the four years of the study; however, 35 per cent of patients had at least one relapse a year, and 28.5 per cent had sustained progression of disability, indicating that they were not responding to the drug.[31]

Filippini and his colleagues concluded in their formal review of the interferon studies that side effects were common and that these side effects had a negative effect on the patients' quality of life. Unlike the interferon studies themselves this study was relatively impartial, in that it was not funded by a drug company and had no vested interest in promoting the effectiveness of interferons. Even in this study, though, all but three of the authors declared at the end of the paper that they had in the past received funding from drug companies, some of which were involved in researching or marketing interferons. It is hard to avoid the insidious effects of drug company sponsorship in this age of high tech pharmaceuticals and marketing.

> There is doubt about the effectiveness of interferons used long term.

A number of neurologists are becoming concerned about what they call the uncritical acceptance of interferons as long-term therapy for MS despite all the trials on its use being short term.[32] They argue that essentially this is an untested approach, extrapolating long-term effectiveness of a therapy from short-term studies. They also argue that there is no convincing evidence that the interferons prevent disease progression, or positively affect common problems such as fatigue, pain, depression and cognitive impairment. We have previously seen that these problems are often the most significant determinants of quality of life for people with MS, and often determine whether people with MS can continue to work.

More recent international collaborative work has suggested that in fact most of the drug trials in MS are too short and do not adequately measure changes in disability progression to allow meaningful decisions to be made about the effectiveness of the drugs.[33] The authors conclude by saying: 'Trials have been too short or degrees of disability change too small to measure the key outcomes. These analyses highlight the difficulty in determining effectiveness of therapy in chronic diseases.'

Concerns about the long-term use of interferons have led to a powerful statement by French neurologists.[34] In response to Filippini's work suggesting there was little evidence that they were effective longer than one year, Clanet and Cucheratt stated: 'If neurologists agree that these compounds have a moderate effect, but that the effect needs to be confirmed in long-term (5–10 year) trials, patients and their doctors deserve an explanation . . .'

CONCERNS ABOUT HARMFUL BRAIN EFFECTS OF INTERFERONS

Dr Russell Blaylock, a US neurosurgeon, has written a number of papers about the harmful effects of interferons on the brain. It is important to note that Blaylock lumps all the interferons together in his assessment, and only some are used in MS. Nevertheless, he paints a disturbing picture of a class of chemicals with significant neurological side effects being used somewhat uncritically for the management of a serious neurological condition.[35]

Interferons injure the brain acutely and also in a more chronic, insidious way. Within hours of treatment, patients often get fever, chills, headache and fatigue, the so-called flu-like side effects. These effects often get gradually better with longer term use. Chronic symptoms can include fatigue, feeling awful, tiredness, sleepiness, headaches, fevers, loss of appetite, cognitive problems and psychiatric disorders.

I am well aware of a number of patients who have stopped their interferons and been amazed at how good they felt. They thought that it was the MS making them feel so bad. There is quite a bit of speculation in the literature about whether the interferons used in MS cause depression,[36] but other interferons certainly can. Generally the higher the dose the worse the brain toxicity, but even at low doses people often feel a lack of drive and disinterest in participating in normal activities. Blaylock estimates that this occurs in 47–80 per cent of patients.

Difficulty thinking clearly can also occur at low doses, and this side effect tends to peak at around one to three months, often with difficulty concentrating and poor short-term memory. Blaylock says that physicians often miss these side effects. This is more likely in a disease like MS, where some of these symptoms are also common to the disease. One systematic review of all studies on IFN-b1a in MS showed that physician-reported depression in the first six months of therapy was significantly associated with the drug, despite patients not reporting symptoms suggestive of depression.[36] The situation is far from clear.

COMPARISON OF INTERFERON THERAPY WITH SWANK'S DIET

I find it fascinating to compare interferon therapy, and what we now know of its likely benefits, with the results of Swank's diet therapy. The relapse rate reduction in the interferon trials has been of the order of one-third. The relapse rate in these treated patients getting optimal benefit is about 0.8 per year at best or about one attack every fifteen months. In some of the other interferon studies, it hasn't even been this good. Compare this with the findings of Swank, who showed in those people consuming under 20g of saturated fat per day a relapse rate of less than one attack every ten years.

This is quite a stunning difference. Further, the interferon trials have had difficulty showing any change in progression of disability, despite demonstrating fewer relapses and fewer new lesions. For Swank, however, the progression of disability was the primary thing he was measuring; he had no difficulty demonstrating a change in progression of disability. Because those were pre-MRI days, we do not know what the relative decrease in the number of MS lesions was. However, as I have previously argued, for people with MS progression of disability is the crucial end-point. Remember that those who started on the low saturated-fat diet before significant disability was present had minimal progression of disability.

So why is interferon 'accepted conventional therapy' for MS and the diet 'alternative or complementary therapy' or, worse still, completely ignored? We go back, of course, to the editorial comment that the diet therapy must remain not 'proven', and what constitutes proof in science. I contend that with a treatment effect of such magnitude, we have to be very careful not to dismiss this therapy simply because the trials were not perfect. We have already discussed the difficulties involved in mounting a trial where one group sticks to a diet. And we have seen that the interferon trials were also far from perfect.

Equally, the drug companies need to shoulder some of the blame here. The interferon studies have been sponsored by drug companies, who clearly have a vested interest in seeing their drug emerge as an effective treatment for MS. Studies of this magnitude are very expensive to run, and this is where the drug companies, with their enormous funds available for research and development, come in. Who would fund a study seeking to explore the role of a very healthy diet in MS? While the case for a low saturated-fat diet may remain unproven, the treatment effect is many times better than for anything yet reported. I believe that this option must be offered to people with MS.

Further, what about a comparison of side effects? The difference is even more staggering. Starting a low saturated-fat diet, and supplementing with essential fatty acids, especially the omega-3 series, is likely to produce the side effects of lower risk of cancer, less heart disease, less depression and improved longevity. Which would you prefer?

OVERVIEW

While interferon has been hailed as exciting new therapy, and it has been said that MS is now a treatable disease, this is only partly true. The studies are all drug company-sponsored, reducing our confidence in their conclusions, and have methodological problems particularly related to blinding and drop-outs. More importantly, the beneficial effect is small, and it may not prevent the progression of disability significantly. Most importantly, side effects are common and can be severe. Indeed, research suggests that the quality of life of patients taking interferon is not improved despite the slowing of disease progression, largely due to side effects[37] and to fatigue and depression.[38]

Nevertheless many people will opt for treatment with disease-modifying agents, either glatiramer or interferon. I believe that these agents should be considered as an addition to the lifestyle changes discussed in this book. And I don't feel that it is a case of one or the other. For people who decide to go with the diet, supplements, meditation and sunlight, a disease-modifying medication like interferon or glatiramer can be commenced in combination right from the beginning; if people opt to start without conventional medicines and the disease progresses, then interferon or glatiramer can be added later. But they should continue with the lifestyle modifications. Although there is no strong evidence to support this, my reading of the literature leads me to believe that the two effects should be complementary. The question of choosing between interferon and glatiramer is explored further in the next chapter and the summary and recommendations section.

14

GLATIRAMER

Extended use of glatiramer is well tolerated and maintains its clinical effect on multiple sclerosis relapse rate and degree of disability

K. Johnson

Glatiramer acetate is another disease-modifying treatment for MS which has been around for quite a while, but is now being considered as a first-line therapy as more and more evidence accumulates of its effectiveness and lack of adverse effects. It was originally called copolymer 1 and has been marketed by the trade name of Copaxone. It was approved for use in Australia towards the end of 1999. The glatiramer story may go down as one of the most fascinating stories in the management of MS. It was discovered by accident by Israeli researchers at the Weizmann Institute of Science in 1968. These researchers were trying to make artificial substances similar to the myelin base protein with which to induce experimental auto-immune encephalomyelitis in experimental animals. Glatiramer was one of a series of mixtures of amino acids, the building blocks of proteins, which were devised to have similar properties to myelin base protein.

Although these substances were found not to cause EAE in the animals, glatiramer somehow stopped mice getting the disease and 'cured'

SUMMARISING THE EVIDENCE

- Glatiramer is modestly effective (30%) in reducing relapse rate in MS.
- Glatiramer appears to work by shifting the immune balance to a Th2 response.
  - It also has neuro-protective effects.
- Clinical trials suggest a similar benefit to the interferons, but the studies were more robust as they were truly blinded.
- Side effects are relatively minor.

EVIDENCE-BASED RECOMMENDATIONS

- Glatiramer offers a safer, better tolerated alternative to the interferons, and is at least as effective.
- Glatiramer should be more often considered as a first-line therapy in MS.

mice that already had the disease. This was a stunning and potentially revolutionary finding. But what works in other animals often does not in humans. So the lengthy process of testing the agent in people with MS began.

HOW DOES GLATIRAMER WORK?

The simple answer to this question is that no one knows. It appears that glatiramer somehow re-educates the immune system because it has a similar structure to the base protein of myelin. This base protein is thought by many to be the part of the nerve which is attacked by the immune system in MS. In effect, glatiramer tricks the immune system into somehow activating certain immune cells which are normally associated with the damage in MS. These cells go into the brain, and upon reaction with myelin base protein reduce the inflammation at the MS lesions. In a sense, it works a bit like the desensitisation injections that people with allergies to bee stings can have. Quite a bit of work now shows that glatiramer shifts the immune system balance from a Th1 to a Th2 response.[1] That means the drug is likely to benefit several other immune-based diseases. Indeed, a 2006 study showed that it was helpful in experimental auto-immune liver disease.[2]

There has now been a very large scientific effort aimed at figuring out how glatiramer works.[3–8] It seems the answer is not going to be simple and that it works in many different ways. At least part of its effect in the animal model of MS is to reduce demyelination and promote remyelination.[9] In humans it appears to induce an anti-inflammatory state in the cerebrospinal fluid surrounding the brain[10] and to reduce free radical formation in blood.[11] Recently there has been considerable interest in its neuro-protective effects.[12, 13] Khan and co-workers have done ingenious studies on patients commencing glatiramer therapy and comparing them over time with people not taking glatiramer.[14] They were able to use special MRI scans which allow assessment of whether or not axons (long nerve connections) degenerate in the brain. They showed that the axons of people taking glatiramer are protected and recover from injury whereas those from people not taking glatiramer tend to die from the injury. Indeed, it has been suggested that because of its neuro-protective effect, glatiramer should be trialled in Parkinson's disease.[15]

Unlike the interferons, glatiramer doesn't appear to have any general effect on the immune system, and it certainly doesn't suppress the immune system. It therefore doesn't make people more susceptible to infections or affect their blood count. And so regular blood tests are unnecessary because it has no measurable effect on any other body system. Again, this is in contrast to the interferons. It also seems to reduce the production of some of the eicosanoids responsible for the inflammation caused by auto-immune activation. Despite considerable scientific study, experts are still not sure exactly how this happens. But happen it does.

GLATIRAMER STUDIES

The glatiramer studies started with enormous optimism. The first major study undertaken by researchers at the Albert Einstein College of Medicine in New York reported astounding improvements in 25 patients treated with glatiramer compared with those treated with placebo injections for two years.[16] Remarkably, the glatiramer treated patients had a 76 per cent reduction in relapse rate, from 1.35 attacks per year to 0.3. The percentage of patients who remained relapse-free over the two years in the treated group was more than double (56 per cent) that of the placebo group (26 per cent).

This was potentially a major breakthrough for MS patients, but clearly more evidence was needed from further studies before authorities would be persuaded to license this drug as therapy for MS. Unfortunately, this appears to be where the process of getting glatiramer to MS patients stalled. Rather unwisely, it was then decided to test the drug on 106 patients with chronic progressive MS, as opposed to relapsing-remitting.[17] This form of MS has been particularly difficult to treat, and glatiramer failed to show any benefit (although in one of the two centres treating patients, there was a significant difference between glatiramer and placebo).

The earlier enthusiasm for the treatment rapidly waned, and it took several years before further studies again confirmed the value of this drug. It was felt that there had perhaps been some problem with the drug's formulation in different batches to explain these discrepancies, and production was standardised to eliminate this possibility before further studies were carried out.

The pivotal study was performed by researchers in Baltimore, using eleven major centres in the United States. They performed a well-constructed RCT in which 251 patients with MS were either treated with glatiramer or inactive placebo for two years.[18] Like the interferon studies, there were about a third (29 per cent) fewer relapses in the treated group (0.59 versus 0.84). The p value was 0.007, so the result was unlikely to have occurred by chance. But more importantly, unlike most of the interferon studies, treatment with glatiramer suggested a slowing of the progression of disability. Although this was not shown with the usual measures of disability, the authors analysed the number of patients who got worse, were unchanged or improved and found significant benefit here for glatiramer. After two years the glatiramer patients had improved EDSS scores by 0.05 points, whereas the placebo patients had worsened by 0.21 points.

Of equal importance was that there were relatively few side effects and no abnormalities detected on blood tests. This is quite unlike the experience with interferon. Most patients developed antibodies to the drug but, unlike the interferons, these antibodies did not interfere with the effect of glatiramer. In an eleven-month extension of the trial the effect of glatiramer improved, with the relapse rate reducing further by a total of 32 per cent. Follow up for more than five years showed that the effects were maintained or even increased over this time. At the end of this period, the relapse rate was reduced to 0.16 a year in those patients taking glatiramer. This represents a relapse only once every six years.

In this study, glatiramer was given by daily injection at a dose of 20mg. However, there has been animal work which strongly suggested that this therapy may be just as effective by mouth.[19] A worldwide multi-centre study was undertaken to investigate this in humans. Results from this trial were, however, disappointing as we will see later.

In 1999, MRI data from the pivotal study showed there was a 35 per cent reduction in the number of brain lesions. A small study of ten patients comparing the rate of new lesions with their rates pre-treatment showed uncertain improvement.[20] For this reason, many neurologists remained unconvinced and unwilling to prescribe glatiramer. They argued that without definitive MRI evidence, which has of course been available for the interferons, they could not be certain of the beneficial effects of the drug. The MS community, researchers and patients alike, eagerly awaited the results of the European–Canadian MRI study on glatiramer. These were published in 2001 in the journal *Neurology*.[21]

This major RCT enrolled 239 patients with relapsing-remitting MS. The patients had had MS for about eight years on average, with a mean EDSS of 2.4 and an average relapse rate in the previous two years of 2.7 per year. Patients had MRI scans every four weeks. After nine months in the study, patients taking glatiramer had 29 per cent fewer new MRI lesions, and about 50 per cent lower total MRI disease burden. The clinical relapse rates, unlike those in the interferon studies, also correlated well with the MRI changes. Patients taking glatiramer had 33 per cent fewer relapses. One particularly interesting feature was that it took some three months before any beneficial effect was seen, and six months before this difference between glatiramer and placebo was significant. The effect seemed to increase the longer patients were on the drug.

> Glatiramer is modestly effective in reducing the number of MS relapses; it remains effective with long-term use.

There has now been considerable experience with glatiramer. Patients from the original 251-patient pivotal study have been followed for six years, with interesting results.[22] A total of 205 of these patients have been studied. The longer patients remained on the drug, the greater the benefit. Patients continually on the drug for six years had an annual relapse rate in the sixth year of 0.23, or roughly one relapse every four to five years. This is markedly less than their starting relapse rate. After ten years, 108 of these patients were still on glatiramer and being followed up, and continued to have sustained falls in relapse rates and severity and accumulation of disability.[23] French researchers have reported similar findings.[24]

Of great interest, approximately 70 per cent of patients continually on the drug for six years were either the same in terms of disability as when they started, or were somewhat better. This is a great result for people with MS and should provide considerable confidence to those people taking glatiramer over an extended period. The same research group looked at patients from the original trial of 251 patients eight years later, and compared those who started on glatiramer and continued with those who started on placebo but at the end of the trial were started on glatiramer. This 30-month delay in starting glatiramer therapy was associated with a significantly smaller proportion of patients remaining stable in terms of their EDSS scores.[25]

Similarly, the European–Canadian study has been followed up long term, now for a mean time of 5.8 years for nearly two-thirds of the original study group.[26] In this study, the control group who originally took placebo were treated with glatiramer after nine months along with those in the treatment group, so effectively this group had a delay of nine months in starting treatment with glatiramer. Researchers then compared at 5.8 years these people with delayed treatment to those who had been receiving glatiramer all along. This group was significantly ($p=0.034$) more likely to be using a walking cane at this stage than those who had been on glatiramer all along. Again this points to a beneficial effect of glatiramer on disease progression.

Researchers in 2000 looking overall at clinical trials to date concluded that the chance of a relapse at one year for a patient on glatiramer was about one-sixth of that for a patient not on glatiramer.[27] A 2005 MRI study showed that for patients in one of the major glatiramer trials, the reduction in lesions after treatment with glatiramer ranged from 20 per cent to 54 per cent.[28] All of these results in combination suggest that glatiramer therapy ought to be more widely prescribed than it is.

As an indication of how difficult the concept of proof is in medicine, despite these trials now over a long period and general acceptance of the benefit of glatiramer by neurologists, a major evidence-based review of the effectiveness of glatiramer by the highly respected Cochrane Collaboration concluded that overall there is no evidence that the drug has any effect on reducing relapses or on disability.[29] Personally, I found the methodology of this review poor in that the reviewers put all studies of glatiramer together for analysis, including trials in primary progressive MS where glatiramer has been shown to be ineffective. Including these trials dilutes the benefit of the other trials where it has been shown to be effective, resulting in the nil benefit conclusion. Others have argued that its effectiveness is equivalent to the interferons, on the basis of reviews of the same studies.[30] If the experts have such trouble agreeing, it is no wonder as patients we find it difficult and confusing when trying to make a decision about what therapy to embark on. More recent work on the cost effectiveness of glatiramer compared with the interferons suggests that glatiramer is the preferred agent.[31]

The most recent news about glatiramer confirms its benefit to people with MS. In this study, the PreCISe study, investigators gave glatiramer to people with a first episode and typical MRI brain lesions suggesting MS (a Clinically Isolated Syndrome or CIS), that is, what may have previously been called transverse myelitis, and compared it to placebo to see if glatiramer would reduce the proportion of people going on to a definite diagnosis of MS. Of the 481 people with CIS randomly assigned to receive glatiramer or inactive placebo, the proportion of patients who developed MS was 43 per cent in the placebo group versus 25 per cent in the glatiramer group. The trial was in fact stopped early because of the clear benefit from glatiramer.[32]

SIDE EFFECTS

Ninety per cent of patients receiving glatiramer in the Baltimore study got skin reactions and 15 per cent a transient flushing feeling, with palpitations and shortness of breath. There were no serious side effects. These rates were somewhat lower in the European–Canadian MRI study, and again there were no serious side effects. In particular, the flu-like symptoms, so commonly seen with the interferons, are not seen with glatiramer. There is no need for regular blood testing, as the drug has not been shown to cause any other abnormalities, and the development of antibodies does not affect the drug's performance.

Although neither the interferons nor glatiramer are recommended for use during pregnancy, we know that the interferons can definitely cause problems. Research reported to the American Academy of Neurology meeting in 2003 suggested that this is unlikely to be the case with glatiramer. Of 215 pregnancies which occurred while patients were on glatiramer, there was no higher incidence of abnormalities than usual. This is at least reassuring for women on glatiramer who unexpectedly fall pregnant. A recent review concluded that glatiramer posed the least risk during pregnancy of the available disease-modifying drugs.[33] It is also safe to breastfeed while taking glatiramer, in contrast with the interferons.

Now that we have longer experience with glatiramer, we are starting to see a few problems related to the effect it has on the balance between Th1 and Th2 lymphocytes. A few uncommon skin conditions related to the change in this balance caused by glatiramer have now been reported, including erythema nodosum (a serious skin rash), and more recently a skin lymphoma.[34] So it is important to keep in mind that even for drugs as apparently innocuous in terms of side effects like glatiramer, it is wise to balance the likely benefit of its use against the potential for side effects, particularly for people who are doing well on the Recovery Program.

Glatiramer has few side effects.

DOSING

The dosing schedule for glatiramer, that is a daily injection, puts some people off and leads them to opt for the interferons, which may be given every second day or even weekly. We are still unsure of the optimal dosing for glatiramer. There is some evidence that injecting every second day is just as effective as daily injection, and this needs to be investigated further.[35] Indeed, given how it works, it may well be that an initial immunising course of, say, nine months injections, followed by periodic boosters, will be all that is necessary. Until we have more evidence, though, daily injection is recommended. For those concerned about this, the advantage of feeling perfectly well while on the medication should outweigh the concerns about the frequency of injection.

A further issue about dosage that has been investigated is doubling the dose. Investigators from Ohio randomised people with MS to standard

dose or double dose glatiramer given in the usual manner, subcuta-
neously, every day.[36] They found evidence suggesting the double dose to
be more effective, with a longer time to first relapse and higher proportion of relapse-free subjects in the double-dose group.

NEW DIRECTIONS WITH GLATIRAMER

Another very interesting possibility is that of combining glatiramer with
interferon. Although there have been some safety concerns about this from
animal studies,[37] and the combination was ineffective in this study, a small,
multi-centre trial in humans is currently underway in the United States to
look at this combination. Reported at the American Academy of Neurology meeting in Toronto in 1999, the trial apparently studied 32 patients,
concentrating on safety issues. I have not seen follow-up results of this
study. More basic research work from the Montreal Neurological Institute
showed that the two therapies may be operating on the immune system
cells in different ways, raising the possibility that they will enhance each
other's effect when used together. This looks extremely promising, although
the side effects caused by interferon remain an issue.

Other combinations with glatiramer are also promising. Researchers
have suggested using mitoxantrone, a chemotherapy drug discussed in
more detail later in the book, to get control of particularly severe MS and
then follow on with glatiramer.[38] This has now been studied in detail
in an RCT of 40 people with MS. The combination of mitoxantrone
followed by glatiramer (M-G) in this study was far superior to glatiramer
alone in all measures of disease activity. Specifically, M-G produced an
89 per cent greater reduction in MRI lesions at six and nine months than
glatiramer alone, and a 70 per cent greater reduction at twelve months;
relapse rates in the M-G group were half that in the glatiramer alone
group. Early work on a combination of minocycline with glatiramer also
looks promising.[39]

Researchers at Harvard University have succeeded in producing other
random copolymers, different from glatiramer, which appear more effective at suppressing EAE in animals.[40] If this finding translates to humans,
we may be on the verge of a considerably more effective treatment for
MS. With advances in immunology, we may see even 'smarter' molecules
which are more stable and more effective than these copolymers.[41] This
has recently been demonstrated in two multi-centre studies of a high

molecular weight copolymer of the same four amino acids as glatiramer, a drug called protiramer.[42] The drug was highly effective at reducing the number of CNS lesions over 36 weeks.

Finally, researchers have for some time been examining the question of whether glatiramer taken by mouth works just as well as it does when injected. This would of course be a huge boon to many thousands of people. Initial work in animals was highly positive, suggesting that oral glatiramer would be equally effective.[19] Unfortunately, a very large clinical trial of around 1100 patients worldwide taking oral glatiramer initially reported interim results which did not support the earlier enthusiasm. Although there was some benefit for patients taking the oral form, it did not reach statistical significance. When finally published in 2006, the study of 1651 patients showed no improvement at either low or high dose oral glatiramer.[43] This effectively rules out oral glatiramer as a therapy for MS.

OVERVIEW

Many authorities are now recommending glatiramer as first-line treatment for MS, equivalent in its effect to the interferons. Given that the side-effect profile is clearly superior to that of interferon, and that the studies on glatiramer were properly blinded and hence more likely to be valid than the interferon studies, my own view is that it should be considered before the interferons. I recommend that people offered interferon because of the number of relapses they have should raise the possibility of taking glatiramer instead. It is certainly likely that it will be better tolerated, and it is likely to be just as or more effective. Interferons appear to take about one to two months to be effective, versus three to six for glatiramer, and this may be an issue if the disease is particularly active, although most patients starting on these therapies have just finished a course of steroids for a relapse or first attack and get some protection from the steroids for a period of time. Overall, glatiramer appears to be a safe and modestly effective therapy for MS, with few side effects.

15

OTHER DRUG THERAPIES AFFECTING IMMUNE SYSTEM FUNCTION

There are options for those experiencing worsening of the disease

National MS Society of the United Kingdom

A number of other therapies have been tried in the treatment of MS. Most of these suppress or otherwise alter the function of the immune system in achieving their effects. These tend to be very aggressive therapies with major side effects. As such, they are generally reserved for those people with established, seriously progressive disease. Some, fortunately, are relatively safe. This is a rapidly developing field in medicine, with many large-scale trials currently either being planned or underway. Given the usual time delays in book publishing, any book on the subject is bound to be somewhat out of date by the time it is published. The Internet is the best way to keep up with the latest on this subject. I suggest Googling what the latest is for a particular therapy. The MS Society of Canada also operates a very well-researched website, with all the latest advances. Many of these therapies are not yet licensed for use in MS in Australia. A neurologist can advise what is available.

SUMMARISING THE EVIDENCE

- Natalizumab is more effective than interferons or glatiramer in reducing (by about two-thirds) the relapse rate in MS; it also reduces progression to disability.
  - Side effects are a serious issue; rarely there have been deaths from progressive multi-focal leukoencephalopathy.
- Mitoxantrone, a chemotherapy agent, causes a similar (about two-thirds) reduction in relapse rate; it also seems effective in secondary progressive MS.
  - Side effects are a serious concern.
- Cladribine, another chemotherapy agent with serious side effects, is effective; it may be effective in oral form.
- Intravenous immunoglobulins (IVIgs) are effective in reducing relapses (by about 60%) with few serious side effects, but are uncommonly prescribed and are not available for use in Australia.
  - IVIgs may be useful in primary progressive MS, a form of MS that has been very difficult to treat.

EVIDENCE-BASED RECOMMENDATIONS

- Natalizumab should be considered when the standard disease-modifying drugs (interferons and glatiramer) have failed, and/or the disease is very active.
- Mitoxantrone has a similar place in MS treatment, but may additionally be useful for secondary progressive disease.
- IVIgs should be used more; they may be useful therapy after childbirth when relapse rates tend to be higher.

NATALIZUMAB

This new drug is an important addition to the therapies available for treating serious, active MS, although there are safety concerns despite its approval in 2006 for use by the FDA in the United States. It was originally marketed under the trade name of Antegren, but more recently Tysabri. Natalizumab works by specifically targeting and inhibiting a protein, alpha 4 integrin, which is present on the surface of immune system cells and helps them attach to blood vessel walls and get into the brain. It has been used in the animal model of MS where it is effective and in a preliminary study in humans. Recent animal work shows that inhibition of alpha integrin allows remyelination to occur, as well as inhibiting demyelination.[1] The difficulty with using drugs of this type is that they don't just affect the immune response in MS, but in all conditions where the immune response is required. As a result, they tend to cause other problems related to underactivity of the immune system.

Initially, an RCT published in 2003 in the prestigious *New England Journal of Medicine*[2] provided strong evidence that this drug is likely to have an important role to play in MS treatment. In this study, 213 patients were randomly assigned to receive a low dose or high dose of natalizumab, or placebo. The drug was given IV and administered once every four weeks for six months. Patients were followed with MRI scanning and clinical assessment. The placebo patients had on average nearly ten new brain lesions at the end of the six months, compared with 0.7 for the low dose group and just over one new lesion for the high dose group. Twice the number of patients in the placebo group had relapses than in either of the treatment groups. Importantly, those taking the drug generally reported improvement in their sense of wellbeing, and those in the placebo group the reverse. This suggests the drug is quite well tolerated and side effects are not too unpleasant.

The natalizumab story has been soured, however, by the events which led to the FDA in America fast tracking the drug to general use in November 2004, only to be forced to remove it three weeks later because of safety concerns. Unexpectedly, two patients who had taken natalizumab in combination with an interferon in MS trials developed a condition called progressive multifocal leukoencephalopathy (PML), an illness similar to very aggressive MS and previously only ever reported in AIDS patients. Shortly after, a third patient, taking natalizumab alone in a trial for inflammatory bowel disease, also died of the illness. Following suspension, there was very careful investigation of all patients who had taken the drug in clinical trials to see if there were other cases of PML which had not been reported.[3] This detailed review revealed no new cases, and concluded that the risk of PML was about 1 in 1000 for patients treated for about eighteen months. The longer term risk was unknown.

Since then, at least two further cases of PML have occurred. In July 2008 it was reported by the manufacturer to the Stock Exchange that two patients taking the drug for MS had developed the disease. At the time, both were still alive. It appears that neither was taking other immuno-suppressive drugs, so the risk is probably now more difficult to quantify as it is not just a risk for those who are otherwise immunosuppressed.

At around the time the first three cases were reported, two further papers were published on the benefits of natalizumab in MS, one with natalizumab alone, the other in combination with an interferon. The former showed that the combination of natalizumab and interferon was significantly better than interferon alone, with the annual relapse rate dropping to 0.34 per year on the combination, compared with 0.75 on the interferon alone, and less progression to disability.[4] In the latter study, 627 patients receiving natalizumab alone had a 68 per cent reduction in annual relapse rate, as well as less progression to disability than those receiving placebo.[5] More recent MRI studies confirm that natalizumab is highly effective at prevent-ing new MRI lesions, with between 76 per cent and 92 per cent fewer lesions (depending on lesion type) in those on natalizumab versus placebo.[6]

> The more profoundly a drug suppresses immune function, the more likely and severe the side effects.

While the studies indicate that natalizumab is likely to be more effective than the currently used disease-modifying drugs in reducing the number of relapses and MRI lesions, the concern about serious side effects has made this drug a much more risky proposition for people with MS. Certainly, taking it in combination with an interferon appears particularly risky at present. Swiss scientists have also raised concerns about taking it long term after deleterious effects in an animal model.[7]

In early 2008, further serious concerns about its toxicity were raised in a letter to the *New England Journal of Medicine*.[8] Two patients receiving the drug who had longstanding benign moles that were being kept under surveillance by their doctors had sudden cancerous change in the moles and developed widespread melanoma. The company marketing the drug followed this by announcing that one earlier similar case had occurred during RCTs of the drug. So some authorities now are suggesting that people with a family history of malignant melanoma should not receive natalizumab.

Several publications have now questioned whether it should be used at all because of toxicity and uncertain benefit in terms of disease progression.[9, 10] Its place is probably as a stand-alone therapy when other disease-modifying drugs do not seem to be working.[11] Some neurologists use it as first-line therapy in aggressive MS before switching to a less toxic drug long term. Tysabri was approved for subsidy under the Pharmaceutical Benefits Scheme in Australia in 2008.

Alemtuzumab and related drugs

At the meeting of the American Academy of Neurologists (AAN) in Honolulu in 2003, findings were presented on a number of related drugs which also proved beneficial for people with MS. The drug alemtuzumab (trade name Campath) was shown to have significant benefit for relapsing-remitting MS although not secondary progressive MS. Unfortunately side effects were a major problem, with a third of patients treated developing a severe auto-immune thyroid disorder, Graves disease. A recent report of this drug's use in 39 people with very aggressive, rapidly progressive MS showed very favourable reductions in relapse rate, from 2.5 to 0.2 annually.[12] Unfortunately, twelve patients developed evidence of auto-immune disease, with two developing frank thyroid disease and one auto-immune skin disease.

More recent work suggests quite marked reductions in relapse rates with this drug, but serious side effects are common and of concern.[13] In this RCT of 334 people with previously untreated, early, relapsing-remitting MS, patients received interferon beta-1a three times per week or annual intravenous cycles of alemtuzumab for three years. The alemtuzumab arm of the trial was stopped early because three people developed an auto-immune disease related to their platelets causing bleeding, and one died. Alemtuzumab-treated patients had significantly fewer relapses (74% less) and less disability (71% less). Somewhat surprisingly, the disability of people taking the alemtuzumab improved on average whereas those taking interferon beta-1a got worse, as has been the case in other disease-modifying drug trials. This was a very widely reported finding that created major news worldwide as no other drug had previously been shown to reverse disability.

The real problem with this drug, however, was in the side effects. Nearly a quarter (23%) of all patients taking alemtuzumab in this study developed auto-immune thyroid disease, 3 per cent auto-immune platelet disease, and two thirds (66%) developed infections. These side effects look to be a serious limitation to the widespread use of this drug in the future.

Another related drug, daclizumab, appears to be a more promising option. At the AAN meeting in 2003, two US groups reported results in ten and eleven patients with relapsing-remitting and secondary progressive MS, either alone or in combination with interferon beta, with dramatic effects on MRI-demonstrated disease activity. One group found no new lesions and the other an over 70 per cent reduction in the number of lesions.

MITOXANTRONE

This drug is a potent agent related to those used in chemotherapy. It is chemically similar to doxorubicin, which is used for acute leukaemias and lymphomas. Mitoxantrone has been used principally for acute leukaemia, but because it powerfully suppresses the immune system it has also been tried in MS. The biggest of the RCTs to date studying this drug in relapsing-remitting MS was from Italy.[14] In this study, 51 patients were randomly allocated to receive mitoxantrone once a month IV or inactive placebo. There was a very major reduction (66%) in the number of relapses in the treated group after two years, and a significant reduction in the proportion of patients with confirmed disease progression at two years. The number of new MRI lesions was also lower, but the p value was not significant. Again, as in the interferon trials, we see the paradox of lack of correlation between number of new MRI lesions and disease progression.

Another study compared the results of patients treated with mitoxantrone plus steroids with a control group of patients treated with just steroids.[15] Forty-two patients with clinically very active, progressive disease were randomly allocated to the two groups. After six months, there were very large differences between the groups. Ninety per cent of the mitoxantrone plus steroid group had no new MRI lesions versus only 31 per cent of the steroid only group. The p value was <0.001. There were also significant improvements in the disability score for patients in the mitoxantrone group at months two to six, with a final mean improvement of more than one point (p<0.001). Additionally, there were significantly fewer relapses (7 compared to 31; p<0.01), and more patients had not relapsed (14 versus 7; p<0.05) in the mitoxantrone group. Five patients in the steroid only group dropped out of the trial because they were deteriorating so badly.

In 2002, *The Lancet* reported a large study of mitoxantrone in patients with secondary progressive MS.[16] This form of MS has been very difficult to treat to date, but some preliminary work had suggested that mitoxantrone may be effective. The study randomly allocated 194 people with secondary progressive MS to treatment with mitoxantrone or to placebo. The drug was given IV every three months for two years. People in the mitoxantrone group had very significant reductions in disease progression, with about one-quarter the worsening of the EDSS measure of disability, about a third fewer relapses, and about a quarter of the worsening of their neurological status. Importantly, there were no serious side effects or cardiac problems, which have been a concern with this drug. A French study followed up 304 people with MS who had been treated with mitoxantrone.[17] It found that the disease activity was markedly reduced for about two years before it became active again, and suggested that other therapies needed to be commenced during that time. These studies together are highly significant. Together they show that even advanced MS can be brought under control with the use of this powerful immunosuppressant drug.

Unfortunately, side effects can be a major problem, as expected. People taking this drug can get some of the effects we regularly see in chemotherapy such as hair falling out, nausea, vomiting and loss of appetite. Bone marrow suppression is common, meaning that people are more susceptible to infections. Indeed, the chemotherapy may itself precipitate cancer and, in the long term, the incidence of cancers in people treated with this drug is likely to be higher than in the general population. Heart muscle toxicity has not yet been seen, although it is often seen in related drugs.

Research reported to the American Academy of Neurologists in Honolulu in 2003 showed some benefit in a study of 64 patients with primary progressive MS in France. While not conclusive, this is extremely important as primary progressive MS has to date proven very resistant to any form of therapy. An influential Cochrane Database Systematic Review in 2005 concluded that mitoxantrone is moderately effective in reducing relapse rate and disease progression in relapsing-remitting, primary progressive and secondary progressive MS in the short terms studied to date (two years), although longer trials are needed.[18] No major side effects related to cancer or cardiotoxicity were reported from the trials studied.

Mitoxantrone therapy opens up an extremely promising avenue for treatment of patients with aggressive forms of MS and secondary progressive MS who would otherwise rapidly deteriorate or have few treatment options. There are obviously concerns about its safety, especially with long-term use. A 2006 review concluded that the benefits of mitoxantrone therapy outweighed the risks, especially for people not responding to the usual disease-modifying therapies.[19] Indeed, a South American study showed that for patients deteriorating despite treatment with interferon beta, mitoxantrone safely stabilised their condition.[20] A 2007 study in 45 people with early but very active MS showed that mitoxantrone also stabilised their condition.[21] One of the patients, however, developed leukaemia shortly after treatment. Further trials are needed, but at this stage it is certainly not a drug that should be considered for the average person with MS. If the disease becomes very active and progressive, at least there is something that can be done, albeit at some cost.

Many neurologists, however, will be concerned about the potential for cardiotoxicity when deciding whether to prescribe this drug. Researchers are currently working on analogues of mitoxantrone which do not possess similar cardiotoxicity. One such drug is pixantrone, which in animal studies appears very promising and may soon be trialled in humans.[22, 23]

CLADRIBINE

This is another drug used in chemotherapy. It has been effective in the treatment of certain leukaemias and lymphomas. Again, it is likely to be of benefit in MS by suppressing the immune system. It was tried in MS because it is relatively less toxic than some of the other anti-cancer agents. The first major study in the literature was performed in California and published in 1996.[24] Fifty-one people were treated in a placebo-controlled RCT. The design was a bit unusual in that patients were crossed over from the placebo to the cladribine treatment group after one year in the study, and patients getting the cladribine first were then given placebo. The drug was given as a weekly course of injections every few months. The study again showed a favourable effect on progression of disability, with patients on cladribine tending to improve while those on placebo deteriorated.

Concerns were raised about side effects, particularly bone marrow suppression, but a more recent study of severely affected people with MS showed that the drug was well tolerated, and that these effects could be diminished by decreasing the dosage.[25] A Californian RCT of 52 people over eighteen months with relapsing-remitting MS showed significant benefits for those treated with cladribine. Patients improved in terms of frequency and severity of relapses and the number of MRI lesions.[26] In fact, by the sixth month of treatment, there were no new lesions at all in the cladribine treated group. The cladribine was given as a five-day course of injections every six months.

Side effects of cladribine are relatively mild considering the class of drug. Bone marrow suppression, decreased platelet count and decreased white cell count have been recorded. Shingles may also occur, as with other immunosuppressant therapies. Overall, these studies are again extremely encouraging for people with MS which is difficult to control with the standard therapies discussed earlier in this book. An advantage I see is that a course of therapy is needed only once every six months, and disease progression is likely to be very significantly slowed. The price in terms of side effects is probably acceptable if the MS is very active.

In January 2005, a large pharmaceutical company announced that it was beginning large-scale trials of an oral formulation of cladribine.[27] This study has now been completed although at the time of writing the results had not yet been peer reviewed or published.[28] This study, the CLARITY study, was a 96-week RCT enrolling 1326 patients with relapsing-remitting MS. A low dose and high dose of cladribine were tested against placebo. The cladribine tablets were taken in two or four treatment four- to five-day courses in the first year, so patients took cladribine tablets for only eight to 20 days in the year. In the second year, all participants took two treatment courses. The relapse rate in the placebo group was 0.33 per year on average; this fell to 0.14 per year in the low dose group, a 58 per cent reduction (p<0.001), and 0.15 in the high dose group, a 55 per cent reduction (p<0.001).

The drug was well tolerated with more patients in the treatment groups finishing the study than those in the placebo groups, and relatively mild side effects according to data released by the drug company. Longer term studies are under way looking at longer term safety, but as a chemotherapy agent there are likely to be some downsides to long-term treatment, especially related to bone marrow suppression and infections. The good news with this study is that the lower dose worked so well, at least as well as the higher dose, and that people tolerated the drug so well and stayed in the study. This compares very favourably to the interferon studies where there was a very high drop-out rate. The other really positive aspect is that the drug is taken orally, and only for a few days each year. It has the potential to really make a difference to the lives of people with MS if it proves in the longer term to be safe, and if it actually makes a difference to disease progression. The drug company is submitting cladribine for approval in mid 2009 in the United States and Europe. It has been granted fast-track status by the Food and Drug Authority.

CYCLOPHOSPHAMIDE

This is a rather toxic anti-cancer drug. It is used, particularly in combination with other chemotherapy agents, for such diseases as lymphomas, multiple myeloma, breast, lung, cervix and ovary cancer, and several childhood cancers. It has the advantage of being able to be given by mouth rather than injection only, unlike most of the other anti-cancer agents. In MS, cyclophosphamide has mostly been used for the chronic progressive form. Several RCTs have not shown any benefit for either cyclophosphamide alone compared with placebo,[29] or different combinations of cyclophosphamide, steroids and other techniques.[30] A later study from Harvard Medical School, however, showed that people who had cyclophosphamide and steroids to induce immunosuppression, and then had booster doses of cyclophosphamide every other month for two years, had slower progression of disease than those without the boosters.[31] This was a large RCT of 256 people with MS. The group who had the booster injections had slower progression of disability at 24 and 30 months, but the effect was confined to those patients under 40 years of age. For this group of patients the effect was very significant.

Another study from Boston in 2005 looked at people who were not responding well to interferon therapy, that is, their disease was still quite active.[32] They randomised patients to receive either monthly cyclophosphamide and steroids or monthly steroids alone in addition to their interferon therapy. The cyclophosphamide group did considerably better, presenting another treatment option for people not responding well to interferons alone. An Italian study monitored ten patients with rapidly progressive MS who were given monthly doses of cyclophosphamide in combination with interferon beta, and then maintained on interferon beta alone.[33] They were quite stable clinically and on MRI at 36 months. One intriguing report from Brazil noted that a 48-year-old woman who had accidentally been given a very high single dose of cyclophosphamide three years after diagnosis had not had any disease activity of any sort seven years later.[34]

Unfortunately cyclophosphamide has major side effects, both short and long term. It causes hair to fall out, nausea and vomiting, ulceration of the mouth and other mucous membranes, dizziness and increased skin pigmentation. More serious effects are bladder irritation with blood in the urine and bone marrow suppression, with increased susceptibility to infections. In the longer term, it can cause a variety of cancers in its own right. These side effects limit its usefulness for people with MS.

INTRAVENOUS IMMUNOGLOBULINS (IVIgs)

Immunoglobulins (Igs) are the natural antibodies made in humans by certain immune system cells in response to infection or a foreign substance. Human Igs have been extracted from plasma and pooled, and used IV to treat several conditions. High dose IVIgs have been used to treat conditions including Guillain-Barré syndrome, chronic inflammatory demyelinating polyneuropathy, multifocal motor neuropathy and MS. Because they are a natural human product they are virtually free of side effects, and so offer advantages over some other therapies which affect the immune system. With human products, there is always the minor risk of transmission of infectious agents through the serum.

A large RCT by the Austrian Immunoglobulin in Multiple Sclerosis Study Group published in 1997 looked at a monthly dose of IVIg for two years compared with inactive placebo.[35] A total of 148 patients with relapsing-remitting MS were enrolled in the study. Results showed that the disability score decreased significantly in the treated group and got worse in the placebo group, and there was a 59 per cent reduction in the number of relapses in the treated group. Best of all, there were no adverse effects. A Danish study of 26 patients looked at MRI lesions during IVIg treatment.[36] There were fewer new MRI lesions with IVIg than on placebo (0.4 versus 1.3). The p value was 0.03. During IVIg treatment, fifteen patients had no relapses compared with only seven on placebo (p=0.02). Although the study was small, this was useful confirmatory evidence of the Austrian study.

Intravenous immunoglobulins are safe and effective.

A 2004 study of 91 Israeli people early after an attack suggestive of MS reported the results of treating with IVIgs every six weeks.[37] The researchers showed that those treated were only one-third as likely as people not treated to progress to definite MS within a year. Further, they had fewer lesions on MRI. There were no significant side effects with the treatment.

Another very interesting study from Iran combined IVIg and an immunosuppressant drug called azathioprine.[38] Although the study was not an RCT, it followed 38 patients with relapsing-remitting MS for three years of this combined therapy. Before starting therapy, patients had been having an average of 1.7 relapses a year. This fell to none by the end of the study, and the disability scale score improved overall.

There has been speculation that some of the benefits seen with IVIgs may be caused not only by immune system effects, but by improved re-myelination of MS lesions. Certainly, at present, the mechanism by which IVIg works is unclear. Nevertheless, the studies show a significant reduction in relapse rates, and improvements in disability scores. Given the low toxicity of this therapy, it makes a very worthwhile addition to our expanding list of agents which can be used for MS when the disease is very active or severe.

However, a large Dutch study of 318 patients with secondary progressive disease found no clinical benefit from IVIgs.[39] There was also no decrease in standard MRI measures of disease progression.[40] A 2005 summary of published work on IVIgs concluded that they are a second-line treatment in relapsing-remitting MS when other treatments are not available, that they have no role in progressive MS or acute attacks, but that they may be useful after childbirth to prevent relapses, and can delay the onset of definite MS after a first attack.[41] Side effects have been documented. These include fever, chills, fatigue, joint and muscle pain, abdominal pain and headache. Serious side effects have included seizures, heart failure and kidney failure, but they have been rare. A 2006 Israeli report on the long-term side effects of IVIg therapy reported 293 people with MS treated for up to ten years.[42] The authors showed that the drug was safe even when given over long periods.

More recently, a large placebo-controlled study in people with primary and secondary progressive MS showed a significant benefit for IVIgs in primary, but not secondary, progressive MS.[43] Given how few effective treatments there are for primary progressive MS, this should be investigated further, and offered to people who are deteriorating with this type of MS, although it is not currently available for use in some countries including Australia.

OTHERS

A number of other therapies which affect the immune system have been tried in MS, mostly with less impressive or doubtful results in comparison with those already discussed. Azathioprine on its own has not been shown conclusively in several trials to have benefit. There is an associated risk as well of cancers developing. A 2005 study did, however, show that azathioprine significantly reduced the number of new lesions.[44] Methotrexate is another immunosuppressant drug used in inflammatory disorders with an immune system basis. Although one study of oral methotrexate in chronic progressive MS showed a reduced rate of progression of disability as assessed by observers, patients in the study noticed essentially no difference.[45] The drug is fairly toxic, with bone marrow depression, liver cirrhosis and kidney damage its main side effects, and regular blood testing is necessary. This reduces the utility of the therapy. A number of other newer drugs affecting the immune system are discussed in the following chapter.

OVERVIEW

Several agents affecting immune system function are now available for use where conventional disease-modifying drugs are not sufficiently effective. Natalizumab and mitoxantrone appear quite effective in reducing relapse rate but are quite toxic. Intravenous immunoglobulins should be used more in countries where they are available.

16

NEWER DRUG THERAPIES ON THE HORIZON

The past is a source of knowledge, and the future is a source of hope

Stephen Ambrose

OESTROGENS AND TESTOSTERONE

Recently there has been a lot of interest in the female hormone oestrogen and its possible effect on the course of MS. Oestrogen is commonly found in oral contraceptive pills. It seems the oestrogens have a modulatory effect on the immune system through a number of mechanisms, including a shift in the Th1 versus Th2 cytokine balance, and its effects on other immune related hormones.[1] It has long been known that there is a decrease in MS activity in late pregnancy when the levels of this hormone are quite high. More recent research shows that relapse rate in MS decreases substantially throughout the whole of pregnancy.[2]

Researchers at the University of Portland, Oregon, found that feeding oestrogen to mice with EAE dramatically reduces the severity of the illness.[3] These researchers suggested that oestrogen may be used as a treatment for MS, perhaps in low doses together with other disease-modifying therapy to minimise side effects.[4] On the negative side, however, the US Nurses

SUMMARISING THE EVIDENCE

- A variety of new drugs is being trialled in MS, many taken orally.
  - The most promising and least toxic appear to be minocycline, an antibiotic, and the statins, which are drugs used to lower cholesterol.
  - Fingolimod, a drug affecting the immune system, is a promising new oral therapy; preliminary work suggests a halving of relapse rate and a reasonable side effect profile.
  - Low dose naltrexone has been widely used but poorly studied, and RCTs are required to assess its value.
- Cannabinoids, derived from cannabis, assist with relief of symptoms, particularly pain, spasticity, muscle cramps and sleep disturbance.
- Bone marrow transplantation is a very risky procedure with significant mortality, but appears potentially helpful in very severe MS not responding to other treatments.

EVIDENCE-BASED RECOMMENDATIONS

- For people with disease that is either rapidly progressing or not responding to standard therapies, there are many therapeutic options being studied.
- None of these newer drugs can currently be definitely recommended.

Health Study failed to show any difference in MS incidence between nurses taking oral contraceptives or the number of pregnancies they had had.[5] This was contradicted by more recent work from the Harvard School of Public Health in 2005.[6] These researchers found a 40 per cent lower incidence of MS in women who had been on the oral contraceptive pill in the previous three years. More human research on oestrogens is needed before we know whether they will be beneficial for people with MS. But at the very least, it is useful for women with MS to know that getting pregnant is not likely to result in an increase in disease activity.

Interestingly, the male sex hormone, testosterone, may also be of benefit to men with MS. Researchers have shown in a study of ten men that with daily application of testosterone gel over twelve months, cognitive ability was improved and there was a slowing of brain atrophy (shrinkage).[7] Larger studies are needed before this can be recommended.

AZATHIOPRINE AND GLATIRAMER/INTERFERONS

An article in *Time* magazine in 2002 sparked worldwide interest in research conducted in Sydney, Australia. It reported that three patients had been treated with a combination of azathioprine, an anti-cancer immune-suppressant drug, and either glatiramer or one of the interferons and that the patients had made dramatic recoveries from quite severe MS, to the point of being able to walk or jog after being confined to wheelchairs. Only one patient to my knowledge was reported in the medical literature by the same neurologist.[8] This was a 24-year-old woman with eye problems and great difficulty walking who was treated with glatiramer and azathioprine and was able to jog again. Another group from Spain reported results from a study of azathioprine and Betaferon in ten people with secondary progressive MS.[9] Only eight stayed in the study, but these people had a 50 per cent reduction in relapse rate and significant improvement in EDSS. There does appear to be some promise here for the treatment of secondary progressive MS, although the combination of drugs is relatively toxic.

Researchers from the Johns Hopkins University in the United States reported in 2005 that the combination of azathioprine and Betaferon, used in patients who had continuing disease activity while on Betaferon, resulted in a 65 per cent reduction in the number of lesions on MRI.[10] As more reports come in on the use of this combination, it appears more likely that it will be an effective treatment for those with very active disease.

PERFENIDONE

This is a drug which has previously been used in the treatment of lung fibrosis. It is one of the few therapies which has been tried and found to be successful for secondary progressive MS, albeit in small studies. After some promising initial work researchers in Texas trialled the agent, which is taken by mouth, in 43 patients in a placebo-controlled RCT.[11] There were significant benefits in clinical disability and bladder function, and patients on perfenidone had far fewer relapses (8% versus 28%). Larger scale studies are underway to confirm this promising work.

MINOCYCLINE

A novel drug approach to treating MS has been reported by Canadian researchers. Minocycline, a widely used antibiotic taken by mouth for acne, also has the effect of reducing the ability of immune cells to get into the CNS, by inhibiting enzymes called matrix metalloproteinases. These enzymes have been shown to be involved in the development of lesions in MS.[12]

These researchers first showed that the drug was effective in EAE in experimental animals,[13] and followed up with a small study in ten patients which they reported to the 2003 AAN meeting. This showed that there was a significant effect on MRI, and that the drug was well tolerated. This research was published in *Annals of Neurology* in 2004.[14] It was found that there was an 84 per cent reduction in the number of MRI lesions while on minocycline. This is substantially higher than other therapies currently available. The same researchers followed the patients for two years and found they remained essentially relapse- and lesion-free, with biochemical tests showing a positive effect of treatment on the immune system.[15] At three years follow-up a further report was published indicating a fall in relapse rate from 1.2 per year to 0.25.[16]

> Minocycline shows the greatest promise for the oral treatment of MS with the least side effects.

Minocycline is now being studied in a large RCT in combination with glatiramer. More recent research in the animal model of MS has shown that in combination with interferons the drug significantly improves immune responses and outcomes.[17] It has also been shown in combination with one of the statins (cholesterol-lowering drugs) to improve the animal form of MS.[18] It may prove to be a very inexpensive and safe treatment option once further studied.[19] It has been used in standard anti-acne doses. Recently a large scale study has commenced in Canada, looking at minocycline versus placebo after a single episode of demyelination to see if minocycline can slow or prevent the progression to definite MS.[20]

It is interesting to note that researchers have shown in the laboratory that like minocycline, polyunsaturated fats also inhibit matrix metallo-proteinases.[21] This is yet another mechanism by which they are likely to be effective in preventing MS progression.

FINGOLIMOD

An extremely promising therapy which is taken daily by mouth has recently been studied. This drug, fingolimod (also called FTY720), has a uniquely novel mechanism of action. It works on the immune system, but rather than suppressing it or modifying its function, it binds to a receptor on a proportion of circulating lymphocytes and temporarily traps them in lymph nodes. This means a lower number of activated T-cells are available to get into the central nervous system, so inflammation and myelin damage in the brain and spinal cord are reduced. Because the lymphocytes are reversibly trapped in lymph nodes, they are potentially available if needed by the immune system.

Results of the first studies into fingolimod were presented at the AAN meeting in 2006. Patients taking both low and high dose fingolimod had a more than 50 per cent reduction in their annual relapse rate during the first six months of the study compared to placebo. During a twelve-month extension this improvement was maintained. After eighteen months, MRI scans showed that most patients were free from lesions which were actively inflamed.

Side effects were not serious, comprising mostly mild infections like colds and flu and headache. A much larger study in 32 centres in Europe and Canada is currently underway, along with two other major studies of the drug.[22] There is every reason to be very optimistic about this new drug for MS. An important positive is that the drug is taken orally, so injections are unnecessary.

LOW DOSE NALTREXONE (LDN)

One of the more contentious but promising new potential therapies for MS is low dose naltrexone. Naltrexone is a drug which reverses the effects of opiates like morphine or heroin. It is used in clinical practice in people trying to rid themselves of addiction to opiates. How it works in MS and other immune-mediated diseases, if it does, is the subject of some conjecture. But there seems to be overwhelming anecdotal evidence that it prevents relapses and also reduces disease progression.[23] It has been suggested that it acts by reducing cell death in oligodendrocytes. There is considerable evidence available of its apparent benefit in individual cases published in a number of sites on the Internet, but to date there are no results from randomised controlled trials, although several are in progress.

The drug does seem to be very promising, though. An important aspect of this treatment is that it is relatively free of side effects, unlike many of the other heavily promoted immune-modulating therapies on the market. In addition, because it is a generic drug that cannot now be patented it is very cheap, far cheaper than other currently available drugs. This may also explain why it hasn't been studied much to date.

There are, however, a number of trials underway at present. A large RCT of 40 patients taking LDN for Crohn's disease is underway at Penn State University after a pilot study showed that two-thirds of seventeen patients taking the medication went into remission.[24] MS research is underway as well, with an Italian study enrolling 40 patients with primary progressive MS. The study reported early results in 2008,[25] showing that LDN is certainly safe and well tolerated by people with MS. It also showed a beneficial effect on spasticity. A further RCT has finished enrolment at University of California, with 80 patients with relapsing-remitting MS randomised. Results should be available soon. The website www.lowdosenaltrexone.org gives periodic updates on progress.

STATINS

As previously discussed, the cholesterol-lowering drugs are being hailed as possible breakthroughs in the treatment of MS. There is already a wealth of evidence from animal studies that they suppress inflammation and reduce the severity of EAE. A study reported in the prestigious journal *Nature* in 2002 showed that atorvastatin, one of this class of drugs, prevented or even reversed paralysis in laboratory animals with EAE.[26] A small pilot study on simvastatin reported to the AAN in 2003 showed a 43 per cent reduction in MRI detected lesions in 30 patients treated for six months. There were no serious side effects reported. Larger studies are underway in several centres. There is also experimental work to show that statins stabilise the blood-brain barrier, and so should be helpful in MS.[27]

Given the experience we have with this group of drugs and their documented safety profile, this is a most promising avenue for treating MS. However, from the work of Swank and others previously discussed, it is likely that a very low saturated-fat diet is considerably more effective than the statins and, of course, is free of negative side effects. It has previously been shown that diet and statins are roughly equivalent in their effects on improving the fat profile in people with raised cholesterol.[28] The fact that diet is very likely to be much more effective than these drugs in MS is probably due to it working in a number of ways to improve MS, including altering the fat profile, causing a shift to a Th2 immune response and neuro-protection, at least.

CANNABIS-RELATED DRUGS

There has long been interest in evaluating drugs which are extracted from cannabis (cannabinoids) in treating certain aspects of MS, particularly pain and spasticity. Indeed, results of clinical trials have been so promising, that a drug consisting of various extracts of the cannabis plant (Sativex) was made available by prescription in Canada in June 2005. The drug is delivered as a spray under the tongue. Perras has summarised the trials involving cannabinoids in MS.[29] He notes that five RCTs have been performed comparing the spray against placebo. Generally, pain, spasticity, muscle cramps and sleep disturbance were all improved. Side effects included dizziness, fatigue and feeling intoxicated.

A recent study, the Cannabinoids in MS (CAMS) Study, examined 630 patients from 33 UK centres.[30] It found some benefit for spasticity, and patients felt the drug was helpful. More detailed study has shown that cannabinoids shift the Th1/Th2 balance towards a Th2 profile, and thus may be of benefit in the immunomodulation of MS. Further, they may have a beneficial effect on the degenerative aspects of the disease.[31, 32]

BONE MARROW TRANSPLANTATION

A number of researchers have suggested that, since MS is effectively an error in the programming of the immune system, then a possible treatment would be to destroy all the bone marrow, either with chemotherapy like some blood cancer treatments or with radiation, and then start again with a 'new' immune system. This is very dangerous therapy and would be reserved for those with very serious rapidly progressive disease. It has been used for various blood cancers such as leukaemia but because the immune system is temporarily knocked out, the individual is susceptible to all sorts of infections, and so a number of patients may die during treatment. Researchers reporting to the AAN in 2003 dampened initial optimism for this therapy. A number of the patients treated to that time had progressed, particularly those with pronounced disability to begin with, just the group likely to be treated with this therapy.

More promising was the report in 2005 from an Italian group.[33] They described 21 patients with very severe MS unresponsive to other treatments who had been transplanted with stem cells from their bone marrow. There was a dramatic improvement, with MRI evidence of brain inflammation virtually disappearing. This is good news indeed for people with severe MS which doesn't respond to other therapies. But it needs to be borne in mind that the procedure is very risky, and that it must be done in highly specialised centres which have experience with the technique.

GOAT SERUM ('AIMSPRO')

This product has been the subject of much discussion and controversy. Goats are apparently injected with inactivated HIV, and the antibodies then produced are claimed to have an anti-inflammatory effect for people with MS. It has been suggested that the drug shifts the immune system balance towards a TH2 response, but also that there is a direct effect on nerves, improving conduction.

Initial results of trials sounded very promising. An Internet report of a trial at St George's Hospital in London noted that in 130 patients receiving the treatment, 85 per cent had improvements in symptoms without any side effects.[34] Since then the situation with Aimspro has soured substantially. *The Sunday Times* in the United Kingdom reported on 26 November 2006 that the company making the drug was under criminal investigation for the way it marketed the drug, noting that the company's chairman and finance directors were both discharged bankrupts. At this point it looks like Aimspro is not the promising therapy it was claimed to be, and may well be ineffective.

T–CELL VACCINATION

As previously discussed, modern medicine is getting very close to manipulating the immune response to produce specific outcomes. Israeli scientists chose a group of twenty people with MS who had not responded to standard disease-modifying drugs, and tried a completely new technique.[35] Here they removed T-cells from these people, activated them with synthetic myelin base protein and myelin oligodendrocyte glycoprotein, the proposed targets of the immune response in MS. They then inactivated the cells and injected them back into the patients. The idea behind this is complex, but basically the body should then develop an immune response to the T-cells, reducing their number and activity and thus reducing the activity of the illness. This is indeed what happened. The annual relapse rate fell from 2.6 to 1.1, a dramatic drop, and there was a reduction in the number of new lesions on MRI. While the long-term consequences of altering the immune response in this way are unknown, the treatment holds promise, certainly at least for those people who do not respond to drug therapies. A 2009 study of this group who had not responded to conventional therapies was very promising, with an 85 per cent reduction in relapse rate by the end of a year of treatment.[36]

DNA VACCINATION

Another very exciting prospect for people with MS is that of DNA vaccination. This basically takes the part of the genetic sequence of a person with MS that codes for myelin base protein and uses it to vaccinate the person, so that they develop an immune response against that part of their own DNA. It is very experimental, but in one study in 2008 from Texas researchers vaccinated a person with MS with this experimental vaccine and found a decrease in inflammatory cytokines as well as decreased antibodies to myelin in the spinal fluid.[37]

This has now been further explored in a large RCT. Using two different doses of the DNA vaccine BHT–3009 compared with placebo in 267 people with MS, the researchers found that after eight weeks there was a statistically significant 61 per cent reduction in the number of new lesions, but only with the lower dose.[38] The method of administration was by intramuscular injection at weeks 0, 2, 4, and every four weeks thereafter. This treatment appears to hold great promise. It is not clear if it will cause any side effects long term, although it appears very safe in the short-term clinical trial.

SYNTHETIC PEPTIDE MBP8298

This is a human-made molecule designed to be very similar to myelin base protein (MBP), one of the likely targets of auto-immunity in MS. In theory, giving a big dose of this peptide periodically should cause the immune system to become tolerant of its own myelin and lessen its attack on it. A major study comparing intravenous injections of MBP8298 every six months with placebo showed that in certain sub-groups of people with MS there was a dramatic (over 75%) reduction in progression of disability in progressive MS.[39] These results are highly impressive and offer great hope for people with progressive MS.

FUMARIC ACID ESTERS

Fumaric acid esters have been used in the treatment of psoriasis, a disease with a known immune basis. In EAE in animals fumaric acid esters had favourable effects,[40] and in a small study of ten patients with relapsing-remitting MS, fumaric acid esters significantly reduced the number and volume of new MS lesions as well as showing positive immune effects.[41] More recently, a Swiss RCT of 257 people with relapsing-remitting MS randomly assigned participants to receive fumarate in three doses versus placebo.[42] The highest dose reduced the mean number of new MRI lesions by 69 per cent but made no significant difference to relapse rate. Side effects unfortunately were common including abdominal pain, flushing, headache, fatigue and hot flushes. The drug is being further studied.

TERIFLUNOMIDE

This new drug has recently been trialled against placebo in 179 people with relapsing-remitting or progressive MS with relapses.[43] Again, it has the advantage of being taken by mouth. It was shown to roughly halve the number of new lesions and to delay disease progression. The drug was well tolerated. There is considerable hope that this new drug may be useful.

OVERVIEW

Overall, the results obtained by using these therapies which either suppress or modulate immune function have been extremely encouraging. For people with relapsing-remitting MS which is very active and doesn't seem to be responding to any of the available therapies (either lifestyle change or drug therapies, or both), these treatment options offer great hope. There is a wealth of other new therapies just around the corner, with minocycline and the statins at this stage appearing the safest and simplest to take, and a number of other newer oral medications likely to become available. People with MS can take a lot of hope from many of these preliminary studies. It is quite possible that the oral medications, once tested adequately, will replace the current injected disease-modifying treatments.

17

VIRUSES AND ANTI-VIRAL TREATMENT

Infection with Epstein-Barr virus has been associated with an increased risk of multiple sclerosis

L.I. Levin

The theory that MS is triggered by a viral infection has been around for a very long time. When I was a medical student the theory was that the measles virus was somehow reactivated later in life to cause MS. Most authorities now feel that viruses are probably involved, but that the story is not straightforward.

EPIDEMIOLOGICAL EVIDENCE

The evidence that viruses play a part in causing MS is largely epidemiological. There has been lots of speculation about the very uneven worldwide distribution of MS. As we have seen, there is good evidence that it is related to diet and exposure to sunlight, but there is also considerable opinion that it relates to viral infections. Probably the most important part of this theory is that people who migrate to other countries change their risk of getting MS.[1] But the age at which they migrate seems to be

SUMMARISING THE EVIDENCE

- A number of viruses have been linked to causing or triggering MS.
  - Human herpes virus 6, Epstein-Barr virus (glandular fever virus), and varicella-zoster virus are the most likely candidates; it is likely that any of these may trigger the disease in susceptible people.
  - Varicella-zoster virus may be a trigger for relapses in MS.
- Anti-viral agents have been inadequately studied despite promising preliminary work.

EVIDENCE-BASED RECOMMENDATIONS

- It is too early to recommend anti-viral agents for the treatment of MS.

critically important, raising the possibility that something happens to them before that age, possibly infection with a certain virus.

In other words, a child under the age of fifteen years going from a country of high incidence, say Denmark, to one of low incidence, say Singapore, acquires the risk of the new area; that is, the chance of getting MS goes down substantially. But an adult doing the same keeps the risk as if staying in Denmark. This strongly suggests some environmental agent, possibly a virus, affects the individual around the age of fifteen. Potentially, this provides the right 'soil' for the later development of MS, precipitated by dietary fats and perhaps lack of sunlight. Recent Australian epidemiological data, however, has disputed these observations about age at migration being important.[2]

Other epidemiological studies have shown a correlation between the incidence of varicella (herpes zoster or shingles) infection and MS.[3] More recent work has shown that this virus is very commonly (95%) present in immune cells of MS patients having relapses compared with other common viruses, but not present commonly in people without MS.[4] There have been regular reports of clusters of cases of MS occurring in particular geographical areas,[1] and several epidemiological studies showing that relapses occur much more frequently after viral infections.[5]

Whether this is due to the particular virus triggering or causing the relapse or a general activation of the immune system is not clear.

HUMAN HERPES VIRUS 6

A lot of work has gone into finding the particular virus which may be causing MS in nervous tissue of people with MS. The most promising leads have related to a type of herpes virus, human herpes virus 6 or HHV-6, and to the Epstein-Barr virus which causes glandular fever. Herpes viruses include herpes simplex, which causes common cold sores and genital herpes, and herpes zoster, which causes shingles. Herpes viruses are good candidates for causing CNS problems, because after an attack of cold sores for example, they persist in the nervous system and are reactivated to again cause infection. HHV-6 causes a common condition in children called roseola. Recently HHV-6 protein and DNA have been found in active MS lesions,[6, 7] and antibodies to HHV-6 have been found in patients after relapses.[8] People with MS have also been found to have higher antibody levels to HHV-6 than those in the general population.[9]

It has been clearly shown that reactivation of HHV-6 infection is closely associated with relapses in MS.[10] This study showed that the risk of relapse in MS was much higher for patients with active HHV-6 infection than for those with inactive infection, again raising potential for suppressing MS activity by suppressing herpes infection with medication. A further study by Scottish researchers in 2005 showed that HHV-6 was present in post-mortem specimens from people with MS at a much higher rate than in the rest of the population,[11] and other autopsy studies have confirmed this finding.[12] A study from New York looked at biopsied lesions from five MS patients who had biopsies because they were thought to have brain tumours.[13] All five had evidence of HHV-6 in all the studied lesions. Another study revealed that treatment with interferon reduced the amount of HHV-6 in people with MS who were having relapses but not in those in remission, suggesting a role for HHV-6 in causing relapses.[14] A Spanish study found HHV-6 in significantly more patients with relapsing-remitting MS than those with secondary progressive disease.[15]

EPSTEIN–BARR VIRUS (EBV)

There is now quite a bit of research implicating the virus known to cause glandular fever, the Epstein-Barr virus (EBV) in the development of MS.[16, 17, 18] One ingenious study looked at blood samples collected from around 3 million US military personnel at their time of enlistment and their subsequent development of MS. Those who had high antibodies to EBV at the time of enlistment, that is, those who had had the viral infection even up to five years before the onset of MS, had a twenty to 30 times higher risk of getting the disease than those with very low antibody levels.[16]

> A number of viruses can cause or trigger MS in susceptible people.

Another study using data from the large US Nurses Health Study showed that nurses who developed MS were 2.5 times as likely to have had EBV in their blood when first enrolled in the study before diagnosis, compared with those who did not develop MS.[19] A further Swedish study showed that people who later develop MS show a heightened immune response to the EBV.[20] A case-control study in children showed that 86 per cent of those with MS showed evidence of EBV infection compared with 64 per cent of matched children without MS (p=0.025).[21] A Canadian population study of over 14,000 people with MS and their spouses as controls showed that those with MS were a little more than twice as likely to have had EBV infection.[22]

These data and others were summarised in a 2009 meta-analysis of all the studies on EBV and MS which concluded that the combined risk of MS after glandular fever from fourteen pooled studies was more than double (2.3) that of the population that had not had EBV infection.[23]

These and other researchers have concluded that EBV infection is associated with the development of MS. Interestingly, it is also implicated in other auto-immune diseases such as rheumatoid arthritis where evidence of EBV infection has been found in affected joints.[24] It is likely that in susceptible people, that is, those with the 'right' genetic make-up and perhaps the right sort of environmental triggers, say lack of sunlight and fish oil, infection with EBV may in some way trigger the onset of auto-immune illness later in life. These factors may also modify the response of the person to EBV and determine whether or not EBV infection results in MS.[25] Whether this will help us determine some way of preventing or treating the disease, however, is another question. Researchers have suggested that vaccination against EBV may prevent MS developing in susceptible individuals,[26] although to date a vaccine has not been developed.

VARICELLA–ZOSTER VIRUS (VZV)

Most recently there has been a resurgence of interest in the varicella-zoster virus (VZV). This virus is one of the herpes family of viruses, and is responsible for measles (varicella) in children and young adults and shingles (zoster) in later life. For many years there was a suspicion that measles infection was somehow related to MS, but recently detailed laboratory work has established a clear link with VZV and MS.

A small Mexican study published in 2005 examined 82 consecutive patients with MS and found that six had either varicella or zoster concurrent with the development or progress of their illness.[27] In 2007, an Italian group published findings of their laboratory detection of VZV in the spinal fluid of people with MS, other neurological illnesses and healthy volunteers.[28] They found that none of the healthy people had the virus, about 10 per cent of those with other neurological diseases had evidence of it, and over 40 per cent of those with MS had it. This suggested that VZV played a part in the development of MS.

Later in 2007, a Mexican group published results of their laboratory studies of immune cells of people with MS and healthy volunteers.[29] They noted that, while none of the healthy people had VZV in their immune cells, 95 per cent of people with MS who were having a relapse had VZV, and 17 per cent of those in remission had evidence of the virus. Demonstrating this close association with relapses added considerable weight to the hypothesis that VZV plays a causal role in the development of MS.

A 2008 study from Mexico provided the strongest possible evidence yet of a direct link between VZV and MS.[30] The researchers used electron microscopy, a method that highly magnifies bodily tisses and fluid so that minute particles are visible, to look at the spinal fluid of people with MS compared with healthy volunteers. They looked at fifteen people with MS during relapse, nineteen with MS during remission, and 28 healthy control subjects. They found particles identical in appearance to VZV in the spinal fluid of the people with MS who were having relapses but none in those in remission or the healthy volunteers. Interestingly, they found the number of particles fell away steadily as people recovered from the relapses.

This is important evidence that VZV is likely to play a direct role in the development of MS and the initiation of relapses. What is most relevant here for people with MS is that VZV is one of the herpes viruses, and hence is able to be prevented and treated with the cyclovir group of antiviral drugs to be discussed shortly.

HOW MIGHT A VIRUS CAUSE MS?

The theory which has recently been put forward is that the virus structure is in parts very similar to the base proteins in myelin which seem to be the target of immune system attack in MS.[31] Why should this happen in some people and not others? It has been suggested that this may only occur in genetically susceptible people, that is, people with the 'right' physical make-up for MS to be triggered. This still leaves a lot of questions unanswered, and most authorities are not convinced this is the answer. From what we have seen, it is also possible that the state of the lipid membranes in the CNS may influence whether the myelin is susceptible to immune attack. Membranes which are flexible and pliable, like those in people who eat mainly polyunsaturated fats, may be less prone to this auto-immune injury.

ANTI-VIRAL AGENTS

Most virus infections are not treatable. While we have really good antibiotics for a whole range of bacterial infections, such as those causing pneumonia, boils and ear infections, rendering many of these diseases a nuisance instead of the lethal diseases of yesteryear, we are still searching for effective antiviral agents. The common cold still lays low millions of people each year, and we are powerless to prevent it. The one virus for which this is not true is the herpes virus. A range of anti-viral agents typified by acyclovir has become available for the treatment of herpes virus infections. These agents are highly effective, and are relatively free from side effects. They are thought to hold great promise for the treatment of MS.

Acyclovir has been used to treat cold sores, shingles and genital herpes, as well as herpes encephalitis. However, it has a relatively short-lived effect in the body and must be taken five times a day for full benefit. A newer range of these drugs has more recently become available. The most commonly prescribed of these is famciclovir. This drug has been shown to suppress genital herpes when taken twice daily in a dose of 250mg. Again, it is very safe and can be taken long term.

RCTS OF ANTI-VIRAL AGENTS FOR MS

Despite the promise of relatively safe anti-viral treatment with acyclovir-like drugs against herpes viruses, there has been little controlled study of this area so far. When researching this for the first book, I could only find one RCT reported in Medline despite suggestions in the literature that these drugs may be effective.[32] Since then another study has reported, this one using the longer acting anti-viral agent of the same family, valacyclovir. Ideally, I would like to see combination therapy tried. Now that we have established both interferon and glatiramer as effective treatments, it should be easy to use one as a control group, with a combination, either of interferon and glatiramer, or one of these plus acyclovir, or even all three, as the treatment group.

The initial RCT in the area was by Lycke and co-workers published in 1996.[33] This study was extremely promising but suffered from having only a small number of patients. As I explained in the discussion on p values earlier, the bigger the number of patients in a trial the more likely the result is to be statistically significant, that is, p<0.05. In other words, if the difference between the treatment and control groups is large, only a small number of patients is required for a significant result. If the difference is small, however, the trial needs to have a lot of patients to achieve significance. This is one of the reasons why the interferon studies have shown a highly significant result, even though the effect of the treatment has been relatively small.

Lycke and co-workers randomised 60 patients to receive either acyclovir 800mg three times a day, or placebo three times a day for two years. Immediately there is a problem with the study. Acyclovir really needs to be given five times a day to ensure adequate levels in the blood. Despite this, treated patients had 34 per cent fewer relapses than the placebo group. They went from a relapse rate of 1.57 per year to 1.03 a year. This is a treatment effect comparable to interferon and glatiramer, yet it hasn't been taken up by the medical profession. Why?

The answer is simple. The p value for the trial was 0.083. After my previous discussion, it's clear that this was most likely due to the small number of patients in the study. In the comparable interferon study the number of patients was 372, hence the lower p value. I imagine it is infuriating for people with MS to read this. You must wonder why the researchers simply didn't enrol more patients in the study so that a significant p value could be reached, and the therapy regarded as definitely of value. It is not that simple.

Research is difficult. For a disease like MS, in a given geographical area, it is often difficult to find enough patients to enrol in a trial. That is why major research tends to be done in so-called multi-centre trials, where patients are recruited from many different areas, perhaps even many different countries, and is usually backed by large drug companies because of the expense involved. This leads to issues of conflict of interest, and we know that the results of trials sponsored by drug companies are less reliable than those not.

One of the problems with publishing the results of a small trial which has a p value just over 0.05, such as this one, is that it tends to act as a deterrent to further study in the area. Doctors reading the publication say that the therapy is not 'proven' and tend not to investigate it further. Fortunately, with the recent basic scientific work on HHV-6 and VZV in MS patients, I suspect much more work on these drugs will now be done.

Lycke and colleagues went back to the data. If they grouped patients according to relapse rates into low (0–2), medium (3–5) and high (6–8) rate groups, the difference between acyclovir and placebo treatment was significant with a p value of 0.017. They went further and looked at only those patients in the study who had had MS for over two years, so that a previous relapse rate could be determined. When they compared the relapse rate while in the trial to the pre-existing relapse rate, the acyclovir-treated group had a much reduced relapse rate, with a p value of 0.024.

This sort of after-the-event data analysis is frowned upon in research circles. It is felt that researchers should declare up front the questions they will be asking of their data at the end of the study. Otherwise, so-called 'data dredging' goes on, where researchers fish through their data, looking for ways of rearranging the numbers so that a significant result will be produced. So the scientific community was still left with the message that anti-viral therapy looks promising but remains 'unproven'.

Friedman and colleagues in 2005 reported results of an RCT using valacyclovir in 58 patients with MS.[34] They too found a trend towards better outcomes but the p value again did not quite reach significance at the 0.05 level. The data really suggest that the studies are too small to detect a significant treatment effect, and that bigger studies are needed. Researchers in Houston, Texas have speculated that some of the effects of the interferons in MS might be due to their anti-viral properties as much as their effects on the immune system.[35] Blood from patients with MS who were on interferon was compared with blood from untreated people with MS and people without MS. It was shown that interferon reduced the activity of HHV-6, and it was felt that this may have contributed to its effect on MS.

OVERVIEW

There is substantial evidence that a virus or viruses are involved in the development of MS. The viruses most implicated at this stage seem to be HHV-6 and EBV. Treatment with anti-virals such as longer acting versions of acyclovir holds great promise for the herpes virus. A few small studies have already suggested treatment may reduce relapse rates by the same degree as the accepted MS treatment drugs interferon and glatiramer. There seems little downside risk to these medications, unlike some of the more accepted therapies, and they can be taken orally. These drugs are, however, costly and are not yet licensed for the treatment of MS.

18

PAIN AND FATIGUE: EVIDENCE-BASED PREVENTION AND MANAGEMENT

Pain is inevitable; suffering is optional

Unknown

PAIN

It is very clear now that MS is not just a disease causing motor and sensory symptoms, and that some of the other symptoms are just as, or more, disabling. Pain appears to be experienced by the majority of people with MS. In one Australian study, 64 per cent of participants reported chronic pain.[1] In this study, pain was closely associated with reduced quality of life. Unlike other forms of pain the pain in MS is often neuropathic, that is, derived from damage to the nervous system. This pain is typically the most difficult pain to treat medically, and is not responsive to the usual pain-killing medications used for other common types of pain.

The medical options used to treat pain in MS are very limited indeed. Doctors typically prescribe antidepressants or anti-epileptic medications, both of which are known to modify the subjective experience of pain. However, there are few if any studies of their effectiveness for this purpose. Italian MS researchers in 2005 looked at the prescription of anti-epileptic

SUMMARISING THE EVIDENCE

- MS is not a painless disease; around two-thirds of people with MS experience chronic pain, often associated with reduced quality of life.
  - Several anti-epileptic agents have been used in managing MS pain, with little success; these medications have many side effects.
  - Meditation offers an important alternative way to manage MS pain.
- Fatigue is very common, affecting over 80 per cent of people with MS; it is often the most troublesome symptom, and can significantly affect quality of life.
  - Fatigue in MS almost certainly has a physical basis.
  - Energy conservation strategies, cognitive behaviour therapy, relaxation therapy and exercise have been used to effectively manage fatigue.
  - Drugs don't help; some commonly used MS medications worsen fatigue.

EVIDENCE-BASED RECOMMENDATIONS

- Drugs are not recommended for the chronic pain of MS and the side effects can be more of a problem than the pain.
  - Meditation can help MS pain.
- Exercise, behaviour therapy and energy conservation strategies can be used to improve fatigue.

drugs in their practice.[2] They found that carbamazepine (Tegretol) was prescribed for 36 people, with adverse effects reported in over half the cases. Gabapentin was prescribed more commonly, for 94 people, with adverse effects in a smaller proportion (sixteen cases). Lamotrigine was prescribed for 22 people, with adverse effects in four.

Really the incidence of side effects was too common, especially for carbamazepine, to suggest that these drugs should be used for pain. Worse, with carbamazepine, a third of patients had significant deterioration of neurological functioning, to the point where the treated patients appeared to be having a relapse. Interestingly, a well-constructed RCT from North Carolina showed that lamotrigine, added to existing drugs for pain in a group of people with neurological pain, made no difference whatsoever to the pain.[3]

Really these anti-epileptic drugs should not be prescribed for pain in MS, or probably in any other condition. Marcia Angell, former editor-in-chief of the *New England Journal of Medicine*, gives a good account of how gabapentin (trade name Neurontin in the United States) was foisted on to an unsuspecting public via 'education' of doctors about its supposed benefits for pain.[4] In fact it was approved by the FDA for a very narrow indication, that is, for epilepsy when other drugs had failed, but was heavily promoted by the drug company for management of chronic pain to the point where it became a blockbuster drug, with sales of over US$2.7 billion in 2003.

In fact there was never any convincing evidence that it had much effect on pain. In May 2004 Pfizer, the drug company marketing gabapentin, pleaded guilty to 'illegal marketing' and was fined US$430 million. But what about all the people, many of them with MS, who remained on the drug, believing it was doing them some good?

It seems clear that we need to focus on other ways of dealing with pain in MS than relying on conventional medication. There is a variety of meditations which specifically focus on pain, and its reduction. Certainly, they offer great advantages over drug therapy, particularly when it comes to side effects. The Gawler Foundation (www.gawler.org) can provide guidance in this area. A 2009 study showed that self-hypnosis was quite effective in managing pain in MS, somewhat more effective than progressive muscle relaxation.[5]

It is interesting to note that Israeli researchers have shown that omega-3 polyunsaturated fats have quite specific effects on pain, apart from their action in decreasing inflammation by lowering the levels of pro-inflammatory cytokines, as we discussed earlier.[6] Specifically they seem to have a direct action on nerve cells, improving neuropathic pain, in addition to their anti-inflammatory effects.

> Drug management of pain in MS has been disappointing; alternative methods offer more hope of relief without side effects.

Other symptoms besides pain such as pins and needles, muscle cramps and spasticity can also be very troublesome for many people with

MS, particularly those who have a large number of lesions. Drug treatments have not been very helpful for these symptoms, hence my focus on preventing them in the first place with lifestyle changes, or taking steroids for relapses very early and for relapses which many doctors do not feel require steroid treatment, such as sensory relapses. One of the few drug therapies to have had any success is botulinum toxin ('Botox') used as an injection into muscles in which there is spasticity.[7] Particularly with early physiotherapy after the injection, there can be substantial relief of symptoms.

A promising option for people who have these troubling symptoms is reflexology. An Israeli study randomised 71 people with MS to a treatment group who received specific reflexology, and a control group who had non-specific massage of the calf.[8] The study found significant benefit in reducing pins and needles and spasticity, but also in improving urinary symptoms. The reduction in pins and needles was still present three months after therapy. Another study found positive psychological and physical benefit from relexology.[9]

Another very interesting possibility is the use of vitamin D to relieve neuropathic pain. Australian researchers have shown in people with type 2 diabetes who have pain caused by nervous system disease that vitamin D improved the pain dramatically, reducing it by up to 50 per cent.[10] This was in people who were vitamin D deficient, but it is quite conceivable that even for people who are not vitamin D deficient, raising the vitamin D level to high normal levels may also improve pain. As previously discussed in the section on sunlight, what is currently considered a normal vitamin D level may not be optimal. And we know that vitamin D has neuro-protective effects.

FATIGUE

Fatigue is the most common serious symptom felt by people with MS. It has been said to affect over 80 per cent of people with MS; in one study, 25 per cent of people said their activities were often or always limited by fatigue;[11] another showed 75 per cent of people with MS had persistent or sporadic fatigue.[12] A large Swedish study showed that 27 per cent of people with MS were persistently fatigued, 19 per cent never fatigued and the remainder varied, being fatigued sometimes and other times not.[13] Some people describe fatigue as their most troublesome symptom,[14] and researchers have shown that fatigue is a good predictor of both mental and physical quality of life for people with MS.[15]

Many researchers have tried to explain fatigue in terms of emotional distress or relate it to depression. US researchers for instance have shown that people with MS who report disabling fatigue are much more likely (76%) to be depressed than those who do not (31%).[11] However, recent studies demonstrate a clear physical basis for fatigue. US researchers showed that fatigue correlated closely with the degree of brain atrophy[16] and researchers in Nottingham in the United Kingdom have shown close correlation with MRI changes in the grey matter of the brain.[14]

A rather unique Norwegian study looked at psychiatric and mood problems in a large group of MS people and compared them with a group of patients with systemic lupus erythematosus (SLE), another auto-immune disorder.[17] The study found that MS people showed very high levels of irritability and apathy compared with the SLE patients, and that these were quite independent of level of disability. Nearly half the MS patients displayed irritability and a third apathy, many more than the SLE patients. The researchers concluded that these features were specific to MS, and were likely due to the underlying brain injury occurring due to the disease. Interestingly, brain lesions have been noted in people with SLE.[18] Researchers found more brain abnormalities were associated with greater levels of fatigue.

I suspect these mood disturbances cross over to some extent with fatigue, and some people with MS, knowing only that fatigue is common in MS, describe these feelings as fatigue. It seems certain that medical professionals are largely unaware of the presence of these features in a large proportion of people with MS. And fatigue is a particularly difficult symptom to manage, as it tends to persist over time. One Spanish study showed that 87 per cent of people who had fatigue at the onset of the study were still fatigued at eighteen months.[19] In this study fatigue did not seem to correlate with progression of disability or relapses, but with the presence of depression. Other studies have also found a close association with depression, and also with level of disability.[12, 13]

It is important to recognise that fatigue in MS can also be secondary to other features of the disease.[20] For instance, many people with MS have trouble sleeping because of pain or spasticity, or anxiety about the condition. Depression is also a very potent cause of insomnia. The insomnia in turn may lead people to being very fatigued. So both the primary form of fatigue, due to the illness itself, and these secondary forms of fatigue need to be looked for when people with MS attend their health carers.

Finding strategies that can prevent or improve fatigue and associated symptoms is clearly very important, but often not seen as a key issue. This is disappointing, as studies have shown that not only is fatigue very common, but that it is the primary reason why people can no longer work full-time. In one study, 90 per cent of people working part-time blamed fatigue as the reason for their change in work status.[21] In this study, employment status was not related to age, sex, the duration of the disease or cognitive functioning.

A number of studies have used psychological or social interventions to modify fatigue successfully.[22, 23, 24] One study used energy conservation techniques and found they significantly reduced fatigue severity and impact.[22] The most helpful strategies were simplifying activities, adjusting priorities, changing body position, resting and planning the day to balance work and rest.

An RCT of 72 people with MS who experienced fatigue compared cognitive behaviour therapy with relaxation therapy, and both in comparison with a control group who did not have fatigue.[25] Both cognitive behaviour therapy and relaxation therapy effectively treated the fatigue, with cognitive behaviour therapy having the greatest effect, but both groups reported levels of fatigue similar to the healthy comparison group, even at six months after treatment. One US RCT showed an improvement in fatigue with yoga and aerobic exercise.[26] Others from Iran[27] and Brazil[28] have shown that fatigue improves after a graded exercise program.

Others have tried drug therapy for fatigue, mostly without success, although a small RCT showed that regular aspirin was significantly better than placebo at improving symptoms of fatigue.[29] A drug used to promote wakefulness, modafinil, which is sometimes used to treat fatigue in clinical practice, has been trialled with mixed results. After promising early work,[30, 31] 72 patients with MS in a US study were started on placebo, then took modafinil, then went back to placebo.[32] The researchers found significantly improved fatigue while on the drug. A more recent RCT was not so promising, with 115 patients being randomised to either modafinil or placebo, but no difference in fatigue between the groups at five weeks.[33] A recent evidence-based review concluded that modafinil had no greater effect than placebo in fatigue.[34] Promoting wakefulness may not be the best strategy for overcoming fatigue, as it has been shown that people with MS commonly have disordered sleep and that this contributes to their fatigue.[35]

> Fatigue in MS has a physical basis.

Other drugs tried include amantadine, which seems to be of help in about a third of cases, and pemoline, a stimulant which has not been shown to be of benefit.[31] It is important to note here that the interferons used in the management of MS seem to worsen fatigue more than the other disease-modifying drugs. Researchers have shown that patients on glatiramer are twice as likely to have reduced fatigue while on therapy than those taking interferon.[36] Further, changing from interferon to glatiramer is very likely to reduce fatigue, while changing the other way has been shown to worsen fatigue.[37] Another study in 2008 of 291 people with MS commenced on glatiramer showed that the drug reduced fatigue significantly, and more than halved the number of sick days taken off work.[38]

It is very likely that diet plays a part in fatigue. Researchers have shown that Th1 cytokines are associated with worse fatigue,[39] and we know that the Swank diet and fish oil shift the immune balance away from the Th1 towards a Th2 response, and that is likely to be beneficial for fatigue. Supplements may also be helpful. One small study showed that gingko biloba supplements improved fatigue and functional performance,[40] although this was not confirmed in a larger study.[41] In general, it appears that these lifestyle and psychosocial changes are more likely to be helpful than drugs.

OVERVIEW

Pain and fatigue are particularly troubling symptoms experienced by the majority of people with MS. Conventional drug treatment options are very limited. It is important that steroids are considered for sensory relapses in MS, so that the later development of neuropathic pain related to these lesions is minimised. Once established, pain may be best approached with a holistic approach, particularly concentrating on meditation, reflexology and psychological support.

Likewise, fatigue responds poorly to drug therapy. However, there is evidence that it is reduced with some lifestyle interventions such as diet and exercise, as well as behaviour therapy and energy conservation techniques.

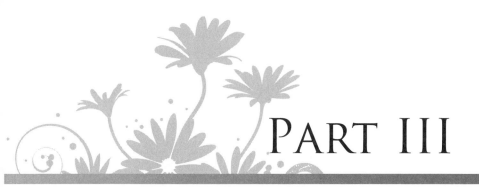

PART III

RECOMMENDATIONS

19

THE RECOVERY PROGRAM:
EVIDENCE-BASED LIFE-STYLE AND THERAPY RECOMMENDATIONS

The natural healing force within each of us is the greatest force in getting well

Hippocrates

Living with MS can be very difficult. From the moment of diagnosis, the whole world changes. It is never the same again. For people like me who are the main breadwinners in the family at the time of diagnosis, the first major concerns often revolve around continuing to provide for the family. But over time a healthy self-interest needs to be added, just like the analogy of putting oxygen masks in a plane emergency on yourself first before others, or you won't be able to help others. MS affects young people, and women in greater numbers than men. I was comparatively lucky. I was 45 when MS struck. Much of my life had already been lived. Today for many young women with MS, the issues are very difficult to balance. Many are trying simultaneously to raise a family and provide an income, often on their own. All of these issues crowd around us as we try to live on as normal.

PRIORITIES

- Accept the diagnosis and express the associated grief.
- Determine to do *whatever it takes* to get well.
- Commit to an ongoing process of exploring and resolving emotional and spiritual 'dis-ease' and resolving unfinished business.
  - This may be facilitated by keeping a diary, talking to friends or counsellors, attending an MS group and meditating.
- Embrace the Recovery Program as a new way of living well.

THE RECOVERY PROGRAM

- *Diet and supplements*
  - A plant-based, wholefood diet, plus seafood, avoiding saturated and altered fats.
  - Omega-3 fatty acids, in 20g (20ml) a day of flaxseed or fish oil or in fish.
  - Optional B group vitamins, or B12 supplement if needed.
- *Vitamin D*
  - Sunlight fifteen minutes daily three to five times a week exposing most of the body.
  - Vitamin D3 supplement of 5000IU daily in winter or if no sun in summer, aiming for a blood level of around 150nmol/L.
- *Meditation*
  - 30 minutes daily.
- *Exercise*
  - Twenty to 30 minutes preferably at least five times a week.
- *Medication*
  - Take one of the disease-modifying drugs regularly.
  - Prednisone or prednisolone (equivalent) 500–1000mg orally for three to five days for distressing relapses.
  - Consider mitoxantrone if the disease is very active, continuing with one of the disease-modifying drugs thereafter.

PRIORITIES

The most important thing is not to deteriorate physically and mentally. This has to be the priority, and the evidence I have assembled strongly suggests that in most cases this is achievable. Once this is achieved, then it is a realistic prospect to hope for genuine healing and recovery. It helps enormously to start as soon after diagnosis as possible with the process of healing emotionally. As we have seen in the chapter on mind–body medicine, failure to express grief and difficult emotions related to the illness can literally make people sicker. Most people when diagnosed with MS are suddenly faced with the loss of many things they have taken for granted for much of their lives; things like the ability to run, walk, look after themselves physically, even go to the toilet. The sense of loss can be profound. Some people feel that the spiritual force in their lives has abandoned them. Naturally, these losses are associated with immense grief.

But many of us find it difficult to express grief. We may have been brought up in families where keeping a stiff upper lip was considered a priority. Or we may find comfort in denial. I feel it is impossible to really start making the changes needed to recover from MS until the diagnosis and the associated potential loss has been faced and accepted, and the grief expressed. This may be through writing or music, keeping a diary, talking to loved ones and friends, seeing a counsellor or attending an MS group. Allowing the emotion to flow without resistance, allowing it to drain away, is really important. Many people find that once they start this process of getting more in touch with their emotions, they find it easier to also confront other emotional problems that are more longstanding. I feel it is useful to commit to a continuous process of exploring and resolving emotional and spiritual 'dis-ease' and unfinished business. Often it is these past, poorly resolved issues that make and keep people sick.

From the day of diagnosis, or the day of reading this book, I feel it is important that you decide to do whatever it takes to stop the disease from progressing. Resolving this moves one from being a passive to an active participant in life after the diagnosis. Adopting the position of waiting for deterioration, as is sometimes recommended, is a very negative, passive place to be and is not conducive to recovery. A major review on brain-immune function in MS has summarised the literature on this, noting that: 'In MS, a problem-focused coping style (e.g. an active effort to change a situation) has often been associated with better adjustment, less disability and less depressive symptoms. A more passive . . . strategy seems to be less adaptive and often goes along with increased psychological distress, increased levels of overall stress and negative mood and depression.'[1]

For me, this was an easy decision to make. I had the experience of seeing first-hand the effects of very aggressive disease on my mother. Many people who haven't had this background, and are unfamiliar with the disease, are tempted to ignore the disease, using denial, as if there will be no problem if they just get on with life.

If there is any doubt about how bad things can get, or if there is temptation to occasionally falter and say it's not worth all the effort, it is important to consider the alternative. Once the damage is done, there is currently considered to be no way of undoing it. For people who feel it's all a bit depressing changing eating habits and lifestyle significantly, and perhaps regularly injecting medication, imagine how much more difficult things would be not being able to walk or pass urine normally. It is extremely important to stop the damage from occurring in the first place, or preventing it from worsening if there is existing damage.

The extensive evidence I have assembled in previous chapters shows clearly that this is now possible for most people using lifestyle changes alone or in combination with drug therapies. At present, drug therapy alone does not purport to offer this possibility. As with most other chronic diseases, lifestyle change offers the greatest potential for sustainable health. Drug therapy alone appears to be the least effective, but is the option most often recommended and is sometimes the only option recommended. At best this is laziness on the part of treating doctors. Many of us in medicine don't realise the extent to which we have been affected by sophisticated drug company marketing; we tend to believe that drugs are the more potent option for many diseases despite abundant evidence to the contrary. As Dr Marcia Angell says, '. . . much published research is seriously flawed, leading doctors to believe new drugs are generally more effective and safer than they actually are'.[2]

> It is now possible for people diagnosed with MS to stay well and live long, happy lives.

For people just diagnosed with MS who follow the recommendations here there is a great chance of living a normal life, well into old age. For those with MS that has already progressed, with some disability, the outlook is also optimistic. The progression of the disease can still be significantly slowed or stopped, and there is often then considerable recovery possible as remyelination occurs and neuroplasticity allows new connections to be made. We are beginning to understand that the nervous system actually has far greater capacity for repair and regeneration than we ever thought possible. There is also the hope that, like all disease, advanced cancer or any other terminal disease, this disease can sometimes be healed. People like Ian Gawler and Joanne Samer can inspire us and show that recovery from any illness, no matter how serious or advanced, is possible. It only has to happen once for it to be possible. And we also know that in many cases, with estimates ranging from 5 to 20 per cent of cases, MS follows a 'benign' course. That is, there is one attack and no or minimal further problems. There is always the real hope of falling into this group.

Further, MS is now considered a treatable disease in the conventional medical sense, albeit partially. With glatiramer, and some of the interferons, we have well studied treatments that should reduce the number of relapses. We also now have a variety of drugs affecting the immune system that can significantly slow even very aggressive MS, although side effects are an issue. And there is a host of new therapies on the horizon, from the statins and minocycline, to more powerful agents, many of them taken by mouth, that are likely to be very effective once adequately tested in clinical trials.

However, there is good evidence that lifestyle change is the most effective way to minimise the health burdens of many chronic diseases,[3-7] and that is one of the reasons why this is my focus. In 2009, my colleague at Monash University Dr Craig Hassed and I published a paper suggesting that many of us in primary care medicine who manage people with MS are neglecting this holistic approach to MS and relying solely on medications; we argued that the best approach in MS is to combine all these facets of treatment, both lifestyle change and medication where appropriate.[8] This holds the greatest promise for continuing good health for people with MS.

Doctors treating people with MS will be familiar with the fact that not all MS is the same. Some people seem to have more aggressive illness than others. While it is important to tailor the pharmaceutical approach to each patient individually, so that those with more aggressive disease are treated with the more potent drugs, it is always important to simultaneously correct as many of the adverse environmental factors that exist for each patient as well. So, it makes no sense to treat someone with aggressive MS with natalizumab but not help them give up smoking, manage stress better, exercise, optimise vitamin D status and so on. This is simply good medicine.

SATURATED FAT

First and foremost, saturated fat must be cut out of the diet. The evidence for dietary change in MS is impressive, as it is for a number of other Western diseases. The evidence is comprehensive, from laboratory bench research, animal research, major epidemiological studies, case-control studies and uncontrolled long-term cohort studies, culminating in randomised controlled trials. The evidence is congruent, consistent and highly persuasive. It strongly suggests that diet is the single most important thing that can be done to facilitate recovery from MS, in that the potential size of the benefit is enormous, at around a 95 per cent reduction in relapse rate with a major effect on progression of disability.

It appears, however, that it is not enough to modify the diet so that the amount of meat and dairy products is cut down. From the evidence available, that may slow the disease a little or not at all. Swank's work shows that the 'bad dieters' reduced their saturated fat intake by about 75 per cent yet this was not enough to alter the disease course. To really arrest it requires a drastic change to a plant-based, wholefood diet supplemented with seafood. For most people that is a major lifestyle change. It is not just a diet, which implies a temporary change; it is a permanently different way of living. And it is much easier if you make a decision to really embrace this lifestyle change, rather than feel it is imposed on you.

For me embracing this lifestyle was easy. I not only felt Mum's deterioration over fifteen years, but as a doctor I saw patient after patient with MS. Naturally, only the ones with problems ever came to my emergency department, so my view was a bit jaundiced. But I needed no convincing that giving up saturated fat was better than the alternative. And although it may seem difficult, we are really only talking about changing habits here. Weighing up the taste of a desirable food against progressive serious disability is no contest in my view. It is essential to learn to live without saturated fat.

ALTERED FATS

But there are worse fats as well. Avoiding saturated fats is extremely important. But evidence from basic science suggests that it is more important to
avoid human-refined and human-made fats. Most of us are unaware of
the extent to which oils are modified in the so-called refining process. In
refining oils we basically turn fragrant nut or seed oil extracts into colour-
less, tasteless, odourless oils which don't really resemble the original food.
Typically this begins with mechanical pressing, which can generate temperatures up to 95 degrees Celsius. This involves cooking the nuts or seeds
for around two hours at high temperature, then mashing and filtering the
oil, and if we are lucky this is all that is done and the oil is sold as natural,
unrefined oil. But mostly, the oils are then subjected to solvent extraction,
in which the oil is treated with powerful acids and alkalis, deodorised and
bleached and sold as pure vegetable oil. By now it is full of trans-fatty acids,
cyclic compounds, dimers and polymers not found in nature.

In manufacturing new fats, we convert liquid oils to semi-solid fats
in order to prolong their shelf life and allow them to be used in products
like biscuits and shortening. These fats are known as hydrogenated fats
and trans-fatty acids. Until last century, these fatty acids did not exist in
our diets. They are the result of major food processing practices which
have transformed our diets. It is likely that MS did not exist either until
fairly recently. In hydrogenation and trans-fatty acid production, commercial processes heat unsaturated fats to high temperatures in the presence
of certain metallic catalysts, and cause chemical changes in the fats to
prolong their shelf life or alter their spreadability.

Trans-fatty acids are like mirror images of the original fat but, unlike
the original, they are hard, have higher melting points and stick together.
It has been reported that as little as 5g a day of trans-fatty acids increases
the risk of heart disease by 25 per cent.[9] There are likely to be similar
effects on other degenerative diseases. The Australian Consumers Association tested a variety of popular fast foods in 2005. They found that
trans-fats made up from 0.8 per cent to 22.5 per cent of total fats, yet
to date no laws require labelling of the trans-fat content of Australian
foods.[9] The effects of all these altered fats in the body are quite unpredictable, although we know they are extremely harmful.

Trans-fatty acids have been implicated in a wide range of Western
diseases such as cancer, heart disease and immune dysfunction. They
make cell membranes even more rigid and dysfunctional than saturated

fats and are to be avoided at all costs. This means margarine is out, and so are pies, biscuits and particularly fast foods like chips and so on. It is important to look carefully at labels. If the words 'hydrogenated vegetable oil' or 'partially hydrogenated vegetable oil' appear, leave the product on the shelf. Indeed, 'vegetable oils' should be avoided, as they are likely to contain the cheaper saturated vegetable oils like coconut and palm oils. The only freely available oil which is not subjected to the above refining processes, and can be used as a general, all-purpose oil, is extra virgin olive oil. It is called extra virgin because it is made from the first cold pressing of the olives. Virgin olive oil is made from later pressings, and olive oil is refined oil.

> The key to good health in MS is avoidance of saturated and altered fats.

In many respects trans-fatty acids and hydrogenated vegetable oils are worse than saturated fats, because many manufacturers try to pass them off as healthy vegetable oils. These fatty acids are the ultimate in processed food. I sometimes joke that if human civilisation ended, biscuits would still be found as relics millennia later, all crisp and ready to eat. Trans-fatty acid and hydrogenated vegetable oils are bad for us in many ways. For a start, the manufacturing process reduces the amount of the good omega-3 and omega-6 fatty acids. They are also bad news for arteries, because of their effects on cholesterol.

But most importantly they compete with the essential fatty acids for inclusion in cell membranes, and in making the eicosanoid chemical messengers. Membranes containing trans-fatty acids are like those made of saturated fats: they are even more rigid and less pliable. Dr Simopoulos, in *The Omega Plan*, estimates that Americans are now consuming 5–10 per cent of all their calories as trans-fatty acids, which seems quite extraordinary. Yet the Food and Drug Administration in the United States recommends that there is no safe level of consumption of trans-fatty acids.

WHAT TO EAT AND WHAT NOT TO EAT

So in many ways it's not a question of what to eat so much as what not to eat. My way of eating is more of a major dietary change than Swank's diet, which can be found in great detail in his marvellous book, *The Multiple Sclerosis Diet Book*. I figure that we get so many hidden saturated fats in foods that we simply have to make a conscious choice to have none at all knowingly. Swank recommends aiming at less than 20g per day of saturated fat, but also points out that those people taking between 5 and 10g do even better. I really aim for no saturated or altered fat in the diet as far as is practicable. Rather than counting fats, I recommend a complete dietary change to a plant-based wholefood diet plus seafood, that is, no meat or dairy and preferably avoiding refined foods, as well as avoiding saturated and altered fats except those that come naturally in plant products (with the exception of coconut and palm oil where the concentration of saturated fats is simply too high).

Foods that should not be eaten

The following foods are not to be eaten:

- Meat, including processed meat, salami, sausages, canned meat
- Eggs except for egg whites
- Dairy products; that is, avoid milk, cream, butter, ice-cream and cheeses. Low-fat milk or yoghurt is not acceptable. Cow's milk and dairy products are best avoided altogether as the protein may be as much of a problem as the saturated fat, given recent evidence. Soy products or rice or oat milk and products made from them are good substitutes.
- Any biscuits, pastries, cakes, muffins, doughnuts or shortening, unless fat-free
- Commercial baked goods
- Prepared mixes (cake mix, pancake mix, etc.)
- Snacks like chips, corn chips, party foods
- Margarine, shortening, lard, chocolate, coconut and palm oil. There is some debate about chocolate's role in good health as it does have some good antioxidants, but most chocolate is also loaded with saturated and altered fat, so it should be avoided. Cocoa, however, is a natural vegetable product (a legume) with only a little saturated fat, and the occasional teaspoon in a glass of soy milk for example, as hot chocolate, is fine. Cocoa is in fact a very healthy vegetable product made into junk food when used to make chocolate.
- Fried and deep fried foods, except those fried without oil or with just a dash of olive oil. It is important not to heat oils if possible, and if

you want to use just a little extra virgin olive oil, the most stable of the oils, it is a good idea to put a little water in with it when frying to keep its temperature down. Things like fish and chips deep fried in, say, sunflower oil, are bad, in that the oil changes its chemical structure when heated in this way and tends to be left in the vat for days, with all sorts of unpredictable chemical changes happening to the fats.

- Most fast foods (burgers, fried chicken, etc.)
- Altered fats and oils

Although this list concentrates on the foods that must be omitted, it overlooks the important point that the foods which are left are incredibly healthy and enjoyable. For instance, the diet then consists of all vegetables, fruits, nuts, seeds and grains (so most pastas and rice), seafood, egg whites and so on, and from these ingredients one can make an enormous variety of tasty, satisfying, and above all healthy meals. I have included a table to summarise these foods to be avoided and the ones that should be eaten (see Table 9). I have also prepared a table to show which foods can be substituted for the unhealthy foods to keep within the nutritional guidelines I advocate here (see Table 10). For recipes using these guidelines, go to my website www.takingcontrolofmultiplesclerosis.org and sign up to the Members Forum where people following this lifestyle exchange recipes.

Table 9: Foods to eat and foods to avoid

As often as desired	In moderation	Occasionally	Never
Vegetables	Oily fish	Alcohol (14g=one standard drink; max. 2 standard drinks/day with min. 2 alcohol-free days/week)	Dairy products
Fruit	Shellfish/other seafood	Coffee, tea	Meat
Grains (wheat, rye, barley, etc.)	Avocado		Egg yolks
Legumes (beans, lentils, etc.)	Olives		Commercial cakes
Soy products White fish	Nuts, seeds		Most fast food Margarine Foods fried in oil Palm oil, 'vegetable oil'

Table 10: Healthy substitutes for unhealthy foods

Food	Substitute food
Cow's milk—drinking, over cereal	Rice milk, oat milk, almond milk, soy milk
——baking, cooking	Soy milk
Dairy yoghurt	Soy yoghurt
Butter—on toast	Flaxseed oil
——baking, cooking	Extra virgin olive oil
Vegetable oils	Extra virgin olive oil
Meat	Tofu, tempeh, fish
Eggs	Egg whites
Refined sugar	Honey
White bread	Wholemeal bread
Commercial biscuits	Fat-free biscuits
Refined cereals	Homemade muesli
Chocolate (in desserts, drinks)	Cocoa
Sweets, lollies	Dried fruit
Potato chips	Nuts
Snacks	Vegetable sticks, dried fruit, nuts
Coffee, tea	Herbal tea
Soft drink	Water, vegetable or fruit juice
Fast food (burgers, etc.)	Sushi, salad wraps (with falafel if desired)
Ice-cream	Sorbet

It is interesting to note that the nutritional approach I describe above has really been taken up and promoted widely by many authorities for many different health conditions. For instance, Dr Sandra Cabot's *Liver Cleansing Diet* is virtually identical to mine.[10] In her book outlining her recovery from advanced breast cancer with secondaries, *Your Life is in Your Hands*, Dr Jane Plant also outlines an identical diet.[11] That book is actually really helpful as it goes into this diet in rather more detail than I have here, with quite a few recipes as well. Similary, Dr Colin Campbell's *The China Study* outlines how a plant-based wholefood diet is the ideal diet for optimal human health.[12] How interesting that there should be so much agreement on what constitutes an optimal diet.

CALCULATING FAT CONSUMPTION

One of the things I probably did not make quite clear in the first book was that Swank's estimation of saturated fat was quite inaccurate. For example, he did not account for the fact that all oils are a mixture of unsaturated and saturated fats. This includes all the so-called 'good' oils like flaxseed and olive oil. A number of people have contacted me because they get very confused when they read on the label of an olive oil bottle, 12 per cent saturated fat, and wonder if they should count that in their daily quota of saturated fat. Any oil bottle label will show that it contains a proportion of saturated fat. Swank did not include these low levels of saturated fat in his calculations of daily intake and I suggest they can be ignored.

Likewise, Swank allowed his patients to consume as much bread as they liked. Most bread has around 2.9–3.4 per cent fat in it, and the ingredients often list 'vegetable oil' rather than one of the recognised oils, meaning this is probably palm oil—that is, saturated fat. Had Swank counted these fats his figure for daily saturated fat consumption would have been quite a bit higher. I think it is sensible to do as Swank suggests and eat bread as and when desired. However, I try to minimise the saturated fat consumption by buying bread either without oil in the ingredients, such as some of the pita breads and sourdough loaves, or bread made with a named oil such as olive oil.

Most supermarket-brand breads, for example, are made with canola oil rather than unnamed vegetable (palm) oil. While canola oil is a refined oil and so has been altered, and is originally low erucic acid rapeseed oil (in fact modified rapeseed oil) and so is not ideal, it is better for health than palm oil. Italian ciabatta loaves use olive oil. Swank really just counted animal fat and palm/coconut oil as saturated fat and nothing else. Swank's 'less than 20g' figure was in fact likely to be much more like 'less than, say, 30g' given all the uncounted saturated fats in vegetables, grains and oils.

So overall, it is probably a waste of effort to spend hours counting up all the grams of saturated fat in the diet and trying to aim for a certain level such as less than 20 grams or less than 10 grams. The crux of the eating change is to cut out animal fat, dairy products and 'hidden' saturated fats in apparently vegetarian products like cakes, pastries, potato chips, etc. If in doubt when buying something, it is important to study the label carefully.

Usually the label will show the saturated fat content. In fact, a packet of potato chips, with a huge fat content (around a third of the weight) and all the problems caused by heating the oil, is a much bigger problem than, say, a thin slice of turkey breast which might have less than 1 per cent saturated fat. My view, though, after reading Colin Campbell's marvellous book is that it is important to cut out all animal products and eat a plant-based, wholefood diet supplemented with seafood. This is the optimal diet for human health.

OMEGA-3 VERSUS OMEGA-6 FATS AS SUPPLEMENTS

As far as fats and oils in general go, this is where I have some minor disagreement with Professor Swank. You may wish to follow his diet exactly, after all, that is the diet he has shown to work in MS. *The Multiple Sclerosis Diet Book* details exactly what needs to be done, and which oils are advised. However, the most recent edition of this book was published in 1987. Most of the current understanding of the omega-3 and omega-6 fatty acids, especially their effects on the immune system, was gained in the 1990s and 2000s. So, I have modified the diet somewhat to take account of this new, important knowledge.

In place of saturated fats in the diet we need to substitute essential fatty acids, with the balance tipped heavily in favour of the omega-3 over the omega-6 fatty acids. The evidence from RCTs is that these supplements, even without cutting out saturated fat, reduce the relapse rate by about as much as the disease-modifying drugs. In combination with the no saturated-fat diet, the effect is considerably greater. Swank recommends between 20–50g a day of these oils. He unfortunately doesn't differentiate much between the omega-3s and omega-6s. I take about 20g of oils, concentrating on omega-3s, as supplements if I haven't eaten oily fish that day, and the rest in my food. I prefer to get the omega-3s in the form of oily fish like sardines or mackerel.

Swank noted that if people did not take in enough unsaturated fats to replace the saturated fat they were omitting from their diets they often got very tired and listless. Although it is important to reduce the amount of fat that is saturated, it is still important to get enough of the essential fatty acids for incorporation into bodily cells and manufacture of chemical messengers. These guidelines are more in line with the Action for Research into MS (ARMS) dietary advice on increasing essential fatty acid intake, but I am much more severe on saturated fats than ARMS. So this diet is not a no-fat diet—there is quite a bit of fat; it is just that the fat is good fat.

Plant versus fish omega-3s

Omega-3 fats can be plant- or fish-based. The best plant source is flaxseed oil, otherwise known as linseed oil. Because it is relatively unstable and prone to oxidation, flaxseed oil needs to be cold pressed and packed in the absence of oxygen and light. Several brands satisfying these conditions are on the market, and most health food stores carry a range in the refrigerator section. It needs to be used within about six weeks of being bought, and stored in the fridge. You can tell when it is time to throw it out because it develops a characteristic bitter taste.

I have found that the flavour is really quite pleasant and look forward to putting it on my salads or pasta, but others may prefer to mix it with orange juice or spoon it over cereal. It is also quite nice on toast before putting on the jam. It is relatively inexpensive. If bought in advance for any reason, it can be frozen without affecting its chemical structure or effectiveness and allowed to thaw out in the fridge when needed. Interestingly, in the fine print in Swank's book, it can be seen that for people who couldn't tolerate cod liver oil, Swank recommended 'raw linseed oil' which is in fact flaxseed oil. One wonders how he stumbled upon this, given how little was known then about omega-3 fatty acids.

Fish oil capsules are available in all good health food shops. They are, however, quite expensive. Cod liver oil is less concentrated in the amount of fish oils it contains; the proportion of omega-3 oils in cod liver oil is around two-thirds lower than in fish oil and the proportion of saturated fat higher, so it is not really a substitute for fish oil. It also contains vitamin D, around 400IU per 5ml dose. I have now omitted cod liver oil from my supplements. I don't think it is a very good product. It is usually found just sitting on the shelf at room temperature, quietly oxidising, and to me always tastes a little rancid.

Cod liver oil is, however, quite inexpensive compared to fish oil, and could be used as an alternative if the budget is tight. Be wary, though, of trying to get all the fish oil omega-3s through cod liver oil. Each 5ml of cod liver oil also contains around 3000 units of vitamin A. While this dose is fine, in high doses vitamin A is very toxic, with skin changes and mental deterioration the commonest effects. Quite a large dose is needed to get these effects, perhaps of the order of over 50,000–500,000 units a day, so it pays to stay under that. And we now know that taking vitamin A as a supplement even in low doses is associated with an increased risk of death.

It is just as inexpensive to get the fish oil in a tin of sardines. John West sardines in springwater, for example, contain 110g of sardines with 16.7 per cent fat, or fish oil. So this is 18.4g of fish oil, or roughly eighteen and a half capsules. It is pretty competitive in cost with capsules, and also provides lunch.

There is a lot of discussion about whether flaxseed oil is 'as good' as fish oil. Given that our oceans are gradually becoming more polluted, particularly with heavy metals like mercury, and that heavy metals are known to cause neurological problems, it would be nice if a plant-based oil like flaxseed oil could provide all our omega-3 needs. The problem is that the fatty acid in flaxseed oil, alpha-linolenic acid (ALA), needs to be converted in the body to the fish oil fatty acids, eicosapenanoic acid (EPA) and then docosahexanoic acid (DHA). I have seen various figures put on this conversion, mostly up to 10 per cent of it being converted, dependent on general health, saturated fat consumption, alcohol consumption and a number of other variables.

In his excellent book *Fats that Heal, Fats that Kill,*[13] Udo Erasmus does the best calculation I have seen on this. Erasmus quotes a figure of 2.7 per cent per day of the ALA being converted to EPA. He says that this figure is likely to be higher for people getting all the essential nutrients from diet and supplements. As most people's fat deposits contain about 2 per cent ALA (quite a bit higher for those following the diet and supplements in this book), this is about 200g of ALA, which could make about 5400mg of EPA (as there is about 180mg of EPA in one 1000mg fish oil capsule, this is equivalent to about 30 of the 1000mg capsules of fish oil). If there is no ALA in your fat deposits at all (if you had been taking no omega-3s in your diet whatsoever), then just taking two tablespoons of flaxseed oil would supply enough ALA to make about 378mg of EPA, equivalent to what is in two 1000mg fish oil capsules.

But as can be seen from the above calculation of body stores, most people have enough stored if they are supplementing every day to make quite adequate amounts of EPA and DHA. The advantage of doing it this way rather than taking it as fish oil is not only related to chemical toxins like mercury in fish oil and to questions about the sustainability of our fish stocks, but also that the EPA made this way is fresher, in the body every day. I prefer to take at least two dessertspoons of flaxseed oil a day (20ml) on the days when I don't eat oily fish. I eat oily fish probably three to four days a week. I have been reassured by a number of reputable authorities that at least at present there doesn't seem to be any traces of mercury found in the major brands of fish oil if that is your preferred way of taking the oil. Some may, however, choose to take all 20ml of the oil supplements a day as flaxseed oil based on the above arguments, and that is a good strategy provided that some fish oil is taken in the first few months (say nine months) until there are adequate fat stores of ALA. Udo Erasmus provides a very good overview of all the issues around plant and animal-based omega-3s, and the problems with altered fats, on his website www.udoerasmus.com.

Evening primrose oil

At one time there was a huge following for evening primrose oil, but that contains only omega-6 fatty acids. After considerable research following publication of the first book, and discussions with reputable authorities, I now avoid this entirely. Most nuts and seeds contain some of the omega-6 oils, as do many vegetables, so there's really no need to supplement them much as there should be significant amounts of omega-6s with this diet. One of the good things about flaxseed oil is that it also contains linoleic acid, about 17 per cent. So there are some omega-6 fatty acids as well. Our modern Western diet, though, is relatively deficient in omega-3s, and that is why I concentrate on supplementing them while getting omega-6s largely through food.

Cooking and oils

As far as cooking goes, I avoid frying with oil at all if I can help it. If it is absolutely necessary, I use a small amount of extra virgin olive oil. The omega-3 and omega-6 oils are too unstable to cook with, particularly flaxseed oil. Heating them rapidly causes oxidation, and conversion to fat breakdown products which are deleterious for health. It is important to avoid the commercial so-called cooking oils altogether. These products are now so refined, bleached, deodorised, heated and tampered with in general that they have little resemblance to the food from which they originally came. For a good account of the terrible refining processes that go on in the making of modern oils, it is worth having a look at Udo Erasmus' book.

Extra virgin olive oil, on the other hand, is relatively stable. Generation upon generation of Mediterranean people have used olive oil for cooking with remarkably low rates of the common degenerative Western diseases, including MS. But avoiding cooking with it altogether is so much better, as all oil degenerates with heat. Olive oil can be used in many other ways. Rather than using margarine, get a small dipping bowl and mix olive oil with balsamic vinegar. The oil sits on top and the black vinaigrette on the bottom. Many restaurants are serving this mix these days. Or extra virgin olive oil can be used alone. There is a wide range of flavours.

> Frying with oils creates very harmful fats and should be avoided.

Lots of people already love the taste of extra virgin olive oil, but for those not used to it it may be worth going for the less strong taste of virgin olive oil. The more expensive extra virgin olive oil has a distinctive flavour that can really be addictive. I love it. It lasts for ages, so it's money well spent. I think the general all-purpose oil around the kitchen should be extra virgin olive oil. It is really the only unrefined vegetable oil that is available commercially. Ordinary olive oil is treated in much the same way as the other refined vegetable oils and is probably best avoided.

I have found that by substituting olive oil for most of the fats in recipes, such as butter and margarine, and by using only the whites of eggs and substituting soy milk for cow's milk I can make a range of cakes and desserts which contain very little saturated fat but taste wonderful. It is sensible to use as little as possible, but while heat causes oil to deteriorate, baking is acceptable in that temperatures get nowhere near as high as when frying. The moistness in cakes can often be achieved by substituting fruit juice for the suggested oil if preferred. Just because saturated fat is out, food doesn't stop being tasty—quite the reverse. It is possible to make a wonderful passionfruit soufflé with egg whites only and olive oil, and a range of cakes like banana cake, chocolate zucchini cake (using cocoa, sugar and a small amount of olive oil instead of chocolate) and so on.

Other oils can be used as well. Sesame oil, for instance, is wonderfully fragrant and can give an Asian dish a superb aroma and taste, but can be simply added over the dish at the end of cooking prior to serving rather than being used in the cooking process. Some people prefer to take their flaxseed oil supplements in this way as well. There are extra virgin oils made of many seeds and nuts and all can be quite tasty, although they should not be heated if possible. The oils should preferably be stored in the fridge, where they will last longer. As I have previously mentioned, all contain some saturated fat, and this is probably the main reason not to use too much of them.

An upper limit of unsaturated oils

Swank advises to only sparingly eat foods which are very rich in the polyunsaturates, so as not to go over 50g per day. Although he doesn't specify why this is so, I suspect it is because all the oils contain saturated fat and this is to minimise the overall load of saturated fat, which could become a problem if the intake of the 'unsaturated' oils like fish oil was not restricted. Typically, oily fish are the ones with the highest unsaturated fat content. As mentioned earlier, a can of sardines containing 110g of fish will have around 18g of fish oil, of which about 4g will be actual omega–3 fatty acids. I don't feel this is too much to worry about, as most people struggle to eat over about 18–20g a day of essential fatty acids unless they supplement their diet. The can of sardines also contains 5–6g of saturated fat. It is good to eat oily fish frequently, at least three times a week. Just imagine how much fish the average Japanese eats, and MS is almost non-existent in Japan. The naturally occurring fish omega-3s will be helping damp down the immune system, and competing with other fats for incorporation into the body's cell membranes.

Incidentally, canned fish seems to be just as good as fresh fish in this regard. Canned sardines with fresh tomato on bread is certainly an inexpensive and tasty way to get essential fatty acids. The fish with the highest omega-3 content are fresh and canned salmon, sardines, canned mackerel, fresh tuna, anchovies and canned herring. Australian salmon has a much lower omega-3 content than Atlantic salmon. It is probably best to avoid the big fish at the top of the food chain, as this is where the pollutants like heavy metals are concentrated. So fish like shark (also known as flake) is better avoided.

Oil supplements

Most days I have a can of sardines or mackerel or similar for lunch, either in a sandwich or salad or on their own. For most common good brands of canned fish this will supply me with close to the required 20g of fish oil. (It is interesting to note that the cheaper the tin of sardines, the lower the fish oil content; I assume they are processed and the fish oil extracted to be sold separately.) There is no need to take any supplement on days when eating fish like this. On other days I take my omega-3 oils as flaxseed oil, so really I have now dispensed with buying fish oil supplements. On top of this I get quite a bit of unsaturated oil, mainly omega-6s, from my food, and omega-9s from the small amount of olive oil in cooking and over salads or for dipping bread.

Most of the unsaturated oil in my diet comes from nuts and grains. Nuts are very high in monounsaturated oil (oleic acid, the same as in olive oil), and to a lesser extent so are some of the grains like oats. Again, I prefer to eat raw nuts rather than cooked nuts because heating oils damages them. Of all the nuts available, the ones with the lowest saturated fat content are raw almonds, and these are the nuts I have mostly. There is actually quite a lot of literature on almonds; typing 'almonds' into PubMed produces a large number of research studies. For instance, increasing almond intake has been shown to progressively improve the profile of fats in the blood of volunteers[14] and people with high blood cholesterol,[15] with quite marked falls in levels of cholesterol and bad fats. We have already seen how important fats are in the progression of MS.

RESTAURANTS AND EATING OUT

All of this can make going out to friends' places or restaurants a little difficult. However, these days many are copying the wonderful eating habits of the low MS areas of southern Europe, focusing on olive oil and vegetables. It may be easiest to describe yourself to your hosts as a seafood-eating vegan. One of the participants at a Gawler Foundation MS Retreat coined the term 'vegaquarian' for seafood-eating vegans. Some people find it easier to say they are allergic to animal products. Everyone seems to understand what an allergy is. If a difficult waiter says a meal wouldn't be the same without the cheese, it may be helpful to ask if anyone in the kitchen staff knows CPR!

When going out to other people's places or to restaurants, I usually ring ahead and tell them my requirements. People can be very accommodating and, of course, restaurants are paid to prepare the desired meals for the customer. My work colleagues now tend to put 'George-friendly' food at my end of the table at functions. It is surprising how many people tend to come down to my end to eat. There can also be a problem with the oil that is used for cooking and it is worth checking closely with the waiter exactly what is used in the restaurant. Most will be quite happy to divulge this, and will be very accommodating if asked that no oil or minimal oil be used. This may be more of a problem if travelling overseas due to language barriers.

Most restaurants have a range of meals that contain no saturated fat. Bruschetta or grilled field mushrooms with garlic and drizzled with olive oil are often found on Italian restaurant menus and are superb. My favourite restaurant knows my order off pat when I come in to get a wood-fired pizza. Spinach, mushrooms, anchovies, olives, no cheese. I have started wondering how I ever ate pizzas with cheese.

One type of cuisine people may really develop a taste for is Japanese. I certainly have. Before getting MS I had eaten Japanese only once, and settled for the Western type dishes. Now I simply love sashimi (thinly sliced raw fish, usually tuna and salmon, with soy sauce), very lightly cooked salmon, and most of their other dishes. Once again it's worth remembering that the Japanese have one of the lowest rates of MS in the world, despite being so far from the equator. The fact that they consume nearly the most fish in the world in their diets is no coincidence. Once hooked on Japanese, it's hard to resist. Fortunately, it's not only delicious, it's doing good. It is worth noting that many Japanese restaurants in Western countries, in their desire to appeal to the Western appetite, now put mayonnaise in their sushi and other dishes. In quite a few I have been to, I have been unable to eat anything because the food is so Westernised. It is worth checking this, and often they will make up the sushi without mayo.

FOODS TO PREPARE AT HOME

It is surprising how easy it is to find tasty, nutritious meals based around a no saturated-fat diet. With Google these days, it is so easy to find recipes. I make my own muesli, for example. It contains rolled oats, other grains as desired such as barley or rye, sultanas, diced dried fruit and linseeds. There is some fat in this but most is unsaturated. It is easy to make really good vegetable soups, using vegetable juices as a stock. Pumpkin, sweet potato, potato and leek—they are all great. I often have a lunch consisting of a bowl of sultanas covered in soy yoghurt, with linseeds sprinkled over the top and passionfruit pulp on top of that. It is absolutely delicious. There are now lots of recipes available using this approach. Vegetable curries, vegetable stir-fries with or without tofu or prawns, using oyster sauce, soy sauce, blackbean sauce or sweet chili sauce depending on the desired flavour, simple pastas with an extra virgin olive oil base and so on.

These days, finding foods which don't contain saturated fats is easy. Foods on the shelf in the supermarket are now labelled with every ingredient, in many cases down to the types of fats contained. It really is easy to find non-fat foods. The unexpected bonus of giving up these saturated fats and substituting omega-3 fatty acids is a longer, healthier life, with less chance of cancer, heart disease and most modern Western style diseases.

OTHER SUPPLEMENTS

For quite some time, I believed it was important to take antioxidants to prevent the highly unsaturated essential fatty acids from oxidising. As I have said, despite many authorities recommending this, I haven't been able to find any evidence that this is helpful. Indeed, we now have convincing evidence about the potentially harmful effects of multivitamin and antioxidant supplements containing vitamins A and E. I have now dropped these supplements. It is obviously preferable to get these essential dietary compounds from this diet that is so rich in vegetables and fruit. I also used to take vitamin E daily. However, none of the studies I have seen in which fish oil supplementation has been used in other diseases, such as heart disease, has shown any difference in the benefit whether vitamin E is added or not,[16, 17] and we now have clear evidence of an increased death rate associated with its use in clinical trials. As a result I have also dropped vitamin E, which is the most expensive of the vitamin supplements.

Vitamin C is a little different. Although there is no definite evidence for taking this vitamin, I have also taken the advice of Ian Gawler and his experience over 21 years with cancer patients. He says that many of his patients have reported great benefit from vitamin C supplementation, so although I don't take this supplement it is very much a personal choice whether to take it or not. If you decide to take it, it has a much shorter duration of effect in the body and should be taken at least twice a day. Some people take mega-doses of this. There is probably no ceiling on how much. There is currently quite a bit of controversy in the medical literature about whether intravenous vitamin C actually has some benefits in cancer. There is no real evidence of any benefit for this supplement in MS. However, there is also no evidence of any harmful effect, unlike vitamins A and E, so this is a personal choice.

The most enjoyable antioxidants for my money come in 750ml bottles with corks. These antioxidants are a bit more expensive than the others, but I am sure you'll enjoy taking them more, too. The recommendation is not to exceed two standard glasses of wine a day, with at least two alcohol-free days a week, otherwise the alcohol can cause health problems. I am reassured by the evidence we saw in the case-control studies that there seems to be no particular risk for people with MS drinking alcohol, apart from the usual general risks, unless they drink too much.

This may be the appropriate place to reiterate the risks of smoking to people with MS, or with the predisposition to get MS. It seems likely that if people with MS smoke it will worsen or aggravate the disease. For anyone who still smokes I suggest very strongly that you stop. Having said that, it seems very unlikely that someone making the sorts of lifestyle changes I am recommending in this book would be poisoning their body with cigarettes. Quite apart from MS, giving up smoking is the single biggest health intervention a person can make in life. In comparison, diet, exercise and so on are all very minor. The benefits of giving up smoking are enormous, in all aspects of health. It is also important to reiterate the importance of family members of people with MS not smoking.

OTHER VITAMINS AND NUTRIENTS

There is a range of other vitamins and nutrients which ought to form part of the daily intake as well. The most important of these are vitamin B12 and folate. Both of these are intimately related to normal nerve cell function. I have presented evidence to show that people with MS are sometimes deficient in these, particularly B12. Additionally, B12 is available mostly through meats, so on a no saturated-fat diet it is possible to miss out. There has been research showing that in high doses, oral B12 gets into the body in adequate amounts and doesn't need to be injected. A dose of at least 25 or 30 micrograms a day orally is really needed if intake is low. This can be achieved by taking the occasional B12 supplement, say one 250 or 1000 microgram tablet a week, or taking B group vitamins. These have not been shown to have the same risks as general multivitamins or the antioxidants.

SUNLIGHT AND VITAMIN D

It is important to make a lifestyle change here that seems to go against current public health advice, and embrace regular sun exposure. The sun is not an enemy. Every bit of life on this planet exists only because of the energy provided by the sun. It makes no sense for nature to have made us unable to tolerate it. Fortunately, public health authorities are starting to shift their recommendations as more and more evidence comes in about the overall health benefits of regular, modest sun exposure. The message is really much more like the message they are giving the community about alcohol consumption. We all know that in excess, alcohol is quite harmful. But in regular low doses it is actually beneficial. The same applies to the sun, but more so.

I recommend getting ten to fifteen minutes of all-over sun, that is, in a bathing suit, three to five times a week. This time estimate is for when the sun's strength is about UV index 7 or higher. If it is lower, more is needed to get the therapeutic amount of vitamin D. For people with a busy work schedule, the best way to do this is to combine sun and exercise. If there is a heated pool nearby, a sensible strategy is to take the occasional lunch break in the sun, doing laps. It is important to emphasise here that getting more sun than this recommended amount will not produce more vitamin D or improve health any further. In fact, it increases the risk of other diseases such as skin cancer.

> Adequate exposure to sunlight is important for people with MS; vitamin D supplements are an alternative if there is little sun available.

For some people it will be well nigh on impossible to get enough sun, no matter how much juggling of work schedules goes on. It's simple in sunny Brisbane, even in winter. But in London, Melbourne or Hobart it is much harder. Fortunately many places still have solariums left over from the days when tanning was all the rage. Solariums have got a lot of bad press. Really, what they offer is just concentrated sunlight, so a lower dose of exposure is needed. A good strategy is, when there are several days in a row of inclement weather, to drop in for a short session in the local solarium. Because the UV radiation is so concentrated, treatment times need to be shorter. There is a variety of different machines, ranging from super-fast tanning machines in which the recommended time is eight minutes to those taking 30 minutes.

The full amount of time recommended in a sun-bed is certainly too much. This will cause most people to burn. Around a third to a half of the recommended times seems to be about right, although it is a bit of trial and error. The right amount is what is called the minimal erythemal dose, that is, the amount that would make the skin just slightly pink. One thing to avoid is exposure to the face. UV radiation certainly causes skin damage. I recommend putting sunscreen on the face when getting UV rays outside, and covering the face if using a solarium. One important point about solariums is to check that the machine used actually puts out UVB, not just UVA. UVB is the form that is needed for vitamin D production, and not all machines produce UVB.

A very good alternative on very overcast days, or days when it's simply not possible to get out and get any sun or visit a solarium, is to take vitamin D supplements. In many places in the world these supplements are easily obtained, in quite high doses, but not in Australia, where the highest dose made is around 1000IU. Goldberg estimated a dose of 3800IU per day to prevent MS. This is about ten to twenty times the recommended daily allowance, determined by the amount needed to prevent rickets in children. Vieth says about 10,000–15,000IU is the most that can be produced naturally by the skin. That is the limit. This dose is useful for maximal immune suppression, and can be achieved by the minimal erythemal dose of UV referred to above.

I take an additional 5000IU of vitamin D3 (not D2, which is synthetic) on really overcast days, or when I miss out on sun altogether, during winter. During summer, there is no need to supplement if sun exposure is adequate. It is possible to easily find 5000IU vitamin D preparations over the Internet. The only recorded toxic effects in the medical literature have been when supplementing at 40,000IU per day, and a dose of 10,000IU has been reported as the safe upper limit of dosing. The literature suggests that a blood level of above 100nmol/L should be aimed for, and this can be checked by the local doctor. I recommend it is checked annually, around the end of winter. I keep mine around 150nmol/L. As

Reinhold Vieth emailed back when I contacted him about the amount of sun needed, 'Enjoy your time in the sun'.

MEDITATION

Meditation is an extremely important part of the healing package. Some, like Ian Gawler, feel it is the most important part. Personally I feel that almost everyone should take time to meditate, given the pace of our lives and the pressures most of us are under. It is doubly important for those with chronic illness. The evidence for the benefits of meditation on health is enormous and growing rapidly. A 2006 review showed that there was clear evidence of benefit for epilepsy, premenstrual syndrome, menopausal symptoms, mood and anxiety disorders, auto-immune illness and emotional disturbance in cancer patients.[18] Given the difficulties associated with 'proof' in medicine, it is likely that meditation is helpful in considerably more conditions.

Many experts recommend meditation twice a day. I find that I simply cannot find time twice a day. The competing demands of work, family and social life just won't allow it. I meditate every day for thirty minutes, and usually after I get home from work, as a kind of circuit-breaker. Some people find they can meditate twice a day or more. The evidence suggests the more it is done, the greater the benefit. We need to focus all the energy we can on healing. If we are wasting energy with our minds being overactive, we are at a disadvantage. There is ample scientific evidence of the value of meditation. But like the diet, it only works if you do it. It is very important to make time every day for this activity.

VISUALISATION

There are a number of good accounts of how to develop a regular practice of visualisation. Both Carolyn Myss' *Why People Don't Heal, and How They Can* and Bernie Siegel's *Peace, Love and Healing* have excellent accounts. The critical step is finding an image that is suitable. For MS, I don't find images of fighting or attacking of much use, although others will I am sure. For me, I like to think of the system being in balance, and trying to stop it tipping towards inflammation and demyelination. Some image related to this may be of help.

By paying careful attention to dreams, an image may arise that is unique and personal (see 'Symbols and dreams', Chapter 11). Images thrown up spontaneously by the subconscious are likely to be of more benefit than those actively developed using the conscious mind. Whatever, finding something suitable and using it regularly, especially something related to balance, is very likely to assist the body in returning to a state of balance. I like to start my meditation sessions off by picturing myself at the controls of my earthmoving machines (white cells). Dania, our former research officer at work, bought me a rather obscure Christmas present a few years ago. At first I had trouble working out why she would buy me a toy earthmover. What a great idea.

COUNSELLING

This can be of great benefit particularly when initially diagnosed, and also later if the disease progresses. Some people find this pretty confronting, and probably it needs to be if anything is really to be achieved. The focus should initially be on practical tips to help develop positivity, resolve conflict and unfinished business and enjoy life. Finding someone you relate to well may be quite difficult. Often, personal recommendation is the best strategy. As time goes on, if the right counsellor is found, the sessions can help with spiritual life. It's wise to shop around, though. Like all professionals, some are good and some not so good. Some people find that close friends or relatives who feel comfortable with talking about difficult issues can be a great source of comfort.

RESOLVING UNFINISHED BUSINESS

I feel it is important not to avoid tackling the unfinished business thrown up by these sessions. Avoiding seems the easier option at times, but I try to remind myself that disease is often a manifestation of unresolved conflict. Resolving these issues may be the harder choice, but it is certainly the healthier. MS is actually a great excuse to deal with issues of the past that still trouble us. Paradoxically, MS can provide a convenient excuse to contact someone with whom there have been difficulties in the past. Avoiding dealing with past issues makes it harder to heal. There is often a great sense of relief when these past issues are confronted, otherwise they remain buried in the subconscious but continue to affect our daily lives. Biography becomes biology; if we live our lives in this way, our bodies will change. The most important skill to learn is that of forgiveness. Forgiving others and ourselves for past mistakes helps healing.

POSITIVITY

Remaining positive in the face of a chronic progressive disease is difficult, although it gets easier when there is a commitment to significant lifestyle change, and the whole process becomes a challenge and a journey. Of course, if this results in continuing health, as it will for many people, positivity can continue to grow. Focusing on positive aspects of what has come out of having the disease is important. It is often difficult for people to see anything positive at all about having MS. But spending some time talking to someone close about the advantages and disadvantages of having MS can be quite illuminating. Not everyone will be able to see the disease as a gift. Keeping focused on the lessons that can be learnt from conflicts and difficulties can help prevent bitterness and negativity. In the end, there is always a choice of how to react to the disease. Reacting positively will almost certainly bring physical benefits as well as mental.

One helpful way of developing positivity is to be surrounded with positive, strong people and environments. Most people with MS find that when they begin to confront the illness and change their way of life, many of their friendships change. Some people will find it difficult to accept the changes, and want people to stay the way they were. Others will relish the opportunity to assist and to change with the person. That is natural, and it is helpful to just accept it and let this re-ordering of friendships happen. A lot of people find it helpful to avoid people who always make them feel negative or down.

I found that it was useful to also surround myself with good stories. Reading about people who have recovered from serious illness or hardship, for example, can really provide some optimism in the face of all the difficulty. Books by Bernie Siegel, Ian Gawler, Lance Armstrong, Nelson Mandela and so on can be really uplifting.

KEEPING A DIARY

I write in my diary a lot, although less than I did when I was going through more difficult times. I'm sure it helps me keep in touch with my feelings better than I used to. At first when things were very difficult I wrote nearly every day. Now I tend to write only when there is something major going on causing me difficulty. And of course it's good to write when things are going really well. The ultimate diary for me has been, of course, this book. Not everyone will feel like writing a book, or will have the opportunity to. I realised that this was something I had to do very early on. Not only did I want to communicate my findings to other people with MS so that I could help them, but I could see that the process of writing it would be extremely good for me. And so it has turned out. The evidence is pretty clear that writing about difficult experiences can make a big difference to the physical expression of chronic illness. It is a simple strategy, but one that can be very liberating.

WORK

I am extremely lucky with the timing of being diagnosed with MS. As someone pointed out quite early, if it had occurred just over two years earlier I would never have accepted my current post of Professor of Emergency Medicine. I would not have had the confidence in my future to start such a major voyage in my life. Further, because I am now in an academic appointment rather than a purely clinical one as I had been, I am expected as part of my work to undertake significant amounts of teaching, research and administration. I can tailor my work life to a certain extent. That wouldn't have been possible had I not taken this appointment. I think it is important to investigate ways of changing our working lives so that they are kinder to us. For some people, this may involve a complete re-appraisal of where work fits into life, resulting potentially in changing career, reducing hours or giving up work altogether. It is important to put ourselves first when faced with such a difficult illness, and that is often something foreign to many of us.

I have found colleagues to be supportive and sympathetic and willing to be flexible in accommodating my needs. I still get incredibly enthused about new developments in the department, initiate new projects, and get actively involved in extracurricular activities such as medical editing, but I have been able to modify my clinical commitments and on-call work in such a way that I feel less pressured. This has certainly made a great difference to my health.

It is common for people with MS to find that they can no longer work full-time. It is commonly said that 80 per cent of people with MS no longer work full-time within five years of diagnosis. I feel it is important to be open and honest with employers about such difficulties. There is legislation to protect the working rights of those with disabling illness, and most employers, even if they are not particularly compassionate, will be aware of this. Colleagues too are often grateful to be told about the illness and about any difficulties it causes, as it gives them the opportunity to help.

Many people following this lifestyle approach feel able to continue working full-time, but make a decision to reduce their hours simply to make life more enjoyable. We are living in a society where busy-ness is regarded as an admirable trait, and it is hard to disengage from that at times. But many people find that a simpler, less pressured life, with fewer hours devoted to work, can be more fulfilling.

RELATIONSHIPS

This is a pretty tricky area. For me, my family and a number of my friends have been really helpful. But I am acutely aware that they have their own lives. While to an extent MS dominates mine, it shouldn't dominate theirs. Not everyone gets a chance to unburden themselves as publicly as I have in writing this book. However it is done, it is worth getting your inner feelings and fears out: a diary, counselling, a group such as one of the MS societies or the MS Residential Retreats we offer through the Gawler Foundation, writing a book. All can be useful outlets. But I try not to bring the conversation at home around to MS. This gets easier all the time the longer I stay well.

WHAT TO DO ABOUT FAMILY MEMBERS GETTING MS

This is a really hard one. Perhaps it was easier for Mum than me, in that she felt there was nothing that a person could do to influence their chances of getting the disease, and the real risk of family members getting

MS was not known. This is no longer true. There are very substantial risks of MS developing in family members of people with MS. So should we put our children on a low saturated-fat diet? Should brothers and sisters go on the diet? What about sunshine and vitamin D?

> The risk of family members getting MS can be greatly reduced with adequate sun exposure or vitamin D supplements.

Professor Swank points out in his book that he placed all family members on the same diet. I imagine this is for two reasons. Firstly, it reduces their chances of getting MS. But it also makes it much easier when preparing meals. Separate meals for the affected family member would then not be an issue. Swank points out that in his experience of over 3500 patients with MS, not one of their relatives has developed the disease, to his knowledge. This is pretty extraordinary, given the statistics we have seen of the high risk in relatives.

I find this question hard. We all know what fussy eaters children can be. We also know how much kids these days like fast food. Rather than eliminating saturated fats from the diets of my children, I have opted to make their diets healthier in general, with more unsaturated essential fats and less saturated fat, but not eliminate it all together. Is this the right approach? I don't know. It is important to reach your own conclusions here. If children are older and understand why their diets are being modified, or very small so that they don't really have a say in it, I can imagine it would be a little easier, although still a difficult issue. For teenage kids, I have found it a lot harder. One day, of course, they will have the prerogative of making their own choice about this. Perhaps this book will help. It may help to discuss the risk figures I have presented here with your partner, and perhaps children if they are old enough, and then make a decision. Alternatively, a service offering genetic counselling may be able to offer advice.

Much more importantly, we now have good data on sunlight and vitamin D preventing MS, and this is now an exciting avenue for disease prevention for relatives of people with MS. Indeed, I feel that all doctors managing people with MS now have a responsibility to advise parents with MS that the evidence is clear that they can greatly reduce the risk of their children getting MS with sun exposure or vitamin D supplements or both. There is now research underway worldwide examining the magnitude of the benefit in supplementing with vitamin D to prevent MS in those at risk. But we already have enough data to know that this will work.

The 2003 Tasmanian study showed a major reduction in risk of MS for those who get adequate sun exposure, particularly in childhood in winter.[19] For those who live in areas where getting adequate sunlight is a problem, or for those who wish to avoid the sun for other health reasons, the US Nurses Health Study has clearly shown that MS risk can be nearly halved by taking a small supplement of vitamin D.[20] From our knowledge of vitamin D effects on the body and immune system, it is likely that a higher dose would have even more significant protective effects. A recent review of the literature concludes that vitamin D supplementation may prevent the development of MS.[21] A 2009 study demonstrated a direct genetic mechanism that may explain why vitamin D prevents MS, by showing its functional interaction with the genes that most influence the onset of MS.[22]

My recommendation is a supplement of 5000IU a day in winter, reduced proportionately for children. So, using 50kg as the adult dose equivalent, for a 25kg child I would give half this dosage. This can be omitted on days when there is adequate sun exposure. It has been suggested that on a population basis, in areas of high MS prevalence, supplementing with vitamin D during pregnancy and early childhood could prevent a great proportion of the MS in the world.[23] The author suggests that, like folic acid, vitamin D supplementation should be routinely recommended in pregnancy. This is supported by a large epidemiological study showing that babies born at the end of winter were more likely to get MS later in life than those born at the end of summer.[24]

So it is important for women with MS not to stop vitamin D supplementation during pregnancy and while breastfeeding. Another important point for women with MS considering pregnancy to be aware of is that breastfeeding also reduces the risk of a relapse after giving birth. A study presented to the 2009 AAN meeting in Seattle showed that those women who didn't breastfeed after childbirth, mostly so that they could re-start their disease-modifying drugs, were more than twice as likely to have a relapse as those who chose to breastfeed for at least two months. This is likely to be due to a hormonal effect on the illness.

EXERCISE

Exercise forms an important part of my formula. There is clear evidence that regular vigorous exercise has many beneficial effects on health in general, and is likely to have similar benefits specifically for people with MS. I have already discussed how important it is to avoid depression, given that it is likely to physically worsen MS, and exercise has been well shown to reduce rates of depression. I prefer to swim in an outdoor pool at around 26–28 degrees Celsius, getting both my exercise and sun in the one session and avoiding the problems that many people get with their MS worsening when they get hot. This would fit nicely into Professor Russell's notion that exercise in the lying down position is the best form.[25]

One thing that has helped my exercise program is to set exercise goals. Not long after being diagnosed with MS, I set myself the goal of running the annual Perth 'City to Surf'. This is a 12-kilometre run from Perth city to the coast. Thousands and thousands of people do it each year, including many disabled people. Having the goal four months away at that stage was a great motivator. It also got my son, now in his twenties but twelve years old at the time, involved in his first ever City to Surf.

The physical effects of exercise are well documented. It improves fitness and bone strength so that osteoporosis and fractures after falls are less frequent. It improves circulation and protects against cardiovascular disease. It also helps with the spasticity problems which can make life with MS a misery later in the disease. The mental effects are not so well studied, but people who regularly exercise simply feel better. They are less prone to depression and are more positive. It appears to have beneficial effects on the immune system. There is also preliminary evidence that regular exercise will slow the progression of disability. I strongly recommend it. It is a great way to get some sun as well.

TAKING SPECIAL CARE AT DIFFICULT TIMES

It seems from analysis of the literature that MS relapses tend to occur between four and eight weeks after a triggering event. Looking at the evidence about stressful events precipitating relapses, the time lag seemed to be about that amount of time, and Embry's data on vitamin D levels and MRI lesions seem to indicate roughly a two-month lag period from a drop in vitamin D levels to new lesions appearing. So, while not wanting to encourage unnecessary dwelling on the possibility of relapses all the time, it is probably wise to take special care in the aftermath of trigger events, like sudden loss, marriage breakdown, major emotional difficulties or even virus infections. By taking special care, I mean being meticulous about diet, sunlight and meditation in particular. It is probably good advice in general to meditate more when things are difficult, but for people with MS this may be particularly so. It may also be worth thinking about getting some help, perhaps from friends or counsellors, when things in life go badly wrong, as they sometimes do. And taking some leave from work may also be a good idea.

DRUG THERAPIES

To this point I have discussed only those things that people with MS can do for themselves. From the evidence I have presented, it should be clear that in many, if not most, cases this should stabilise the illness. Some people, though, will decide that the dietary and other changes are too much to ask. And there will be those who, despite sticking to the diet and making all the other changes, have a relapse. This happened to people in Swank's original study at about the rate of one relapse every ten to twenty years. Some people just have a more aggressive form of the disease. And many people will just want to take no chances and cover every base.

No matter what the reason, one or more of the drug therapies may need to be considered. These include steroids, glatiramer, interferon and others. Despite the large amount of evidence presented on the sometimes serious side effects of many of the medications used in MS, I hope this doesn't discourage their use if needed. Steroids are effective in reducing the impact and aftermath of relapses, and the disease-modifying drugs have been 'proven' in large trials to be modestly effective at reducing relapses. These medications should be seriously considered by anyone wanting to do everything possible to stabilise the illness, particularly early on after diagnosis.

Anti–virals

Before discussing these therapeutic agents in detail, one of the as yet 'unproven' therapies is treatment with anti-viral agents. The chapter on viruses showed that human herpes virus 6 has been implicated in causing MS. And small studies have shown a trend towards lower relapse rates with regular acyclovir and other anti-herpes medications. The drugs are safe, with very few side effects. Acyclovir needs to be taken five times a day for maximal effect. But famciclovir and other newer agents in the same class have much longer duration of action. Famciclovir, for instance, has been shown to suppress genital herpes equally effectively whether given twice or three times a day.

I feel the treatment holds great promise. Unfortunately we must wait for more definitive studies before recommending these drugs. But there is great potential here for the future use of combination therapy of these anti-virals taken orally along with one or more of the injectable disease-modifying agents.

Steroids, interferon and glatiramer

As far as steroids, interferon, glatiramer and others go, again these potent medicines can only be prescribed by a doctor, either a general practitioner or a specialist neurologist. In general, a short one-off course of steroids is extremely safe, and effective at improving recovery after a relapse. As discussed previously, they should be considered for all but the most minor relapse, so as to minimise the chances of long-term symptoms from the relapse. The UK National Institute for Health and Clinical Excellence (NICE) has recommended that at this stage there is insufficient evidence of clinical benefit or cost benefit for either interferon or glatiramer to recommend their routine use in the National Health Service.[26] Much of their reluctance to endorse these therapies is that, while there is much evidence that they modestly reduce relapse rate, there has been difficulty showing they have much effect on progression of disabililty, and that is the key in MS. And they are extremely expensive. They have, however, withheld a definitive recommendation until they reconsider all available evidence.

One of the drawbacks of the currently available drugs, and indeed those being prepared for study, is that they all seem to target the immune system. The problem as we have seen is that MS is both auto-immune in nature as well as degenerative, and when it becomes secondary, if it does, it is mainly degenerative. For a long time Western society has been looking for some drug that will prevent or reverse the degeneration that comes with living our unhealthy lifestyle. To date no one has come up with much, except perhaps the statins. Nothing apart from living and eating well seems to really prevent or treat degenerative disease. So the lifestyle changes we have been discussing so far are by far the best way to tackle MS, as they affect both immune function and degeneration. Drugs are a modestly effective, narrowly focused, additional therapy.

For those deciding to take the drugs, there are a number of issues. A study from Italy showed that 30 per cent of patients taking either interferons or glatiramer stopped them for one reason or another within five years, but around half shifted to another agent. For people who stayed on the medications, relapse rates declined each year. They also showed that there was no difference in effectiveness between any of the interferon preparations or glatiramer over that time.[27] In contrast, a German study showed that people taking glatiramer had greater reductions in relapse rates than patients on any of the interferons, and the drop-out rate due to side effects was also lower with glatiramer.[28] A US study showed that for patients switching from interferon therapy to glatiramer due to lack of effectiveness of the interferon, the relapse rate dropped dramatically on glatiramer.[29] A good study from Argentina in 2008 showed that people who not only switched from interferons to glatiramer but vice versa actually did really well, with annual relapse rates falling by about half to three-quarters in the three years after switching.[30] This has been confirmed by more recent work from the United States.[31] It is important for people with MS and their doctors to be aware that if the chosen drug is not working, there are always other options.[32]

These were not randomised controlled trials, but the data support the view that the drugs do have a place in MS management, although they really make only a modest difference. We can expect much greater benefit from the lifestyle changes I have outlined, according to the available evidence. It is important when considering whether to commence these agents that the situation is discussed carefully with the doctor, weighing up the pros and cons and considering the side effects. Then there is the question of choosing between the agents.

> Glatiramer is better tolerated than the interferons and may be more suitable for many people.

On the balance of evidence, if taking one of these disease-modifying therapies is recommended, I believe that glatiramer offers the best bet in terms of safety and lack of side effects. Further, it appears to remain effective with extended use. It is possible that the beneficial effects increase with continued use of the drug. There is more doubt about the rigour of the clinical trials and the safety profile of the interferons, about whether neutralising antibodies formed in the body against them reduce their effectiveness over time and whether they will prove to be effective or safe when used for many years. We don't yet have a long enough track record to judge these things. But head to head research published in 2008 showed that in a large cohort of 845 people with MS taking glatiramer or interferon in Kansas City, United States, using 'intention to treat' analysis (that is, ignoring the drop-outs and analysing everyone who started on the drugs), the two-year risk of relapse with glatiramer was nearly half that for the interferon (5.9% vs 10.9%, p=0.03).[33] In those who used the drug continuously for the period, the difference was even greater in favour of glatiramer (1.9% vs 9.1%, p=0.005). Another head to head RCT of glatiramer versus Rebif showed comparable efficacy for the two treatments[34] and similarly for glatiramer versus Betaferon.[35]

Many neurologists and much drug company marketing claim that the interferons are superior to glatiramer, but this does not seem be borne out by the medical literature. There is also the definite negative of the side effects with the interferons to consider when choosing. Research suggests for example that glatiramer is more than twice as likely as the interferons to reduce fatigue from MS.[36]

Nevertheless, the interferons appear to be effective, at least initially, and should be considered if necessary. Many neurologists appear to favour the interferons if the disease is very active because the evidence suggests they are effective more quickly than glatiramer. This may be a sensible strategy, although if steroids have been given for a relapse they usually confer protection for some time, allowing time for glatiramer to exert its effect. So glatiramer should not necessarily be avoided just because the disease is particularly active. Certainly in my experience people with MS seem to find glatiramer more acceptable than the interferons in terms of side effects.

Most neurologists will offer disease-modifying therapy once there has been more than one attack. There is evidence accumulating that even in the absence of attacks damage is continuing, and many authorities are arguing that patients should start disease-modifying therapy as soon as they are diagnosed. I feel this is an important consideration; if a decision is made to use one of the drug therapies as well as the lifestyle changes, then the earlier it is started the better. This means confronting the issue of regular, lifelong self-injection. For people without a medical background, or even for those with one, this can be extremely daunting. Worse, many will feel that to have to begin injecting medicine regularly represents a failure in some sense. Again, I feel it is important to resolve to do whatever it takes to control this disease. It may put the situation in perspective to know that diabetics have to self-inject twice or more a day. With glatiramer it is only once a day, and for the interferons between once every second day and once a week. Once self-injection becomes a routine, it is hard to imagine how it could have been so daunting.

It is important to reiterate that if the particular disease-modifying medication that you have started on does not seem to be working, it is sensible to change to a different class of medication. This is often overlooked as a way of dealing with deterioration should it occur. It is worth mentioning this to the treating doctor if things aren't going well on one of the medications.

Above all, the drug therapies and the lifestyle changes are not mutually exclusive. Starting drug therapy doesn't mean that the lifestyle changes can't be made in addition. Indeed, there is every reason to expect that they will complement each other. It may happen, for example, that there hasn't been long enough for the lifestyle changes to take effect before a second attack occurs, and you feel you have to do something to stop getting another. Swank's work suggested that the effects of the diet were not fully realised until at least three years after starting it, and probably more like five years. It may be worth considering starting one of the interferons at the beginning when the disease is particularly active and before lifestyle changes have had much time to have an effect, and then stopping the drug once stable. It is important that these issues are discussed with the neurologist or general practitioner. Forming a partnership with the doctor provides the best chance of taking control of the disease. Keeping secrets from your doctor is likely to be counterproductive.

Some people will have very active, progressive disease. This may not have happened for any particular reason, such as diet or lifestyle. Some forms of MS are just more aggressive than others. But there is still a range of therapies that can potentially slow down or even halt the illness. That is of course the key at this stage. While there are promising leads in remyelination therapy, answers still look quite a way off, so preventing damage in the first place is the key.

Others

The interferons and glatiramer are probably not much use for advanced progressive disease. However, the therapies that affect the immune system may be of more value here, balanced against the risk of side effects. Mitoxantrone alone or with steroids seems to be able to halt the disease progression for many patients. The cost in terms of side effects is quite high, however. And it seems that a disease-modifying therapy like glatiramer ought to be started at the same time, as the beneficial effects probably only last two years or so.

Combinations of interferon or glatiramer with azathioprine may prove to be helpful for active progressive disease. Intravenous immuno-globulins appear to be effective with few side effects, even for primary progressive MS. These therapies offer hope even for quite aggressive disease. Natalizumab is now also available in several countries including Australia and may be offered to those with aggressive or progressive forms of the disease.

THE WHOLE PACKAGE

In April 2002, Ian Gawler and I began a series of live-in retreats for people with MS at the Gawler Foundation, about an hour south-east of Melbourne. Ian has been running residential retreats for people with cancer for over 21 years. After he wrote the foreword for the first book, he and I got together and decided to set up retreats for people with MS along the same lines. The retreats last one week, and combine all the elements I have discussed in the book. These include daily meditations in the Meditation Sanctuary, communication exercises, education sessions about the techniques presented in this book, inspiring sessions with a range of counsellors and facilitators, and of course wonderful food prepared by the experienced cooks at the Gawler Foundation. I cannot recommend this more highly for a kick-start to help tackle this disease. Equally a number of people with quite advanced disease, including several in wheelchairs or beds, have attended the retreats and benefited enormously. For further information contact the Gawler Foundation or go to the website www.gawler.org. My wife Sandra and I also run retreats annually in New Zealand (see www.msakl.org.nz) and periodically in other parts of Australia for people unable to get to Victoria. For further information on all these retreats that I run see my website, www.takingcontrolofmultiplesclerosis.org.

A live-in retreat is a good way of kick-starting recovery from MS.

RECOVERY

So, after all this clear evidence that lifestyle change can make a great difference to the progression of MS, and indeed to a range of other degenerative Western diseases, we come to the question of recovery. Is it possible to recover from MS? The conventional response to this question of course is no. The abstract of a 2008 review in *Journal of Neurology* starts with the sentence: 'Multiple sclerosis is a lifelong, immune-mediated progressive disorder.'[37] That is the current medical paradigm; it is not possible to recover from MS. Once you have MS, you always have MS.

But then, the conventional answer to whether people can do anything themselves to slow or stop the progression of MS has also been no. I have even heard it said from reputable authorities that 'MS has a mind of its own', as if MS is some kind of external invader in the body, like a virus or bacterium, and not part of us. But even with a virus or bacterium we know there are all sorts of 'host' factors that interact with the organism and change the way it behaves in a particular person.

So, if the conventional response is that recovery from MS is not possible, what do we make of people who make the whole raft of changes I have outlined here and stay well? Let's say, like me, they stay well for a decade. Or twenty years. Or more. Or like some of Swank's patients, for 50 years! We know if they had cancer, for example, they would be considered cured if there had been no relapse after five years. So why is MS different? The consequences of it being considered different is that people with MS can never really feel they are over it and get on with a new life free of illness. Surely there must come a point when someone who commits to all these changes and stays well, and commits to keeping on with the lifestyle program permanently, is considered to have re-covered. But what is that point?

I submit that it is probably an individual thing, but that for the sake of starting a discussion about this why don't we take the ten-year mark, relapse-free, as signifying recovery? My strong feeling is that this would be an enormously liberating thing for people with MS to aim for and achieve. And as long as they didn't then abandon all the things that have kept them well, I feel there is nothing to lose and everything to gain from considering themselves recovered.

If you ask Ian Gawler if he has recovered from cancer, 30 years after being given three weeks to live,[38] he will say, tongue in cheek, 'I don't know; I'll know when I die of something else!' But of course he knows, as we do, that he has recovered. And he lives life as if he has recovered. But for people with MS, there is often the feeling that no matter how long they remain well they still live under the cloud of MS, that it could return at any time, that it is a lifelong disease. For a sense of how debilitating this way of living can be, just read Lance Armstrong's book and how he became so dispirited as every little odd symptom triggered the feeling that the cancer had returned.

But recovery from MS may in fact be just as possible as recovery from cancer. Recent work by Dr Dean Ornish in the United States shows that people who adopt an intensive lifestyle approach to prostate cancer similar to the Recovery Program actually change the way their genes are expressed.[39] Like Ian Gawler's recovery from 'terminal' bone cancer, where presumably his DNA actually changed so that the cancer was no longer expressed, it must be possible for people with MS who adopt a similar approach to Ornish and Gawler to change the way their genetic structure is expressed so they literally no longer have MS.

My own experience and that of many of the people who are following the Recovery Program and staying well is that it is well and truly possible to remain well after a diagnosis of MS, and that after a period of time this constitutes recovery from the illness. I know for me, it took a long time to accept that this was a reasonable position to take. But I believe the benefits of looking at it that way are that a great weight is lifted off my shoulders. I don't jump at every little symptom, thinking I am going to have a relapse. Mind you, I am never tempted to go back to my old way of life, and I pay great attention to getting the detail of the lifestyle right, such as keeping my vitamin D levels in the right range.

So I propose that a good goal to have to begin with is to get to two years as a first milestone, then ten years relapse-free. At that point, I feel it is quite appropriate to consider yourself recovered. And quite appropriate to celebrate that wonderful event, and look forward to a long, healthy and happy life! To get some sense of how well people are doing who are following the Recovery Program, go to my website www.takingcontrolofmultiplesclerosis.org and read the testimonials under 'What others say about us'.

OVERVIEW

People with MS have a wide range of choices about how to tackle the disease. The scientific evidence is now very clear. Starting with diet and getting adequate sunshine or vitamin D, there are many simple lifestyle changes that can significantly slow or halt the progression of the disease. Exercise, meditation, the management of stress and difficult emotions and avoiding depression are also important. In combination, this exceptionally healthy lifestyle is very likely to result in sustainable wellbeing for people with MS, and indeed for people without MS.

One bonus of getting the disease under control with these interventions is the sense of positivity and achievement it brings. If that doesn't help, for whatever reason, or in combination, there is now a range of medical therapies, some more toxic than others, that have been clearly shown to be effective in MS, albeit modestly, even in very active disease. There is no conflict here; it is not a case of one or the other, lifestyle change or drugs. They are likely to be optimally effective in combination.[8] Although despair is an understandable initial response to diagnosis, the outlook is far from bleak. Armed with the information now available, people should be able to make an informed choice from the lifestyle changes and therapies offered, and live long, healthy and happy lives. MS is now a treatable disease, regardless of type or severity. And recovery from MS is now a realistic possibility; overcoming multiple sclerosis is possible.

EPILOGUE

Be realistic: plan for a miracle

Osho

RIPPLES IN A POND

I liken what followed on from my diagnosis of MS to ripples in a pond. It was as if MS was a rock being thrown into the middle of a pond, sending out shock waves which touched the lives of many around me. Take the case of my old friend, Mike Galvin. Mike was director and sole special-ist in the ED at Fremantle Hospital when I started there in 1985. He is now retired, but for many years has been battling a chronic neurological disease for which the doctors can find no name. One of the first things I did when I was diagnosed with MS was to organise a regular Friday morning walk with him while I was off work. This ended up being thera-peutic for both of us.

Mike is a friendly, outgoing guy. He had an extraordinary medical career. He started off doing science at university, but after graduating decided he wanted to pursue his passion for medicine. He went back to uni and graduated as a doctor. He also developed a parallel career in the military, working his way up the ladder in the regular air force and later the reserve. The combination of his officer training and medical practice made him a formidable leader in medicine, and that is how his career worked out. His path and mine crossed when I was a bit out of control, having quit specialist anaesthesia training suddenly, realising it was driving me crazy. After I was 'parked' in the emergency department to allow me to find my feet again, I found Mike running the department.

That fateful association led me down the path that culminated in my present appointment. But it also began a friendship I have valued very highly. His path led to acting as Chief Executive Officer of a teaching hospital in Perth, and climbing to the rank of Group Captain in the air force, before he was suddenly ill. Whether his many overseas attachments in New Guinea and Asia and his brushes with malaria and hepatitis had anything to do with it is conjecture, but he developed an extremely unusual neurological disease in which areas of his brain began to 'disappear' in MRI scanning. The neurologists could find no explanation.

When we first started walking, I didn't feel as if I was very good company. My thoughts were focused in those first few weeks on finances, children's schooling, how long I could work, mortgages, insurance and so on. Mike's disease had affected him somewhat later in life, perhaps ten years further on, and his finances were secure. But it soon became clear that, unlike me, he was having trouble finding hope. Every day, as I scoured Medline for further information, hunted through the medical journals and worked on my positivity and focus, I felt stronger. Mike didn't have 19,000 articles to look through. No one could tell him what might happen to him. I started to see how hard it must have been for him.

Our walks were great. We would always pick a spot where there were natural highlights to look at, like walking along the beachfront at Cottesloe or alongside the Swan River. We saw dolphins out at sea, chatted about life and friends. I kept dropping into the conversation interesting things I was starting to pick up about omega-3 fatty acids, or sunlight. It came as something of a surprise to me when one day he said that he had started taking fish oil supplements. His rationale was simple. The doctors hadn't been able to offer him anything at all, so what did he have to lose. Some time after that, I asked him how he was. The first thing he did was make a fist. 'See that', he said. 'I've been getting regular steroid injections into this hand to combat arthritis, and I haven't been able to make a fist for years.' The fish oil had improved his arthritis so dramatically (as it has been shown to do in a series of RCTs) that he had stopped needing the steroids. He felt much better in himself as well, and also put that down to the supplements. I was pleased to see that physically he had improved so much.

But there was more to it. It wasn't easy to put my finger on. He seemed to radiate optimism. I thought back to those early walks, and realised what the difference was. The hope was back. A major ripple. And the really good news is that, after being given a very grim prognosis initially, my great friend continues to remain well and very active a decade on, much to the surprise of his neurologists.

Another series of ripples began when word started geting around that I was coming up with some answers in my search. I became the local referral centre amongst my friends and colleagues for the newly diagnosed. I was astonished at how many people were being diagnosed with MS. Within weeks of my illness, two clerical people at work were diagnosed, the sister of a work colleague, another colleague's babysitter. I seemed to be developing a small clientele of people who wanted to know what, if anything, they could do to heal their illness. That was at least one of the reasons why I chose to write this book. Since then of course I have been contacted by many, many people, have met all sorts of people with MS and their families, and have been involved with the residential retreats at the Gawler Foundation in Victoria and a series of MS support and residential groups in Perth, Canberra and Auckland, New Zealand. I have many hundreds of people with MS who regularly keep in touch with me and who have adopted my lifestyle suggestions, most of whom remain remarkably well.

It seemed to me that the shock waves emanating from my life spread out and touched so many other people's lives. Many of the waves provided enough energy for others to make changes to their own lives that they saw as beneficial. But I also got a lot back. I really enjoyed this newfound ability to help people. This may sound strange. It may seem that as a doctor I would regularly get satisfaction from helping people. But this seemed different. While as an emergency physician I could intervene and perhaps relieve pain or save a limb, or sometimes even save a life, this seemed more meaningful. It seemed that these changes in other people's lives that were emanating from my changes were all the more profound and satisfying, coming as they did from adversity.

And I got other things too. One day, early on after diagnosis, I was down at the local heated pool, swimming. I'd just finished my laps when I noticed a woman of about my age being lowered into the water by a hoist. She was obviously paralysed from the waist down. Having MS makes you bold in these situations. Another positive.

I swam over and introduced myself, told her I had MS, and asked if that was what she had too. She said that she had been diagnosed with transverse myelitis some four years earlier. One of the clear difficulties with this is that people don't then really know what they are dealing with. (I think in my case, because of my medical background, the neurologist felt he could be more frank, and so told me this. It certainly enabled me to deal with things a lot earlier than if I had thought of it as transverse myelitis. In fact, it was only a few days later that I saw him again to go over the MRI report, and that showed another five lesions in my brain, making the diagnosis certain.)

In Hilary's case, she had been on a conference trip to Japan when she developed weakness in her legs. This progressed rapidly to paraplegia. We started talking and have been in regular contact since. Specialists have now found another plaque in her brain, so the diagnosis is confirmed, but Hilary had already started making changes to try to avoid any more relapses. What I got from Hilary, though, was worth more than I can say. Hilary radiates optimism. Whenever I have seen her at the pool, being lowered in by the hoist or having a bucket of warm water tipped over her head to rinse herself after a swim, she is laughing or joking. I have never heard a negative comment from her. And yet she was paralysed with her very first lesion. She did a personal best the other day, 32 laps of the pool. I find her a great inspiration.

Many other ripples have emanated from the shock of MS in my life. My real hope is that this book will start another series of ripples, the world over. These ripples, I hope, can change the courses of many, many people's lives.

THE JOURNEY

I grew up in a family very traumatised from the experience of our mother having MS, and taking her own life. While we didn't really understand this at the time, all of us in the family were badly affected. It affected our view of the world, our relationships, our life choices. Watching someone so dearly loved deteriorate, and feeling completely powerless in the face of the disease, coloured our perception of the world and engendered in all of us a sense of resignation and lack of control.

It goes without saying that our mothers shape our lives. They are probably the most important people we ever have in our lives. I look back at my own life and see the profound influence Mum had on who I am, what I feel, how I interact and the people I choose to be with. Much of this was in place before she had MS. The fact that she developed MS, and I lived those years of physical deterioration with her, also dramatically affected my life and who I have become. Would I have become a doctor without this influence? Would I have made the relationship choices I made? I don't know. I know I can't change any of it, and will never know what life would have been like without MS in it. But I also know where my passion and motivation comes from for investigating the science behind possible treatments for MS.

Motivation is a very important issue. The same act can be seen completely differently depending on the motivation behind it. Sometimes it is easy to see someone's motivation. In my own case, I am very grateful that my motivation for the work I do for people with MS is quite clear. Given my experience of my mother's suffering, and now being very directly affected by the illness myself, I feel I almost have no choice but to make public the findings of my research into what is possible for people with MS. I am driven to do this by irresistible forces that have shaped my whole life.

Sometimes motivation can be a little more murky. My mother's suicide for example could be seen as a selfish act. While there is no doubt she wanted to end her suffering, I feel she was also motivated by wanting to end the suffering of her family, watching and living through her deterioration. Yet, undoubtedly, in attempting to alleviate her suffering and the suffering of those she loved, her suicide also caused much suffering. Our mother gone. While we were all so young. My siblings and I look with envy at other people who have their mothers well into their older years. Yet we understand the motivation behind our mother's action, and of course, in an intellectual sense, forgive her. And I of course would do anything possible to avoid other people finding themselves in the same position.

But the contradictory emotions around understanding my mother's dilemma and motivation, while repressing feelings of abandonment and anger, are hard to reconcile. They undoubtedly contribute to a chronic sense of dis-ease in my life. And knowing how important emotions are to the development of illness, I can see how easily this translates into chronic disease, like MS. As Carolyn Myss says, biography becomes biology. Often people spend their whole lives trying to repress these powerful emotions while attempting to forgive people for things they have every reason to feel deeply upset about. Actually accepting those contradictory feelings is a necessary first step before resolution and forgiveness can occur.

***

I am sure all of us with MS hope that we never find ourselves in a position like my mother did. But while hope is crucial, the reality is that there is much more than hope now. There is a highly credible and coherent body of scientific research indicating that recovery is now within the reach of a great proportion of people with MS. This is simply the truth of it. The research is clear. And we are also, with adequate exposure to sunlight or vitamin D supplements, in a position to prevent the disease occurring in our children, so that they never find themselves in the position my mother did and I have.

But while the physical tools of correct nutrition, adequate sunlight, exercise and meditation are critical to remaining well with MS, my firm belief is that this is only part of the story. Healing illness really requires fundamentally healing ourselves. The lifestyle changes outlined in this book can dramatically slow or stop the progress of the disease. The evidence for that is quite clear. But for real healing to occur, the under-lying dis-ease needs to be sorted out. This is where keeping a diary, counselling, talking to family and friends, meditating and being honest with ourselves about our innermost fears and emotions are necessary.

Many people with MS and other major illnesses actually see the disease as bringing many gifts into their lives. MS can be a good excuse to begin a more profound inner exploration and spiritual journey. The journey ultimately becomes an end in itself. Many times I have felt that without the illness, I would never have had the stimulus to stop what I was frantically doing with my life and really examine what was going on inside, and where my life was going. I am grateful to have been given the opportunity, despite the many difficult and painful times I have experi-enced since diagnosis.

For me, MS was to trigger a series of big changes. Having passed ten years since diagnosis, and remaining well, I feel my life beginning to stabilise. A medical colleague I had not seen for some time said to me recently that she thought my health was a miracle. In many respects she is right. To have remained free of relapses despite the enormously unsettling events of the last decade sometimes astounds me. It is really a testament to the strength of the whole package I describe in this book. But equally, had I not followed my heart and gone with the changes, had I fought them and resisted them, I suspect the package may not have been enough to keep me well, even though the changes were so dramatic and potentially damaging to my health. The changes were necessary if I was to heal.

MS has caused me to reconsider everything about my life. It has brought very considerable pain, but also major insights and a gradual reshaping of my emotional life. I have been tested, and forced to face fears I have carried with me since early childhood. I have learnt an enormous amount about rejection, abandonment, compassion, being judgmental and about myself. I have come closer to understanding my own true nature, and being comfortable with it. I know I will be much better for it. And I have had the opportunity to meet and get close to some wonderful people, many of whom also have MS.

My conviction is that the immune balance which is disrupted in MS is a very subtle one. For most people, rebalancing involves relatively minor fine-tuning with a commitment to improved diet, sunlight, meditation and personal growth. While drug therapies can be helpful, they represent a much more heavy handed approach to the problem, and don't claim to make much difference to the progression of the disease. I have no reservations about urging people with MS to adopt these lifestyle approaches rather than relying exclusively on conventional medicines. Equally, I think it is important to seriously consider taking the medicines. There really is no dichotomy here. My rationale from the beginning has been to do whatever it takes to overcome the illness.

There is every reason for people with MS to be hopeful about the future. A very large, coherent body of research suggests that those who adopt the lifestyle changes outlined in this book can reasonably hope to stabilise the illness where it is. And there is always the possibility of profound healing and recovery for some. In the process of making the effort to really look after ourselves, and understanding the underlying disease that may have precipitated the illness, for many another bigger journey will unfold. I wish you well on the journey.

FURTHER INFORMATION

THE INTERNET

At the start of the new millennium, we are extremely fortunate to live in the information age. When Mum got MS in 1967, the world's first computers were taking shape. Some of them took up whole rooms, and could do little more than modern calculators. Today, at the click of a mouse we can be surfing the web, getting access to the most sophisticated, up to the minute information about anything you care to name. This is great. But there is a downside. Nothing on the web is censored or evaluated for its truth or scientific integrity. Particularly in areas where disease is incurable, charlatans abound. It is important to be careful and analyse everything carefully.

Fortunately there are many reputable websites to visit. I would start of course with my website www.takingcontrolofmultiplesclerosis.org, where you will find continually updated information. You can join as a member and get newsletter updates on the latest about MS, as well as exchange recipes and comments in the Forum. The best of the others is, I think, the website for the Multiple Sclerosis Resource Centre in the United Kingdom at www.msrc.co.uk. This is a really comprehensive website with information from a variety of sources for people with MS. For more technical information, the MS Society of Canada has a good website at www.mssoc.ca. They have a very useful section summarising the most recent research papers on MS where it is possible to keep up to date with new therapies, and get a reputable opinion on the latest fad. They also have pre-release data from some of the clinical trials of new drugs. They occasionally shoot down a charlatan who comes up with a 'cure for MS'. The site is very well balanced, although extremely traditional and conservative in philosophy. There is nothing here about faith or visualisation. But to find out, for example, whether natalizumab has been approved for the treatment of MS in the United States, this is the site.

Another useful one is the International Federation of Multiple Sclerosis Societies (IFMSS). They can be found at www.msif.org or by typing MSIF into a web search engine. Things change so quickly in cyberspace. The best engine to find anything on the web of course is now Google (www.google.com). It is possible to Google almost any question and rapidly get up to date information on it.

If you wish to do as I did and search the Medline-indexed medical literature, then Pubmed is the place. This can be found at www.ncbi. nlm.nih.gov. The rules are pretty simple, and very soon you can be looking through up to 250-word summaries of medical articles just as they appeared in the medical journals. I hope that some of the information I have provided in this book will provide you with enough scientific background to at least have a reasonable idea about the worth of many of these studies.

If you have a real interest in the omega-3 fatty acid story and all the research showing its widespread benefits to health, the best website is www.udoerasmus.com. Here there is detailed information on all things fatty and their roles in conditions as diverse as cancer, depression, auto-immunity, arthritis, asthma and so on. There are also links to other omega-3 sites. *The Omega Plan* now has its own website as well, which you can find in the book. The website set up by Professor Swank is at www.swankmsdiet.org and his book is still available, and can be ordered from www.amazon.com.

Another website I have found really useful is www.netrition.com. To find out exactly how much fat is in a given food, and what it is composed of in terms of saturated and unsaturated fats, this is the website. For instance, when skimming the nutritional information on a packet of rolled oats, I noticed that oats are 6.9 per cent fat. A quick look at this website under 'Info' and 'Food nutrients' allows you to type in 'oats' and get an immediate breakdown of all its constituents. It is extremely reassuring to find that rolled oats are only 1.2 per cent saturated fat, and the rest of the fat is mono- and polyunsaturated.

BOOKS

I have found a number of books most useful. Most of them I have already mentioned under each chapter heading where applicable. The best self-help book on MS is *Multiple Sclerosis: A self-help guide to its management* by Judy Graham, a UK journalist. She has had MS herself for over fifteen years, and has used a combination of diet and other therapies to maintain her physical condition. She writes well and in an open-minded and unbiased way about available therapies. The book is out of date now though, being published in 1987, missing out all the recent advances such as interferon, glatiramer and so on. It may be found in libraries or second-hand on the Internet.

Professor Swank's *Multiple Sclerosis Diet Book* is wonderful. For those interested in finding out in detail about his study, this is the book. It has far more detail than any of the journal articles he has published. Further, it has many, many recipes for healthy, low-fat meals. I recommend it highly. Again it is a little out of date now, with the most recent edition being published in 1987. Hence, a lot of the more recent advances in understanding the balance between omega-3 and omega-6 fatty acids don't get a mention. But this man is the pioneer, and his book should certainly be read.

For general dietary advice on fatty acids, the best-selling *The Omega Plan* by Artemis Simopoulos and Jo Robinson is extremely informative and easy reading. Again, there are many recipes which can easily be translated into an MS diet. It's fascinating to see how many Western diseases can be improved with a low saturated-fat, high omega-3 diet.

For those wanting to follow the mind–body connection, or who have been prompted by this illness to explore a spiritual path, the possibilities are endless. Any good modern bookstore will usually have racks of books under the heading of self-improvement or new age, or some such. I must, however, recommend much of the work of Carolyn Myss. For some people, *Anatomy of the Spirit* will be too much to start with. It is a heavy book, but provides the clearest signposts, I think, to the spiritual journey which awaits you. *Why People Don't Heal and How They Can* is a good follow-up. I am less taken with the book she co-wrote with Dr Norman Shealy, *The Creation of Health*. I found the description of the personality type of people with MS a little insulting. (Incidentally, I think this applied to many of the other descriptions as well.) It did not seem terribly sensitively written, and I don't recommend it.

The same cannot be said, though, of the outstanding work of Dr Deepak Chopra. You could pick up almost anything this great man has written and be enlightened. *Quantum Healing* is a pretty good place to start, but any or all of the others would be worthwhile.

Unreservedly, I say that the most liberating book to read for a doctor who is ill is Bernie Siegel's *Love, Medicine and Miracles*. *Peace, Love and Healing* is also fantastic. This exquisitely compassionate and caring surgeon deserves all the plaudits he has received for these wonderful books. I found Dan Millman's *The Laws of Spirit* a good short read after the comparatively heavy going of Carolyn Myss, but with similarly strong messages.

And *Tuesdays with Morrie* is a good book to read for those with advanced MS who find the disability hard to live with. Morrie's insights are profound. And for a story of true inspiration, try Lance Armstrong's self-titled book.

I have since gotten into the collection of books written by Pema Chodron, starting with *Start Where You Are*, *The Places That Scare You* and *The Wisdom of No Escape*. These led me on to the wonderful work of Osho, including his books *Courage*, *Intuition*, *Freedom* and others. These writings have been a source of enormous inspiration for me.

I could go on, but the spiritual journey is an individual one. One book will lead to another, and the unique signposts along the way will be yours, and yours alone, to follow.

A great place to find other books related to any of these or any you have found yourself is at www.amazon.com, www.amazon.co.uk, the UK version or www.amazon.ca, the Canadian version. This hugely successful website allows one not only to find and order a particular book, but it will show, for instance, what the last few people who bought that book also bought. You can be led into areas you may not have otherwise found. Of course, having found a book, there is no compulsion to buy it. I am now an avid reader, and get most of my books, where possible, from the local libraries.

SOCIETIES AND GROUPS

Each area has its own MS society. Most have only a nominal joining fee and provide access to a range of services, from counselling to newsletters, physiotherapy or accommodation. Many are now getting more in touch with what their members with MS actually want, rather than just being places to meet others with the same disease or assisting late in the disease with wheelchairs and accommodation. Some, like the MS Society of Auckland in New Zealand (www.msakl.org.nz), are quite progressive, and offer a full range of complementary therapies as well as workshops for the newly diagnosed. Some may also wish to join a meditation or yoga group or other gathering of like-minded people who have in common their spiritual path rather than disease. This may be a very good way of keeping things in perspective. There is often information on such groups through MS societies. Alternatively, the Gawler Foundation runs meditation retreats and offers a range of CDs and tapes. See www.gawler.org.

OVERVIEW

I am so grateful I was diagnosed with my disease in 1999, and not in 1967. Mum knew only that she had an incurable illness. In this age, you and I can find almost any piece of information we need, whether it be the latest theory on causes of MS, the latest advance in treatment or just a letter from someone else with MS. Become an expert on MS. There is no better way to sort out the vast array of information that surrounds people after diagnosis. It will also provide the strength to deal with the illness in your journey to recovery.

NOTES

Chapter 2

1. Barnard ND, Cohen J, Jenkins DJ, et al. A low-fat vegan diet improves glycemic control and cardiovascular risk factors in a randomized clinical trial in individuals with type 2 diabetes. Diabetes Care 2006; 29:1777–83

2. Gillies CL, Abrams KR, Lambert PC, et al. Pharmacological and lifestyle interventions to prevent or delay type 2 diabetes in people with impaired glucose tolerance: systematic review and meta-analysis. BMJ 2007; 334:299

3. Sinha K. The Kalam way to a healthy heart. Times of India. New Delhi, 30 September 2006; 15

4. Ornish D, Scherwitz LW, Billings JH, et al. Intensive lifestyle changes for reversal of coronary heart disease. JAMA 1998; 280:2001–2007.

5. Ornish D, Weidner G, Fair WR, et al. Intensive lifestyle changes may affect the progression of prostate cancer. J Urol 2005; 174:1065–9; discussion 1069–70

6. Daubenmier JJ, Weidner G, Marlin R, et al. Lifestyle and health-related quality of life of men with prostate cancer managed with active surveillance. Urology 2006; 67:125–30

7. Frattaroli J, Weidner G, Kemp C, et al. Clinical events in prostate cancer lifestyle trial: results from two years of follow-up. Urology 2008; 72:1319–23

8. Jelinek GA. Lifting the veil on the editorial process. Emerg Med 1997; 9:275–6.

9. Sackett DL, Rosenberg WM, Gray JA, et al. Evidence based medicine: what it is and what it isn't. BMJ 1996; 312:71–2

10. Kurtzke JF. Rating neurological impairment in multiple sclerosis: an expanded disability scale. Neurology 1983; 33:1444–52

11. Bodenheimer T. Uneasy alliance: clinical investigators and the pharmaceutical industry. N Engl J Med 2000; 342:1539–44

12. Als-Nielsen B, Chen W, Gluud C, et al. Association of funding and conclusions in randomized drug trials: a reflection of treatment effect or adverse events? JAMA 2003; 290:921–8

13. Stelfox HT, Chua G, O'Rourke K, et al. Conflict of interest in the debate over calcium-channel antagonists. N Engl J Med 1998; 338:101–106

14. Campbell EG, Gruen RL, Mountford J, et al. A national survey of physician-industry relationships. N Engl J Med 2007; 356:1742–50

15. Angell M. The Truth About the Drug Companies: How they deceive us and what to do about it. Carlton North: Scribe Publications, 2005

Chapter 3

1. Chopra D. Journey Into Healing. Sydney: Random House, 1994

2. Patani R, Balaratnam M, Vora A, et al. Remyelination can be extensive in multiple sclerosis despite a long disease course. Neuropathol Appl Neurobiol 2007; 33: 277–87

3. Kerschensteiner M, Bareyre FM, Buddeberg BS, et al. Remodeling of axonal connections contributes to recovery in an animal model of multiple sclerosis. J Exp Med 2004; 200:1027–38

4. Atkins EJ, Biousse V, Newman NJ. Optic neuritis. Semin Neurol 2007; 27:211–20

5. Milonas I, Georgiadis N. Role of optic neuritis diagnosis in the early identification and treatment of MS. Int MS J 2008; 15:69–79

6. Optic neuritis study group. Multiple sclerosis risk after optic neuritis: final optic neuritis treatment trial follow-up. Arch Neurol 2008; 65:727–32

7. Swanton JK, Fernando KT, Dalton CM, et al. Early MRI in optic neuritis: the risk for disability. Neurology 2009; 72:542–50

8. Gilbert ME, Sergott RC. New directions in optic neuritis and multiple sclerosis. Curr Neurol Neurosci Rep 2007; 7:259–64

9. Optic Neuritis Study Group. Visual function 15 years after optic neuritis: a final follow-up report from the Optic Neuritis Treatment Trial. Ophthalmology 2008; 115:1079–82 e1075

10. Pelidou SH, Giannopoulos S, Tzavidi S, et al. Multiple sclerosis presented as clinically isolated syndrome: the need for early diagnosis and treatment. Ther Clin Risk Manag 2008; 4:627–30

11. Costello F. Optic neuritis: the role of disease-modifying therapy in this clinically isolated syndrome. Curr Treat Options Neurol 2007; 9:48–54

12. Vedula SS, Brodney-Folse S, Gal RL, et al. Corticosteroids for treating optic neuritis. Cochrane Database Syst Rev 2007:CD001430

13. Hirtz D, Thurman DJ, Gwinn-Hardy K, et al. How common are the 'common' neurologic disorders? Neurology 2007; 68:326–37

14. Wesler IS. Statistics of multiple sclerosis. Am Med Assoc Arch Neurol Psych 1922; 8:59–63

15. Swank RL, Dugan BB. The Multiple Sclerosis Diet Book: A low fat diet for the treatment of MS. New York: Doubleday, 1987

16. Pugliatti M, Riise T, Sotgiu MA, et al. Increasing incidence of multiple sclerosis in the province of Sassari, northern Sardinia. Neuroepidemiology 2005; 25:129–34

17. Warren SA, Svenson LW, Warren KG. Contribution of incidence to increasing prevalence of multiple sclerosis in Alberta, Canada. Mult Scler 2008; 14:872–9

18. Houzen H, Niino M, Hata D, et al. Increasing prevalence and incidence of multiple sclerosis in northern Japan. Mult Scler 2008; 14:887–92

19. Gray OM, McDonnell GV, Hawkins SA. Factors in the rising prevalence of multiple sclerosis in the north-east of Ireland. Mult Scler 2008; 14:880–6

20. Brotherson G. Editorial. MS Society of Western Australia Bulletin, April 2007; 2

21. Simopoulos A, Robinson J. The Omega Plan. Hodder: Rydalmere, 1998

22. Orton SM, Herrera BM, Yee IM, et al. Sex ratio of multiple sclerosis in Canada: a longitudinal study. Lancet Neurol 2006; 5:932–6

23. Debouverie M, Pittion-Vouyovitch S, Louis S, et al. Increasing incidence of multiple sclerosis among women in Lorraine, eastern France. Mult Scler 2007; 13:962–7

24. Hansen T, Skythe A, Stenager E, et al. Concordance for multiple sclerosis in Danish twins: an update of a nationwide study. Mult Scler 2005; 11:504–10

25. Sadovnick AD, Ebers GC, Dyment DA, et al. Evidence for genetic basis of multiple sclerosis. The Canadian Collaborative Study Group. Lancet 1996; 347:1728–30

26. Ebers GC, Sadovnick AD, Risch NJ. A genetic basis for familial aggregation in multiple sclerosis. Canadian Collaborative Study Group. Nature 1995; 377:150–51

27. Dyment DA, Yee IM, Ebers GC, et al. Multiple sclerosis in step-siblings: recurrence risk and ascertainment. J Neurol Neurosurg Psychiatry 2006; 77:258–9

28. Ebers GC, Sadovnick AD, Dyment DA, et al. Parent-of-origin effect in multiple sclerosis: observations in half-siblings. Lancet 2004; 363:1773–4

29. Kantarci OH, Barcellos LF, Atkinson EJ, et al. Men transmit MS more often to their children vs women: the Carter effect. Neurology 2006; 67:305–10

30. Herrera BM, Ramagopalan SV, Orton S, et al. Parental transmission of MS in a population-based Canadian cohort. Neurology 2007; 69:1208–12

31. Ebers GC, Kukay K, Bulman DE, et al. A full genome search in multiple sclerosis. Nat Genet 1996; 13:472–6

32. Olsson T, Hillert J. The genetics of multiple sclerosis and its experimental models. Curr Opin Neurol 2008; 21:255–60

33. Svejgaard A. The immunogenetics of multiple sclerosis. Immunogenetics 2008; 60:275–86

34. Sadovnick AD, Yee IM, Ebers GC, et al. Effect of age at onset and parental disease status on sibling risks for MS. Neurology 1998; 50:719–23

35. Ponsonby AL, van der Mei I, Dwyer T, et al. Exposure to infant siblings during early life and risk of multiple sclerosis. JAMA 2005; 293:463–9

36. Amato MP, Zipoli V, Goretti B, et al. Benign multiple sclerosis: cognitive, psychological and social aspects in a clinical cohort. J Neurol 2006; 253:1054–9

37. Jenkins TM, Khaleeli Z, Thompson AJ. Diagnosis and management of primary progressive multiple sclerosis. Minerva Med 2008; 99:141–55

38. Paty DW, Oger JJF, Kastrukoff LF, et al. Magnetic resonance imaging in the diagnosis of multiple sclerosis (MS): a prospective study of comparison with clinical evaluation, evoked potentials, oligoclonal banding, and CT. Neurology 1988; 38:180–85

39. Rovira A, Leon A. MR in the diagnosis and monitoring of multiple sclerosis: An overview. Eur J Radiol 2008; 67:409–14

40. Tedeschi G, Lavorgna L, Russo P, et al. Brain atrophy and lesion load in a large population of patients with multiple sclerosis. Neurology 2005; 65:280–85

41. Scott TF, Kassab SL, Singh S. Acute partial transverse myelitis with normal cerebral magnetic resonance imaging: transition rate to clinically definite multiple sclerosis. Mult Scler 2005; 11:373–7

42. Elian M, Dean G. To tell or not to tell the diagnosis of multiple sclerosis. Lancet 1985; 6:27–8

43. Papathanasopoulos PG, Nikolakopoulou A, Scolding NJ. Disclosing the diagnosis of multiple sclerosis. J Neurol 2005; 252:1307–1309

44. NICE. Multiple Sclerosis: Management of multiple sclerosis in primary and secondary care. London: National Institute for Clinical Excellence, 2003

45. Fawcett TN, Lucas M. Multiple sclerosis: living the reality. Br J Nurs 2006; 15:46–51

46. Solari A, Acquarone N, Pucci E, et al. Communicating the diagnosis of multiple sclerosis: a qualitative study. Mult Scler 2007; 13:763–9

47. Bogosian A, Moss-Morris R, Yardley L, et al. Experiences of partners of people in the early stages of multiple sclerosis. Mult Scler 2009; Epub 27/01/2009

48. Kremenchutzky M, Rice GP, Baskerville J, et al. The natural history of multiple sclerosis: a geographically based study 9: Observations on the progressive phase of the disease. Brain 2006; 129:584–94

49. Tremlett H, Paty D, Devonshire V. The natural history of primary progressive MS in British Columbia, Canada. Neurology 2005; 65:1919–23

50. Tremlett H, Paty D, Devonshire V. Disability progression in multiple sclerosis is slower than previously reported. Neurology 2006; 66:172–7

51. Whiting P, Harbord R, Main C, et al. Accuracy of magnetic resonance imaging for the diagnosis of multiple sclerosis: systematic review. BMJ 2006; 332:875–84

52. Pittock SJ, Mayr WT, McClelland RL, et al. Disability profile of MS did not change over 10 years in a population-based prevalence cohort. Neurology 2004; 62:601–606

53. Confavreux C, Vukusic S. Natural history of multiple sclerosis: a unifying concept. Brain 2006; 129:606–616

54. Confavreux C, Vukusic S. Age at disability milestones in multiple sclerosis. Brain 2006; 129:595–605

55. Simons LA, Simons J, McCallum J, et al. Lifestyle factors and risk of dementia: Dubbo Study of the elderly. Med J Aust 2006; 184:68–70

56. Kuzniarz M, Mitchell P, Cumming RG, et al. Use of vitamin supplements and cataract: the Blue Mountains Eye Study. Am J Ophthalmol 2001; 132:19–26

57. Mowry EM, Pesic M, Grimes B, et al. Demyelinating events in early multiple sclerosis have inherent severity and recovery. Neurology 2009; 72:602–608

58. Hammond SR, McLeod JG, Macaskill P, et al. Multiple sclerosis in Australia: prognostic factors. J Clin Neurosci 2000; 7:16–19

59. Bronnum-Hansen H, Koch-Henriksen N, Stenager E. Trends in survival and cause of death in Danish patients with multiple sclerosis. Brain 2004; 11:11

60. Hirst CL, Swingler R, Compston A, et al. Survival and cause of death in multiple sclerosis: A prospective population based study. J Neurol Neurosurg Psychiatry 2008; 79:1016–21

61. Optic Neuritis Treatment Group. Neurologic impairment 10 years after optic neuritis. Arch Neurol 2004; 61:1386–9

62. Stefferl A, Schubart A, Storch M, et al. Butyrophilin, a milk protein, modulates the encephalitogenic T cell response to myelin oligodendrocyte glycoprotein in experimental autoimmune encephalomyelitis. J Immunol 2000; 165:2859–65

63. Winer S, Astsaturov I, Cheung RK, et al. T cells of multiple sclerosis patients target a common environmental peptide that causes encephalitis in mice. J Immunol 2001; 166:4751–6

64. Westall FC. Molecular mimicry revisited: gut bacteria and multiple sclerosis. J Clin Microbiol 2006; 44:2099–2104

65. Arnold DL. Changes observed in multiple sclerosis using magnetic resonance imaging reflect a focal pathology distributed along axonal pathways. J Neurol 2005; 252 Suppl 5:v25–v29

66. Chaudhuri A, Behan PO. Treatment of multiple sclerosis: beyond the NICE guidelines. QJM 2005; 98:373–8

67. Hauser SL, Oksenberg JR. The neurobiology of multiple sclerosis: genes, inflammation, and neurodegeneration. Neuron 2006; 52:61–76

68. Riise T, Moen BE, Kyvik KR. Organic solvents and the risk of multiple sclerosis. Epidemiology 2002; 13:718–20

69. Poser CM. The multiple sclerosis trait and the development of multiple sclerosis: genetic vulnerability and environmental effect. Clin Neurol Neurosurg 2006; 108:227–33

70. De Stefano N, Cocco E, Lai M, et al. Imaging brain damage in first-degree relatives of sporadic and familial multiple sclerosis. Ann Neurol 2006; 59: 634–9

71. Ebers GC. Environmental factors and multiple sclerosis. Lancet Neurol 2008; 7:268–77

72. Zamboni P, Galeotti R, Menegatti E, et al. Chronic cerebrospinal venous insufficiency in patients with multiple sclerosis. J Neurol Neurosurg Psychiatry, 2009; 80:392–9

Chapter 4

1. Mosmann TR, Coffman RL. TH1 and TH2 cells: different patterns of lymphokine secretion lead to different functional properties. Annu Rev Immunol 1989; 7:145–73

2. Hedegaard CJ, Krakauer M, Bendtzen K, et al. T helper cell type 1 (Th1), Th2 and Th17 responses to myelin basic protein and disease activity in multiple sclerosis. Immunology 2008; 125:161–9

3. Weinstock JV, Summers RW, Elliott DE. Role of helminths in regulating mucosal inflammation. Springer Semin Immunopathol 2005; 27:249–71

4. Calder PC. n–3 polyunsaturated fatty acids and cytokine production in health and disease. Ann Nutr Metab 1997; 41:203–34

5. Simopoulos A, Robinson J. The Omega Plan. Hodder: Rydalmere, 1998

6. Gallai V, Sarchielli P, Trequattrini A, et al. Cytokine secretion and eicosanoid production in the peripheral blood mononuclear cells of MS patients undergoing dietary supplementation with n–3 polyunsaturated fatty acids. J Neuroimmunol 1995; 56:143–53

7. Calabrese V, Bella R, Testa D, et al. Increased cerebrospinal fluid and plasma levels of ultraweak chemiluminescence are associated with changes in the thiol pool and lipid-soluble fluorescence in multiple sclerosis: the pathogenic role of oxidative stress. Drugs Exp Clin Res 1998; 24:125–31

8. Toshniwal PK, Zarling EJ. Evidence for increased lipid peroxidation in multiple sclerosis. Neurochem Res 1992; 17:205–207

9. Norris JM, Yin X, Lamb MM, et al. Omega-3 polyunsaturated fatty acid intake and islet autoimmunity in children at increased risk for type 1 diabetes. JAMA 2007; 298:1420–28

10. Hafstrom I, Ringertz B, Spangberg A, et al. A vegan diet free of gluten improves the signs and symptoms of rheumatoid arthritis: the effects on arthritis correlate with a reduction in antibodies to food antigens. Rheumatology (Oxford) 2001; 40:1175–9

11. Kaartinen K, Lammi K, Hypen M, et al. Vegan diet alleviates fibromyalgia symptoms. Scand J Rheumatol 2000; 29:308–313

12. Skoldstam L, Hagfors L, Johansson G. An experimental study of a Mediterranean diet intervention for patients with rheumatoid arthritis. Ann Rheum Dis 2003; 62:208–214

13. Hagfors L, Nilsson I, Skoldstam L, et al. Fat intake and composition of fatty acids in serum phospholipids in a randomized, controlled, Mediterranean dietary intervention study on patients with rheumatoid arthritis. Nutr Metab (Lond) 2005; 2:26

14. Chrysohoou C, Panagiotakos DB, Pitsavos C, et al. Adherence to the Mediterranean diet attenuates inflammation and coagulation process in healthy adults: the ATTICA Study. J Am Coll Cardiol 2004; 44:152–8

15. Stamp LK, James MJ, Cleland LG. Diet and rheumatoid arthritis: a review of the literature. Semin Arthritis Rheum 2005; 35:77–94

16. McCarty MF. Upregulation of lymphocyte apoptosis as a strategy for preventing and treating auto-immune disorders: a role for wholefood vegan diets, fish oil and dopamine agonists. Med Hypotheses 2001; 57:258–75

17. McCarty MF. A moderately low phosphate intake may provide health benefits analogous to those conferred by UV light: a further advantage of vegan diets. Med Hypotheses 2003; 61:543–60

18. Flower RJ, Perretti M. Controlling inflammation: a fat chance? J Exp Med 2005; 201:671–4

19. Das UN, Ramos EJ, Meguid MM. Metabolic alterations during inflammation and its

modulation by central actions of omega-3 fatty acids. Curr Opin Clin Nutr Metab Care 2003; 6:413–19

20. Zampelas A, Panagiotakos DB, Pitsavos C, et al. Fish consumption among healthy adults is associated with decreased levels of inflammatory markers related to cardiovascular disease: the ATTICA Study. J Am Coll Cardiol 2005; 46:120–24

21. Holmoy T. The immunology of multiple sclerosis: disease mechanisms and therapeutic targets. Minerva Med 2008; 99:119–40

22. Chaudhuri A, Behan PO. Treatment of multiple sclerosis: beyond the NICE guidelines. QJM 2005; 98:373–8

23. Shea TB, Lyons-Weiler J, Rogers E. Homocysteine, folate deprivation and Alzheimer neuropathology. J Alzheimers Dis 2002; 4:261–7

24. Ramsaransing GS, Fokkema MR, Teelken A, et al. Plasma homocysteine levels in multiple sclerosis. J Neurol Neurosurg Psychiatry 2006; 77:189–92

25. Teunissen CE, van Boxtel MP, Jolles J, et al. Homocysteine in relation to cognitive performance in pathological and non-pathological conditions. Clin Chem Lab Med 2005; 43:1089–1095

26. Triantafyllou N, Evangelopoulos ME, Kimiskidis VK, et al. Increased plasma homocysteine levels in patients with multiple sclerosis and depression. Ann Gen Psychiatry 2008; 7:17

27. Scott TM, Tucker KL, Bhadelia A, et al. Homocysteine and B vitamins relate to brain volume and white-matter changes in geriatric patients with psychiatric disorders. Am J Geriatr Psychiatry 2004; 12:631–8

28. Mattson MP, Kruman, II, Duan W. Folic acid and homocysteine in age-related disease. Ageing Res Rev 2002; 1:95–111

29. Lehmann M, Regland B, Blennow K, et al. Vitamin B12-B6-folate treatment improves blood-brain barrier function in patients with hyperhomocysteinaemia and mild cognitive impairment. Dement Geriatr Cogn Disord 2003; 16:145–50

30. Filippi M, Rovaris M, Inglese M, et al. Interferon beta-1a for brain tissue loss in patients at presentation with syndromes suggestive of multiple sclerosis: a randomised, double-blind, placebo-controlled trial. Lancet 2004; 364:1489–96

31. Filippi M, Rocca MA. MRI evidence for multiple sclerosis as a diffuse disease of the central nervous system. J Neurol 2005; 252 Suppl 5:v16–v24

32. Bruck W. The pathology of multiple sclerosis is the result of focal inflammatory demyelination with axonal damage. J Neurol 2005; 252 Suppl 5:v3–v9

33. Bruck W. Inflammatory demyelination is not central to the pathogenesis of multiple sclerosis. J Neurol 2005; 252 Suppl 5:v10–v15

34. Coles AJ, Cox A, Le Page E, et al. The window of therapeutic opportunity in multiple sclerosis: evidence from monoclonal antibody therapy. J Neurol 2005; 253:98–108

35. Zipp F, Aktas O. The brain as a target of inflammation: common pathways link inflammatory and neurodegenerative diseases. Trends Neurosci 2006; 29:518–27

36. Zamaria N. Alteration of polyunsaturated fatty acid status and metabolism in health and disease. Reprod Nutr Dev 2004; 44:273–82

37. Das UN, Vaddadi KS. Essential fatty acids in Huntington's disease. Nutrition 2004; 20:942–7

38. Das UN. Long-chain polyunsaturated fatty acids in memory formation and consolidation: further evidence and discussion. Nutrition 2003; 19:988–93

39. Das UN. Can memory be improved? A discussion on the role of ras, GABA, acetylcholine, NO, insulin, TNF-alpha, and long-chain polyunsaturated fatty acids in memory formation and consolidation. Brain Dev 2003; 25:251–61

40. Das UN, Fams. Long-chain polyunsaturated fatty acids in the growth and development of the brain and memory. Nutrition 2003; 19:62–5

41. de Lau LM, Bornebroek M, Witteman JC, et al. Dietary fatty acids and the risk of Parkinson disease: the Rotterdam study. Neurology 2005; 64:2040–45

42. Hogyes E, Nyakas C, Kiliaan A, et al. Neuroprotective effect of developmental docosahexaenoic acid supplement against excitotoxic brain damage in infant rats. Neuroscience 2003; 119:999–1012

43. Wang X, Zhao X, Mao ZY, et al. Neuroprotective effect of docosahexaenoic acid on glutamate-induced cytotoxicity in rat hippocampal cultures. Neuroreport 2003; 14:2457–61

44. Wu A, Molteni R, Ying Z, et al. A saturated-fat diet aggravates the outcome of traumatic brain injury on hippocampal plasticity and cognitive function by reducing brain-derived neurotrophic factor. Neuroscience 2003; 119:365–75

45. Walford RL. The clinical promise of diet restriction. Geriatrics 1990; 45:81–3

46. Johnson JB, Laub DR, John S. The effect on health of alternate day calorie restriction: eating less and more than needed on alternate days prolongs life. Med Hypotheses 2006; 67:209–11

47. Sanna V, Di Giacomo A, La Cava A, et al. Leptin surge precedes onset of auto-immune encephalomyelitis and correlates with development of pathogenic T-cell responses. J Clin Invest 2003; 111:241–50

Chapter 5

1. Esparza ML, Sasaki S, Kesteloot H. Nutrition, latitude, and multiple sclerosis mortality: an ecologic study. Am J Epidemiol 1995; 142:733–7

2. Swank RL, Dugan BB. The Multiple Sclerosis Diet Book: A low fat diet for the treatment of MS. New York: Doubleday, 1987

3. Knox EG. Foods and diseases. Br J Prev Soc Med 1977; 31:71–80

4. Agranoff BW, Goldberg D. Diet and the geographical distribution of multiple sclerosis. Lancet 1974; 2:1061–6

5. Bernsohn J, Stephanides LM. Aetiology of multiple sclerosis. Nature 1967; 215:821–3

6. Malosse D, Perron H, Sasco A, et al. Correlation between milk and dairy product consumption and multiple sclerosis prevalence: a worldwide study. Neuroepidemiology 1992; 11:304–12

7. Malosse D, Perron H. Correlation analysis between bovine populations, other farm animals, house pets, and multiple sclerosis prevalence. Neuroepidemiology 1993; 12:15–27

8. Stefferl A, Schubart A, Storch M, et al. Butyrophilin, a milk protein, modulates

the encephalitogenic T cell response to myelin oligodendrocyte glycoprotein in experimental autoimmune encephalomyelitis. J Immunol 2000; 165:2859–65

9. Winer S, Astsaturov I, Cheung RK, et al. T cells of multiple sclerosis patients target a common environmental peptide that causes encephalitis in mice. J Immunol 2001; 166:4751–6

10. Mana P, Goodyear M, Bernard C, et al. Tolerance induction by molecular mimicry: prevention and suppression of experimental auto-immune encephalomyelitis with the milk protein butyrophilin. Int Immunol 2004; 16:489–99

11. TRIGR Study Group. Study design of the Trial to Reduce IDDM in the Genetically at Risk (TRIGR). Pediatr Diabetes 2007; 8:117–37

12. Akerblom HK, Virtanen SM, Ilonen J, et al. Dietary manipulation of beta cell auto-immunity in infants at increased risk of type 1 diabetes: a pilot study. Diabetologia 2005; 48:829–37

13. Chen H, Zhang SM, Hernan MA, et al. Diet and Parkinson's disease: a potential role of dairy products in men. Ann Neurol 2002; 52:793–801

14. Campbell TC, Campbell TM. The China Study. New York: Benbella Books, 2006

15. Ghadirian P, Jain M, Ducic S, et al. Nutritional factors in the aetiology of multiple sclerosis: a case-control study in Montreal, Canada. Int J Epidemiol 1998; 27: 845–52.

16. Lauer K. The risk of multiple sclerosis in the USA in relation to sociogeographic features: a factor-analytic study. J Clin Epidemiol 1994; 47:43–8

17. Sepcic J, Mesaros E, Materljan E, et al. Nutritional factors and multiple sclerosis in Gorski Kotar, Croatia. Neuroepidemiology 1993; 12:234–40

18. Gusev E, Boiko A, Lauer K, et al. Environmental risk factors in MS: a case-control study in Moscow. Acta Neurol Scand 1996; 94:386–94

19. Zhang SM, Willett WC, Hernan MA, et al. Dietary fat in relation to risk of multiple sclerosis among two large cohorts of women. Am J Epidemiol 2000; 152: 1056–64

20. Hutter C. On the causes of multiple sclerosis. Med Hypotheses 1993; 41:93–6

21. Hutter CD, Laing P. Multiple sclerosis: sunlight, diet, immunology and aetiology. Med Hypotheses 1996; 46:67–74

22. Ben-Shlomo Y, Davey Smith G, Marmot MG. Dietary fat in the epidemiology of multiple sclerosis: has the situation been adequately assessed? Neuroepidemiology 1992; 11:214–25

Chapter 6

1. Swank RL. Multiple sclerosis: a correlation of its incidence with dietary fat. Am J Med Sci 1950; 220:421–30

2. Swank RL, Dugan BB. The Multiple Sclerosis Diet Book: A low fat diet for the treatment of MS. New York: Doubleday, 1987

3. Swank RL, Dugan BB. Effect of low saturated fat diet in early and late cases of multiple sclerosis. Lancet 1990; 336:37–9

4. Swank RL. Multiple sclerosis: fat-oil relationship. Nutrition 1991; 7:368–76

5. Swank RL, Goodwin J. Review of MS patient survival on a Swank low saturated fat diet. Nutrition 2003; 19:161–2

6. Das UN. Is there a role for saturated and long-chain fatty acids in multiple sclerosis? Nutrition 2003; 19:163–6

7. Das UN. Estrogen, statins, and polyunsaturated fatty acids: similarities in their actions and benefits: is there a common link? Nutrition 2002; 18:178–88

8. Wald NJ, Law MR. A strategy to reduce cardiovascular disease by more than 80%. BMJ 2003; 326:1419

9. Franco OH, Bonneux L, de Laet C, et al. The Polymeal: a more natural, safer, and probably tastier (than the Polypill) strategy to reduce cardiovascular disease by more than 75%. BMJ 2004; 329:1447–50

10. Ben-Shlomo Y, Davey Smith G, Marmot MG. Dietary fat in the epidemiology of multiple sclerosis: has the situation been adequately assessed? Neuroepidemiology 1992; 11:214–25

11. Anonymous. Lipids and multiple sclerosis. Lancet 1990; 336:25–6

12. Nordvik I, Myhr KM, Nyland H, et al. Effect of dietary advice and n–3 supplementation in newly diagnosed MS patients. Acta Neurol Scand 2000; 102:143–9

13. Weinstock-Guttman B, Baier M, Park Y, et al. Low fat dietary intervention with omega-3 fatty acid supplementation in multiple sclerosis patients. Prostaglandins Leukot Essent Fatty Acids 2005; 73:397–404

14. Schwarz S, Leweling H. Multiple sclerosis and nutrition. Mult Scler 2005; 11:24–32

15. Holman RT, Johnson SB, Kokmen E. Deficiencies of polyunsaturated fatty acids and replacement by nonessential fatty acids in plasma lipids in multiple sclerosis. Proc Natl Acad Sci USA 1989; 86:4720–24

16. Cunnane SC, Ho SY, Dore-Duffy P, et al. Essential fatty acid and lipid profiles in plasma and erythrocytes in patients with multiple sclerosis. Am J Clin Nutr 1989; 50:801–806

17. Nightingale S, Woo E, Smith AD, et al. Red blood cell and adipose tissue fatty acids in mild inactive multiple sclerosis. Acta Neurol Scand 1990; 82:43–50

18. Harbige LS, Sharief MK. Polyunsaturated fatty acids in the pathogenesis and treatment of multiple sclerosis. Br J Nutr 2007; 98 Suppl 1:S46–53

19. Millar JH, Zilkha KJ, Langman MJ, et al. Double-blind trial of linoleate supplementation of the diet in multiple sclerosis. Br Med J 1973; 1:765–8

20. Paty DW, Cousin HK, Read S, et al. Linoleic acid in multiple sclerosis: failure to show any therapeutic benefit. Acta Neurol Scand 1978; 58:53–8

21. Bates D, Fawcett PR, Shaw DA, et al. Polyunsaturated fatty acids in treatment of acute remitting multiple sclerosis. Br Med J 1978; 2:1390–91

22. Meade CJ, Mertin J, Sheena J, et al. Reduction by linoleic acid of the severity of experimental allergic encephalomyelitis in the guinea pig. J Neurol Sci 1978; 35:291–308

23. Dworkin RH, Bates D, Millar JH, et al. Linoleic acid and multiple sclerosis: a reanalysis of three double-blind trials. Neurology 1984; 34:1441–5

24. NICE. Multiple Sclerosis: Management of multiple sclerosis in primary and secondary care. London: National Institute for Clinical Excellence, 2003

25. Fitzgerald G, Harbige LS, Forti A, et al. The effect of nutritional counselling on diet and plasma EFA status in multiple sclerosis patients over 3 years. Hum Nutr Appl Nutr 1987; 41:297–310

26. Graham J. Multiple Sclerosis: A self-help guide to its management. Northamptonshire: Thorsons, 1987

27. Fitzgerald G, Briscoe F. Multiple Sclerosis: Healthy menus to help in the management of multiple sclerosis. Northamptonshire: Thorsons, 1989

28. Bates D, Cartlidge NE, French JM, et al. A double-blind controlled trial of long chain n–3 polyunsaturated fatty acids in the treatment of multiple sclerosis. J Neurol Neurosurg Psychiatry 1989; 52:18–22

29. van Meeteren ME, Teunissen CE, Dijkstra CD, et al. Antioxidants and polyunsaturated fatty acids in multiple sclerosis. Eur J Clin Nutr 2005; 59:1347–61

30. Allison RS. Survival in disseminated sclerosis: a clinical study of a series of cases first seen twenty years ago. Brain 1950; 73:103–120

31. Maclean A, Berkson J. Mortality and disability in multiple sclerosis. JAMA 1951; 146:1367–9

32. Miller R. Studies of disseminated sclerosis. Acta Medical Scandinavia 1949; 222:1–214

33. Veterans Administration Multiple Sclerosis Study Group. Five year follow-up on multiple sclerosis. Arch Neurol 1964; 11:583–92

34. Lauritzen I, Blondeau N, Heurteaux C, et al. Polyunsaturated fatty acids are potent neuroprotectors. Eur Mol Biol Org J 2000; 19:1784–93

35. Blondeau N, Widmann C, Lazdunski M, et al. Polyunsaturated fatty acids induce ischemic and epileptic tolerance. Neuroscience 2002; 109:231–41

36. Mayer M. Essential fatty acids and related molecular and cellular mechanisms in multiple sclerosis: a new look at old concepts. Folia Biologica (Praha) 1999; 45:133–41

37. McCarty MF. Upregulation of lymphocyte apoptosis as a strategy for preventing and treating auto-immune disorders: a role for wholefood vegan diets, fish oil and dopamine agonists. Med Hypotheses 2001; 57:258–75

Chapter 7

1. Bermejo Vicedo T, Hidalgo Correas FJ. Antioxidants: the therapy of the future? Nutr Hosp 1997; 12:108–120

2. Calabrese V, Bella R, Testa D, et al. Increased cerebrospinal fluid and plasma levels of ultraweak chemiluminescence are associated with changes in the thiol pool and lipid-soluble fluorescence in multiple sclerosis: the pathogenic role of oxidative stress. Drugs Exp Clin Res 1998; 24:125–31

3. Toshniwal PK, Zarling EJ. Evidence for increased lipid peroxidation in multiple sclerosis. Neurochem Res 1992; 17:205–207

4. van der Veen RC, Hinton DR, Incardonna F, et al. Extensive peroxynitrite activity during progressive stages of central nervous system inflammation. J Neuroimmunol 1997; 77:1–7

5. Vivekananthan DP, Penn MS, Sapp SK, et al. Use of antioxidant vitamins for the prevention of cardiovascular disease: meta-analysis of randomised trials. Lancet 2003; 361:2017–23

6. Bjelakovic G, Nikolova D, Simonetti RG, et al. Antioxidant supplements for preventing gastrointestinal cancers. Cochrane Database Syst Rev 2004:CD004183

7. Bjelakovic G, Nikolova D, Simonetti RG, et al. Antioxidant supplements for prevention of gastrointestinal cancers: a systematic review and meta-analysis. Lancet 2004; 364:1219–28

8. Miller ER, 3rd, Pastor-Barriuso R, Dalal D, et al. Meta-analysis: high-dosage vitamin E supplementation may increase all-cause mortality. Ann Intern Med 2005; 142:37–46

9. Bleys J, Miller ER, 3rd, Pastor-Barriuso R, et al. Vitamin–mineral supplementation and the progression of atherosclerosis: a meta-analysis of randomized controlled trials. Am J Clin Nutr 2006; 84:880–87

10. Lawson KA, Wright ME, Subar A, et al. Multivitamin use and risk of prostate cancer in the National Institutes of Health-AARP Diet and Health Study. J Natl Cancer Inst 2007; 99:754–64

11. Bjelakovic G, Nikolova D, Gluud LL, et al. Mortality in randomized trials of antioxidant supplements for primary and secondary prevention: systematic review and meta-analysis. JAMA 2007; 297:842–57

12. Millen AE, Dodd KW, Subar AF. Use of vitamin, mineral, nonvitamin, and nonmineral supplements in the United States: The 1987, 1992, and 2000 National Health Interview Survey results. J Am Diet Assoc 2004; 104:942–50

13. Bjelakovic G, Gluud C. Surviving antioxidant supplements. J Natl Cancer Inst 2007; 99:742–3

14. Marchioli R, Barzi F, Bomba E, et al. Early protection against sudden death by n–3 polyunsaturated fatty acids after myocardial infarction: time-course analysis of the results of the Gruppo Italiano per lo Studio della Sopravvivenza nell'Infarto Miocardico (GISSI)-Prevenzione. Circulation 2002; 105:1897–1903

15. Flood VM, Smith WT, Webb KL, et al. Prevalence of low serum folate and vitamin B12 in an older Australian population. Aust NZ J Public Health 2006; 30:38–41

16. Butler CC, Vidal-Alaball J, Cannings-John R, et al. Oral vitamin B12 versus intramuscular vitamin B12 for vitamin B12 deficiency: a systematic review of randomized controlled trials. Fam Pract 2006; 23:279–85

17. Bial AK. Review: Limited evidence from 2 randomised controlled trials suggests that oral and intramuscular vitamin B12 have similar effectiveness for vitamin B12 deficiency. Evid Based Med 2006; 11:9

18. Rabunal Rey R, Monte Secades R, Pena Zemsch M, et al. Should we use oral replacement for vitamin B12 deficiency as the first option of treatment? Rev Clin Esp 2007; 207:179–82

19. Miller A, Korem M, Almog R, et al. Vitamin B12, demyelination, remyelination and repair in multiple sclerosis. J Neurol Sci 2005; 233: 93–7

20. Pitkin RM. Folate and neural tube defects. Am J Clin Nutr 2007; 85:285S–8S

21. Kaneko S, Wang J, Kaneko M, et al. Protecting axonal degeneration by increasing nicotinamide adenine dinucleotide levels in experimental auto-immune encephalo-myelitis models. J Neurosci 2006; 26:9794–804

22. Serafini M. Red wine, tea and antioxidants. Lancet 1994; 344:626

23. Zhang X, Haaf M, Todorich B, et al. Cytokine toxicity to oligodendrocyte precursors is mediated by iron. Glia 2005; 52: 199–208

24. Abo-Krysha N, Rashed L. The role of iron dysregulation in the pathogenesis of multiple sclerosis: an Egyptian study. Mult Scler 2008; 14: 602–8

25. Zhang GX, Yu S, Gran B, et al. Glucosamine abrogates the acute phase of experimental auto-immune encephalomyelitis by induction of Th2 response. J Immunol 2005; 175:7202–7208

26. Marracci GH, McKeon GP, Marquardt WE, et al. Alpha-lipoic acid inhibits human T-cell migration: Implications for multiple sclerosis. J Neurosci Res 2004; 78: 362–70

27. Morini M, Roccatagliata L, Dell'Eva R, et al. Alpha-lipoic acid is effective in prevention and treatment of experimental auto-immune encephalomyelitis. J Neuroimmunol 2004; 148:146–53

28. Schreibelt G, Musters RJ, Reijerkerk A, et al. Lipoic acid affects cellular migration into the central nervous system and stabilizes blood-brain barrier integrity. J Immunol 2006; 177:2630–37

29. Yadav V, Marracci G, Lovera J, et al. Lipoic acid in multiple sclerosis: a pilot study. Mult Scler 2005; 11:159–65

30. Zhang SM, Hernan MA, Olek MJ, et al. Intakes of carotenoids, vitamin C, and vitamin E and MS risk among two large cohorts of women. Neurology 2001; 57:75–80

Chapter 8

1. Grant WB, Strange RC, Garland CF. Sunshine is good medicine. The health benefits of ultraviolet-B induced vitamin D production. J Cosmet Dermatol 2003; 2:86–98

2. Holick MF. Sunlight and vitamin D for bone health and prevention of auto-immune diseases, cancers, and cardiovascular disease. Am J Clin Nutr 2004; 80:1678S–88S

3. Holick MF. The vitamin D epidemic and its health consequences. J Nutr 2005; 135:2739S–48S

4. Ebeling PR. Megadose therapy for vitamin D deficiency. Med J Aust 2005; 183:4–5

5. Holick MF, Chen TC. Vitamin D deficiency: a worldwide problem with health consequences. Am J Clin Nutr 2008; 87:1080S–1086S

6. Grant WB, Garland CF, Holick MF. Comparisons of estimated economic burdens due to insufficient solar ultraviolet irradiance and vitamin D and excess solar UV irradiance for the United States. Photochem Photobiol 2005; 81:1276–86

7. Grant WB, Holick MF. Benefits and requirements of vitamin D for optimal health: a review. Altern Med Rev 2005; 10:94–111

8. Flicker L, Mead K, MacInnis RJ, et al. Serum vitamin D and falls in older women in residential care in Australia. J Am Geriatr Soc 2003; 51:1533–8

9. Pasco JA, Henry MJ, Kotowicz MA, et al. Seasonal periodicity of serum vitamin D and parathyroid hormone, bone resorption, and fractures: the Geelong Osteoporosis Study. J Bone Miner Res 2004; 19:752–8

10. Bischoff HA, Stahelin HB, Dick W, et al. Effects of vitamin D and calcium supplementation on falls: a randomized controlled trial. J Bone Miner Res 2003; 18:343–51

11. Zittermann A. Vitamin D in preventive medicine: are we ignoring the evidence? Br J Nutr 2003; 89:552–72

12. Grimes DS, Hindle E, Dyer T. Sunlight, cholesterol and coronary heart disease. Qjm 1996; 89:579–89

13. Ponsonby AL, McMichael A, van der Mei I. Ultraviolet radiation and auto-immune disease: insights from epidemiological research. Toxicology 2002; 181–2:71–8.

14. Ponsonby AL, Lucas RM, van der Mei IA. UVR, vitamin D and three auto-immune diseases—multiple sclerosis, type 1 diabetes, rheumatoid arthritis. Photochem Photobiol 2005; 81:1267–75

15. Arnson Y, Amital H, Shoenfeld Y. Vitamin D and auto-immunity: new aetiological and therapeutic considerations. Ann Rheum Dis 2007; 66:1137–42

16. Mohr SB, Garland CF, Gorham ED, et al. The association between ultraviolet B irradiance, vitamin D status and incidence rates of type 1 diabetes in 51 regions worldwide. Diabetologia 2008; 51: 1391–8

17. Zipitis CS, Akobeng AK. Vitamin D supplementation in early childhood and risk of type 1 diabetes: a systematic review and meta-analysis. Arch Dis Child 2008; 93:512–17

18. Grant WB. Ecologic studies of solar UVB radiation and cancer mortality rates. Recent Results Cancer Res 2003; 164:371–7

19. Autier P, Gandini S. Vitamin D supplementation and total mortality: a meta-analysis of randomized controlled trials. Arch Intern Med 2007; 167:1730–37

20. Melamed ML, Michos ED, Post W, et al. 25-hydroxyvitamin D levels and the risk of mortality in the general population. Arch Intern Med 2008; 168:1629–37

21. Cherniack EP, Levis S, Troen BR. Hypovitaminosis D: a stealthy epidemic that requires treatment. Geriatrics 2008; 63:24–30

22. Esparza ML, Sasaki S, Kesteloot H. Nutrition, latitude, and multiple sclerosis mortality: an ecologic study. Am J Epidemiol 1995; 142:733–7

23. Llorca J, Guerrero P, Prieto-Salceda D, et al. Mortality of multiple sclerosis in Spain: demonstration of a north-south gradient. Neuroepidemiology 2005; 24:135–40

24. Kampman MT, Wilsgaard T, Mellgren SI. Outdoor activities and diet in childhood and adolescence relate to MS risk above the Arctic Circle. J Neurol 2007; 254:471–7

25. Hutter C. On the causes of multiple sclerosis. Med Hypotheses 1993; 41:93–6

26. Hutter CD, Laing P. Multiple sclerosis: sunlight, diet, immunology and aetiology. Med Hypotheses 1996; 46:67–74

27. Kampman MT, Brustad M. Vitamin D: A candidate for the environmental effect in multiple sclerosis: observations from Norway. Neuroepidemiology 2008; 30:140–46

28. Dumas AM, Jauberteau-Marchan MO. The protective role of Langerhans' cells and sunlight in multiple sclerosis. Med Hypotheses 2000; 55:517–20

29. Goldberg P. Multiple sclerosis: vitamin D and calcium as environmental determinants of prevalence (a viewpoint). Part 1: sunlight, dietary factors and epidemiology. Int J Environ Studies 1974; 6:19–27

30. Heaney RP, Davies KM, Chen TC, et al. Human serum 25-hydroxycholecalciferol response to extended oral dosing with cholecalciferol. Am J Clin Nutr 2003; 77:204–210

31. Hayes CE, Cantorna MT, Deluca HF. Vitamin D and multiple sclerosis. Proc Soc Exp Biol Med 1997:21–7

32. Deluca HF, Cantorna MT. Vitamin D: its role and uses in immunology. Faseb J 2001; 15:2579–85

33. Nataf S, Garcion E, Darcy F, et al. 1 25 Dihydroxyvitamin D3 exerts regional effects in the central nervous system during experimental allergic encephalomyelitis. J Neuropathol Exp Neurol 1996; 55:904–914

34. Garcion E, Wion-Barbot N, Montero-Menei CN, et al. New clues about vitamin D functions in the nervous system. Trends Endocrin Metab 2002; 13:100–105

35. May E, Asadullah K, Zugel U. Immunoregulation through 1, 25-dihydroxyvitamin d3 and its analogs. Curr Drug Targets Inflamm Allergy 2004; 3:377–93

36. Goldberg P, Fleming MC, Picard EH. Multiple sclerosis: decreased relapse rate through dietary supplementation with calcium, magnesium and vitamin D. Med Hypotheses 1986; 21:193–200

37. Embry AF, Snowdon LR, Vieth R. Vitamin D and seasonal fluctuations of gadolinium-enhancing magnetic resonance imaging lesions in multiple sclerosis. Ann Neurol 2000; 48:271–2

38. Lansdowne AT, Provost SC. Vitamin D3 enhances mood in healthy subjects during winter. Psychopharmacology (Berl) 1998; 135:319–23

39. Soilu-Hanninen M, Airas L, Mononen I, et al. 25-hydroxyvitamin D levels in serum at the onset of multiple sclerosis. Mult Scler 2005; 11:266–71

40. Soilu-Hanninen M, Laaksonen M, Laitinen I, et al. A longitudinal study of serum 25-hydroxy-vitamin D and intact PTH levels indicate the importance of vitamin D and calcium homeostasis regulation in multiple sclerosis. J Neurol Neurosurg Psychiatry 2007; 79:152–7

41. Correale J, Ysrraelit MC, Gaitan MI. Immunomodulatory effects of vitamin D in multiple sclerosis. Brain 2009; 132: 1146–60

42. Ozgocmen S, Bulut S, Ilhan N, et al. Vitamin D deficiency and reduced bone mineral density in multiple sclerosis: effect of ambulatory status and functional capacity. J Bone Miner Metab 2005; 23:309–13

43. Faulkner MA, Ryan-Haddad AM, Lenz TL, et al. Osteoporosis in long-term care residents with multiple sclerosis. Consult Pharm 2005; 20:128–36

44. VanAmerongen BM, Dijkstra CD, Lips P, et al. Multiple sclerosis and vitamin D: an update. Eur J Clin Nutr 2004; 58:1095–9

45. Munger KL, Zhang SM, O'Reilly E, et al. Vitamin D intake and incidence of multiple sclerosis. Neurology 2004; 62:60–65

46. Munger KL, Levin LI, Hollis BW, et al. Serum 25-hydroxyvitamin D levels and risk of multiple sclerosis. JAMA 2006; 296:2832–8

47. Freedman DM, Dosemeci M, Alavanja MC. Mortality from multiple sclerosis and exposure to residential and occupational solar radiation: a case-control study based on death certificates. Occup Environ Med 2000; 57:418–21

48. Westberg M, Feychting M, Jonsson F, et al. Occupational exposure to UV light and mortality from multiple sclerosis. Am J Ind Med 2009; 52:353–7

49. Goldacre MJ, Seagroatt V, Yeates D, et al. Skin cancer in people with multiple sclerosis: a record linkage study. J Epidemiol Community Health 2004; 58:142–4

50. van der Mei IA, Ponsonby AL, Blizzard L, et al. Regional variation in multiple sclerosis prevalence in Australia and its association with ambient ultraviolet radiation. Neuroepidemiology 2001; 20:168–74

51. Lucas RM, Ponsonby AL. Ultraviolet radiation and health: friend and foe. Med J Aust 2002; 177:594–8

52. van der Mei IA, Ponsonby AL, Dwyer T, et al. Past exposure to sun, skin phenotype, and risk of multiple sclerosis: case-control study. BMJ 2003; 327:316

53. Islam T, Gauderman WJ, Cozen W, et al. Childhood sun exposure influences risk of multiple sclerosis in monozygotic twins. Neurology 2007; 69:381–8

54. Tremlett H, van der Mei IA, Pittas F, et al. Monthly ambient sunlight, infections and relapse rates in multiple sclerosis. Neuroepidemiology 2008; 31:271–9

55. Garland FC, White MR, Garland CF, et al. Occupational sunlight exposure and melanoma in the US Navy. Arch Environ Health 1990; 45:261–7

56. Constantinescu CS. Melanin, melatonin, melanocyte-stimulating hormone, and the susceptibility to auto-immune demyelination: a rationale for light therapy in multiple sclerosis. Med Hypotheses 1995; 45:455–8

57. Balashov KE, Olek MJ, Smith DR, et al. Seasonal variation of interferon-gamma production in progressive multiple sclerosis. Ann Neurol 1998; 44:824–88

58. Bisgard C. Seasonal variation in disseminated sclerosis. Ugeskr Laeger 1990; 152:1160–61

59. Panitch HS. Influence of infection on exacerbations of multiple sclerosis. Ann Neurol 1994; 36:S25–S28

60. Vieth R. Vitamin D supplementation, 25-hydroxyvitamin D concentrations, and safety. Am J Clin Nutr 1999; 69:842–56

61. Working Group of the Australian and New Zealand Bone and Mineral Society Endocrine Society of Australia Osteoporosis Australia. Vitamin D and adult bone health in Australia and New Zealand: a position statement. Med J Aust 2005; 182:281–5

62. Ness AR, Frankel SJ, Gunnell DJ, et al. Are we really dying for a tan? BMJ 1999; 319:114–16

63. Holick MF. Vitamin D: A millenium perspective. J Cell Biochem 2003; 88:296–307

64. Vieth R. Why the optimal requirement for Vitamin D(3) is probably much higher than what is officially recommended for adults. J Steroid Biochem Mol Biol 2004; 89–90:575–9

65. Pasco JA, Henry MJ, Nicholson GC, et al. Vitamin D status of women in the Geelong Osteoporosis Study: association with diet and casual exposure to sunlight. Med J Aust 2001; 175:401–405

66. Moan J, Porojnicu AC. The photobiology of vitamin D, a topic of renewed focus. Tidsskr Nor Laegeforen 2006; 126:1048–52

67. Ursell MR, Vieth R, O'Connor PW, et al. A phase I dose escalation study of vitamin D3 with calcium supplementation in patients with multiple sclerosis. Colchester, Essex: Multiple Sclerosis Resource Centre, 2002

68. Kimball SM, Ursell MR, O'Connor P, et al. Safety of vitamin D3 in adults with multiple sclerosis. Am J Clin Nutr 2007; 86:645–51

69. Wingerchuk DM, Lesaux J, Rice GP, et al. A pilot study of oral calcitriol (1, 25-dihydroxyvitamin D3) for relapsing-remitting multiple sclerosis. J Neurol Neurosurg Psychiatry 2005; 76:1294–6

70. van der Mei IA, Ponsonby AL, Dwyer T, et al. Vitamin D levels in people with multiple sclerosis and community controls in Tasmania, Australia. J Neurol 2007; 254:581–90

71. Diamond TH, Ho KW, Rohl PG, et al. Annual intramuscular injection of a megadose of cholecalciferol for treatment of vitamin D deficiency: efficacy and safety data. Med J Aust 2005; 183:10–12

72. Barnes MS, Bonham MP, Robson PJ, et al. Assessment of 25-hydroxyvitamin D and 1, 25-dihydroxyvitamin D3 concentrations in male and female multiple sclerosis patients and control volunteers. Mult Scler 2007; 13:670–72

73. Hathcock JN, Shao A, Vieth R, et al. Risk assessment for vitamin D. Am J Clin Nutr 2007; 85:6–18

74. Kimball S, Vieth R. Self-prescribed high-dose vitamin D(3): effects on biochemical parameters in two men. Ann Clin Biochem 2008; 45:106–110

75. Owusu W, Willett WC, Feskanich D, et al. Calcium intake and the incidence of forearm and hip fractures among men. J Nutr 1997; 127:1782–7

76. Feskanich D, Willett WC, Stampfer MJ, et al. Milk, dietary calcium, and bone fractures in women: a 12-year prospective study. Am J Public Health 1997; 87:992–7

77. Lanou AJ, Berkow SE, Barnard ND. Calcium, dairy products, and bone health in children and young adults: a reevaluation of the evidence. Pediatrics 2005; 115:736–43

78. New SA. Nutrition Society Medal lecture. The role of the skeleton in acid-base homeostasis. Proc Nutr Soc 2002; 61:151–64

79. McCarty MF. A moderately low phosphate intake may provide health benefits analogous to those conferred by UV light: a further advantage of vegan diets. Med Hypotheses 2003; 61:543–60

80. Heaney RP, Dowell MS, Hale CA, et al. Calcium absorption varies within the reference range for serum 25-hydroxyvitamin D. J Am Coll Nutr 2003; 22:142–6

81. Bolland MJ, Barber PA, Doughty RN, et al. Vascular events in healthy older women receiving calcium supplementation: randomised controlled trial. BMJ 2008; 336:262–6

82. Reid IR, Bolland MJ, Grey A. Effect of calcium supplementation on hip fractures. Osteoporos Int 2008; 19:1119–23

83. Bischoff-Ferrari HA, Dawson-Hughes B, Baron JA, et al. Calcium intake and hip fracture risk in men and women: a meta-analysis of prospective cohort studies and randomized controlled trials. Am J Clin Nutr 2007; 86:1780–90

84. Bischoff-Ferrari HA, Dawson-Hughes B. Where do we stand on vitamin D? Bone 2007; 41:S13–19

Chapter 9

1. Russell WR. Multiple Sclerosis: Control of the disease. Oxford: Pergamon Press, 1976

2. Holmes MD, Chen WY, Feskanich D, et al. Physical activity and survival after breast cancer diagnosis. JAMA 2005; 293:2479–86

3. Das UN. Anti-inflammatory nature of exercise. Nutrition 2004; 20:323–6

4. Brown TR, Kraft GH. Exercise and rehabilitation for individuals with multiple sclerosis. Phys Med Rehabil Clin N Am 2005; 16:513–55

5. Bjarnadottir OH, Konradsdottir AD, Reynisdottir K, et al. Multiple sclerosis and brief moderate exercise. A randomised study. Mult Scler 2007; 13:776–82

6. White LJ, McCoy SC, Castellano V, et al. Resistance training improves strength and functional capacity in persons with multiple sclerosis. Mult Scler 2004; 10:668–74

7. White LJ, Dressendorfer RH. Exercise and multiple sclerosis. Sports Med 2004; 34:1077–1100

8. Rietberg M, Brooks D, Uitdehaag B, et al. Exercise therapy for multiple sclerosis. Cochrane Database Syst Rev 2005:CD003980

9. Kileff J, Ashburn A. A pilot study of the effect of aerobic exercise on people with moderate disability multiple sclerosis. Clin Rehabil 2005; 19:165–9

10. Romberg A, Virtanen A, Ruutiainen J, et al. Effects of a 6-month exercise program on patients with multiple sclerosis: a randomized study. Neurology 2004; 63:2034–8

11. Romberg A, Virtanen A, Ruutiainen J. Long-term exercise improves functional impairment but not quality of life in multiple sclerosis. J Neurol 2005; 252:839–45

12. Gutierrez GM, Chow JW, Tillman MD, et al. Resistance training improves gait kinematics in persons with multiple sclerosis. Arch Phys Med Rehabil 2005; 86:1824–9

13. Sutherland G, Andersen MB. Exercise and multiple sclerosis: physiological, psychological, and quality of life issues. J Sports Med Phys Fitness 2001; 41: 421–32

14. Kerdoncuff V, Durufle A, Le Tallec H, et al. Multiple sclerosis and physical activities. Ann Readapt Med Phys 2005; 49:32–6

15. McCullagh R, Fitzgerald AP, Murphy RP, et al. Long-term benefits of exercising on quality of life and fatigue in multiple sclerosis patients with mild disability: a pilot study. Clin Rehabil 2008; 22:206–214

16. Fragoso YD, Santana DL, Pinto RC. The positive effects of a physical activity program for multiple sclerosis patients with fatigue. NeuroRehabilitation 2008; 23:153–7

17. Motl RW, Gosney JL. Effect of exercise training on quality of life in multiple sclerosis: a meta-analysis. Mult Scler 2007; 14:129–35

18. van den Berg M, Dawes H, Wade DT, et al. Treadmill training for individuals with multiple sclerosis: a pilot randomised trial. J Neurol Neurosurg Psychiatry 2006; 77:531–3

19. Surakka J, Romberg A, Ruutiainen J, et al. Effects of aerobic and strength exercise on motor fatigue in men and women with multiple sclerosis: a randomized controlled trial. Clin Rehabil 2004; 18:737–46

20. Rampello A, Franceschini M, Piepoli M, et al. Effect of aerobic training on walking capacity and maximal exercise tolerance in patients with multiple sclerosis: a randomized crossover controlled study. Phys Ther 2007; 87:545–55

21. Gold SM, Schulz KH, Hartmann S, et al. Basal serum levels and reactivity of nerve growth factor and brain-derived neurotrophic factor to standardized acute exercise in multiple sclerosis and controls. J Neuroimmunol 2003; 138:99–105

22. Schulz KH, Heesen C. Effects of exercise in chronically ill patients. Examples from oncology and neurology. Bundesgesundheitsblatt Gesundheitsforschung Gesundheitsschutz 2005; 48:906–913

23. Dalgas U, Stenager E, Ingemann-Hansen T. Multiple sclerosis and physical exercise: recommendations for the application of resistance-, endurance- and combined training. Mult Scler 2008; 14:35–53

24. Brown RF, Valpiani EM, Tennant CC, et al. Longitudinal assessment of anxiety, depression, and fatigue in people with multiple sclerosis. Psychol Psychother 2008; 82:41–56

25. Gallien P, Nicolas B, Robineau S, et al. Physical training and multiple sclerosis. Ann Readapt Med Phys 2007; 50:369–72, 373–6

26. Nortvedt MW, Riise T, Maeland JG. Multiple sclerosis and lifestyle factors: the Hordaland Health Study. Neurol Sci 2005; 26:334–9

27. Motl RW. Physical activity and its measurement and determinants in multiple sclerosis. Minerva Med 2008; 99:157–65

28. Heesen C, Romberg A, Gold S, et al. Physical exercise in multiple sclerosis: supportive care or a putative disease-modifying treatment. Expert Rev Neurother 2006; 6:347–55

29. White LJ, Castellano V. Exercise and brain health: implications for multiple sclerosis: Part 1—neuronal growth factors. Sports Med 2008; 38:91–100

30. White LJ, Castellano V. Exercise and brain health: implications for multiple sclerosis: Part II—immune factors and stress hormones. Sports Med 2008; 38:179–86

31. Stuifbergen AK, Blozis SA, Harrison TC, et al. Exercise, functional limitations, and quality of life: a longitudinal study of persons with multiple sclerosis. Arch Phys Med Rehabil 2006; 87:935–43

32. Gold SM, Mohr DC, Huitinga I, et al. The role of stress-response systems for the pathogenesis and progression of MS. Trends Immunol 2005; 26:644–52

33. Lalive PH, Burkhard PR, Chofflon M. TNF-alpha and psychologically stressful events in healthy subjects: potential relevance for multiple sclerosis relapse. Behav Neurosci 2002; 116:1093–97

34. Ackerman KD, Stover A, Heyman R, et al. Relationship of cardiovascular reactivity, stressful life events, and multiple sclerosis disease activity. Brain Behav Immun 2003; 17:141–51

35. Mohr DC, Goodkin DE, Bacchetti P, et al. Psychological stress and the subsequent appearance of new brain MRI lesions in MS. Neurology 2000; 55:55–61

36. Mohr DC, Goodkin DE, Nelson S, et al. Moderating effects of coping on the relationship between stress and the development of new brain lesions in multiple sclerosis. Psychosom Med 2002; 64:803–809

37. Mohr DC, Pelletier D. A temporal framework for understanding the effects of stressful life events on inflammation in patients with multiple sclerosis. Brain Behav Immun 2006; 20:27–36

38. Strenge H. The relationship between psychological stress and the clinical course of multiple sclerosis. An update. Psychother Psychosom Med Psychol 2001; 51:166–75

39. Buljevac D, Hop WC, Reedeker W, et al. Self reported stressful life events and exacerbations in multiple sclerosis: prospective study. BMJ 2003; 327:646

40. Golan D, Somer E, Dishon S, et al. Impact of exposure to war stress on exacerbations of multiple sclerosis. Ann Neurol 2008; 64:143–8

41. Mitsonis CI, Zervas IM, Mitropoulos PA, et al. The impact of stressful life events on risk of relapse in women with multiple sclerosis: A prospective study. Eur Psychiatry 2008; 23:497–504

42. Sadovnick AD, Remick RA, Allen J, et al. Depression and multiple sclerosis. Neurology 1996; 46:628–32

43. Galeazzi GM, Ferrari S, Giaroli G, et al. Psychiatric disorders and depression in multiple sclerosis outpatients: impact of disability and interferon beta therapy. Neurol Sci 2005; 26:255–62

44. Figved N, Klevan G, Myhr KM, et al. Neuropsychiatric symptoms in patients with multiple sclerosis. Acta Psychiatr Scand 2005; 112:463–8

45. Khan F, McPhail T, Brand C, et al. Multiple sclerosis: disability profile and quality of life in an Australian community cohort. Int J Rehabil Res 2006; 29:87–96

46. McGuigan C, Hutchinson M. Unrecognised symptoms of depression in a community-based population with multiple sclerosis. J Neurol 2005; 253:219–23

47. Sollom AC, Kneebone, II. Treatment of depression in people who have multiple sclerosis. Mult Scler 2007; 13:632–5

48. Patten SB, Williams JV, Metz L. Anti-depressant use in association with interferon and glatiramer acetate treatment in multiple sclerosis. Mult Scler 2007; 14:406–11

49. D'Alisa S, Miscio G, Baudo S, et al. Depression is the main determinant of quality of life in multiple sclerosis: a classification-regression (CART) study. Disabil Rehabil 2006; 28:307–14

50. Benedict RH, Wahlig E, Bakshi R, et al. Predicting quality of life in multiple sclerosis: accounting for physical disability, fatigue, cognition, mood disorder, personality, and behavior change. J Neurol Sci 2005; 231:29–34

51. Goldman Consensus Group. The Goldman Consensus statement on depression in multiple sclerosis. Mult Scler 2005; 11:328–37

52. Arnett PA, Barwick FH, Beeney JE. Depression in multiple sclerosis: review and theoretical proposal. J Int Neuropsychol Soc 2008; 14:691–724

53. Sutcigil L, Oktenli C, Musabak U, et al. Pro- and anti-inflammatory cytokine balance in major depression: effect of sertraline therapy. Clin Dev Immunol 2007; 2007:76396

54. Mohr DC, Goodkin DE, Islar J, et al. Treatment of depression is associated with suppression of nonspecific and antigen-specific T(H)1 responses in multiple sclerosis. Arch Neurol 2001; 58:1081–6

55. Gold SM, Irwin MR. Depression and immunity: inflammation and depressive symptoms in multiple sclerosis. Neurol Clin 2006; 24:507–19

56. Ytterberg C, Johansson S, Holmqvist LW, et al. Longitudinal variations and predictors of increased perceived impact of multiple sclerosis, a two-year study. J Neurol Sci 2008; 270:53–9

57. Even C, Friedman S, Dardennes R, et al. Prevalence of depression in multiple sclerosis: a review and meta-analysis. Rev Neurol (Paris) 2004; 160:917–25

58. White CP, White MB, Russell CS. Invisible and visible symptoms of multiple sclerosis: which are more predictive of health distress? J Neurosci Nurs 2008; 40:85–95, 102

59. Morgan AJ, Jorm AF. Self-help interventions for depressive disorders and depressive symptoms: A systematic review. Ann Gen Psychiatry 2008; 7:13

60. Dinan T, Siggins L, Scully P, et al. Investigating the inflammatory phenotype of major depression: focus on cytokines and polyunsaturated fatty acids. J Psychiatr Res 2008; 43:471–6

61. Su KP. Mind–body interface: the role of n-3 fatty acids in psychoneuroimmunology, somatic presentation, and medical illness comorbidity of depression. Asia Pac J Clin Nutr 2008; 17 Suppl 1:151–7

62. Adams PB, Lawson S, Sanigorski A, et al. Arachidonic acid to eicosapentanoic acid ration in blood correlates positively with clinical symptoms of depression. Lipids 1996; 31:S157–S161

63. da Silva TM, Munhoz RP, Alvarez C, et al. Depression in Parkinson's disease: A double-blind, randomized, placebo-controlled pilot study of omega-3 fatty-acid supplementation. J Affect Disord 2008; 111:351–9

64. Lansdowne AT, Provost SC. Vitamin D3 enhances mood in healthy subjects during winter. Psychopharmacology (Berl) 1998; 135:319–23

65. Gloth FM, 3rd, Alam W, Hollis B. Vitamin D vs broad spectrum phototherapy in the treatment of seasonal affective disorder. J Nutr Health Aging 1999; 3:5–7

66. Stumpf WE, Privette TH. Light, vitamin D and psychiatry. Role of 1, 25-dihydroxyvitamin D3 (soltriol) in etiology and therapy of seasonal affective disorder and other mental processes. Psychopharmacology (Berl) 1989; 97:285–94

67. Jorde R, Waterloo K, Saleh F, et al. Neuropsychological function in relation to serum parathyroid hormone and serum 25-hydroxyvitamin D levels: the Tromso study. J Neurol 2005; 253:464–70

68. Hernan MA, Oleky MJ, Ascherio A. Cigarette smoking and incidence of multiple sclerosis. Am J Epidemiol 2001; 154:69–74

69. Riise T, Nortvedt MW, Ascherio A. Smoking is a risk factor for multiple sclerosis. Neurology 2003; 61:1122–4

70. Hawkes CH. Smoking is a risk factor for multiple sclerosis: a meta-analysis. Mult Scler 2007; 13:610–15

71. Hernan MA, Jick SS, Logroscino G, et al. Cigarette smoking and the progression of multiple sclerosis. Brain 2005; 128:1461–5

72. Sundstrom P, Nystrom L. Smoking worsens the prognosis in multiple sclerosis. Mult Scler 2008; 14:1031–5

73. Mikaeloff Y, Caridade G, Tardieu M, et al. Parental smoking at home and the risk of childhood-onset multiple sclerosis in children. Brain 2007; 130:2589–95

74. Di Pauli F, Reindl M, Ehling R, et al. Smoking is a risk factor for early conversion to clinically definite multiple sclerosis. Mult Scler 2008; 14:1026–30

75. Ascherio A, Munger KL. Environmental risk factors for multiple sclerosis. Part II: Noninfectious factors. Ann Neurol 2007; 61:504–13

76. Savettieri G, Messina D, Andreoli V, et al. Gender-related effect of clinical and genetic variables on the cognitive impairment in multiple sclerosis. J Neurol 2004; 251:1208–14

77. Simioni S, Ruffieux C, Bruggimann L, et al. Cognition, mood and fatigue in patients in the early stage of multiple sclerosis. Swiss Med Wkly 2007; 137:496–501

78. Wallin MT, Wilken JA, Kane R. Cognitive dysfunction in multiple sclerosis: Assessment, imaging, and risk factors. J Rehabil Res Dev 2006; 43:63–72

79. Schulz D, Kopp B, Kunkel A, et al. Cognition in the early stage of multiple sclerosis. J Neurol 2006; 253:1002–10

80. Nilsson P, Rorsman I, Larsson EM, et al. Cognitive dysfunction 24–31 years after isolated optic neuritis. Mult Scler 2008; 14:913–18

81. Haase CG, Tinnefeld M, Faustmann PM. The influence of immunomodulation on psycho-neuroimmunological functions in benign multiple sclerosis. Neuro-immunomodulation 2004; 11:365–72

82. Kleeberg J, Bruggimann L, Annoni JM, et al. Altered decision-making in multiple sclerosis: a sign of impaired emotional reactivity? Ann Neurol 2004; 56:787–95

Chapter 10

1. Graham J. Multiple Sclerosis: A self-help guide to its management. Northamptonshire: Thorsons, 1987

2. Ludvigsson JF, Olsson T, Ekbom A, et al. A population-based study of coeliac disease, neurodegenerative and neuroinflammatory diseases. Aliment Pharmacol Ther 2007; 25:1317–27

3. Salvatore S, Finazzi S, Ghezzi A, et al. Multiple sclerosis and celiac disease: is there an increased risk? Mult Scler 2004; 10:711–12

4. Pengiran Tengah CD, Lock RJ, Unsworth DJ, et al. Multiple sclerosis and occult gluten sensitivity. Neurology 2004; 62:2326–7

5. Borhani Haghighi A, Ansari N, Mokhtari M, et al. Multiple sclerosis and gluten sensitivity. Clin Neurol Neurosurg 2007; 109:651–3

6. Nicoletti A, Patti F, Lo Fermo S, et al. Frequency of celiac disease is not increased among multiple sclerosis patients. Mult Scler 2008; 14:698–700

7. Di Marco R, Mangano K, Quattrocchi C, et al. Exacerbation of protracted-relapsing experimental allergic encephalomyelitis in DA rats by gluten-free diet. Apmis 2004; 112:651–5

8. Alonso A, Jick SS, Hernan MA. Allergy, histamine 1 receptor blockers, and the risk of multiple sclerosis. Neurology 2006; 66:572–5

9. Ingalls TH. Epidemiology, etiology, and prevention of multiple sclerosis. Am J Forensic Med Pathol 1983; 4:55–61

10. Ingalls TH. Clustering of multiple sclerosis in Galion, Ohio, 1982–1985. Am J Forensic Med Pathol 1989; 10:213–15

11. McGrother CW, Dugmore C, Phillips MJ, et al. Multiple sclerosis, dental caries and fillings: a case-control study. Br Dent J 1999; 187:261–4

12. Bangsi D, Ghadirian P, Ducic S, et al. Dental amalgam and multiple sclerosis: a case-control study in Montreal, Canada. Int J Epidemiol 1998; 27:667–71

13. Casetta I, Invernizzi M, Granieri E. Multiple sclerosis and dental amalgam: case-control study in Ferrara, Italy. Neuroepidemiology 2001; 20:134–7

14. Wahl MJ. Amalgam: resurrection and redemption. Part 2: The medical mythology of anti-amalgam. Quintessence Int 2001; 32:696–710

15. Mitchell RJ, Osborne PB, Haubenreich JE. Dental amalgam restorations: daily mercury dose and biocompatibility. J Long Term Eff Med Implants 2005; 15:709–21

16. Aminzadeh KK, Etminan M. Dental amalgam and multiple sclerosis: a systematic review and meta-analysis. J Public Health Dent 2007; 67:64–6

17. Geier DA, Geier MR. A case-control study of serious auto-immune adverse events following hepatitis B immunization. Autoimmunity 2005; 38:295–301

18. Hernan MA, Jick SS, Olek MJ, et al. Recombinant hepatitis B vaccine and the risk of multiple sclerosis: a prospective study. Neurology 2004; 63:838–42

19. Geier MR, Geier DA. A case-series of adverse events, positive re-challenge of symptoms, and events in identical twins following hepatitis B vaccination: analysis of the Vaccine Adverse Event Reporting System (VAERS) database and literature review. Clin Exp Rheumatol 2004; 22:749–55

20. Comenge Y, Girard M. Multiple sclerosis and hepatitis B vaccination: Adding the credibility of molecular biology to an unusual level of clinical and epidemiological evidence. Med Hypotheses 2005; 66:84–6

21. Bogdanos DP, Smith H, Ma Y, et al. A study of molecular mimicry and immunological cross-reactivity between hepatitis B surface antigen and myelin mimics. Clin Dev Immunol 2005; 12:217–24

22. Kleijnen J, Knipschild P. Hyperbaric oxygen for multiple sclerosis. Review of controlled trials. Acta Neurol Scand 1995; 91:330–34

23. Bennett M, Heard R. Hyperbaric oxygen therapy for multiple sclerosis. Cochrane Database Syst Rev 2004:CD003057

24. Kindwall EP, McQuillen MP, Khatri BO, et al. Treatment of multiple sclerosis with hyperbaric oxygen. Results of a national registry. Arch Neurol 1991; 48:195–9

25. Schuhfried O, Mittermaier C, Jovanovic T, et al. Effects of whole-body vibration in patients with multiple sclerosis: a pilot study. Clin Rehabil 2005; 19:834–42

26. Wesselius T, Heersema DJ, Mostert JP, et al. A randomized crossover study of bee-sting therapy for multiple sclerosis. Neurology 2005; 65:1764–8

27. Castro HJ, Mendez-Lnocencio JI, Omidvar B, et al. A phase I study of the safety of honeybee venom extract as a possible treatment for patients with progressive forms of multiple sclerosis. Allergy Asthma Proc 2005; 26:470–76

Chapter 11

1. Siegel BS. Love, Medicine And Miracles. New York: HarperCollins, 1990

2. Dyer W. Becoming a waking dreamer. In: Carlson R, Shield B, eds. Handbook for the Soul. Sydney: Transworld Publishers, 1995

3. Mackereth PA, Booth K, Hillier VF, et al. Reflexology and progressive muscle relaxation training for people with multiple sclerosis: a crossover trial. Complement Ther Clin Pract 2009; 15:14–21

4. Kern S, Ziemssen T. Review: brain–immune communication psychoneuroimmunology of multiple sclerosis. Mult Scler 2007; 14:6–21

5. Armstrong L. Lance Armstrong. It's Not About the Bike: My journey back to life. Sydney: Allen & Unwin, 2000

6. Isaksson AK, Gunnarsson LG, Ahlstrom G. The presence and meaning of chronic sorrow in patients with multiple sclerosis. J Clin Nurs 2007; 16:315–24

7. Shinto L, Yadav V, Morris C, et al. The perceived benefit and satisfaction from conventional and complementary and alternative medicine (CAM) in people with multiple sclerosis. Complement Ther Med 2005; 13:264–72

8. Smyth JM, Stone AA, Hurewitz A, et al. Effects of writing about stressful experiences on symptom reduction in patients with asthma or rheumatoid arthritis: a randomized trial. JAMA 1999; 281:1304–1309

9. Spiegel D. Healing words: emotional expression and disease outcome. JAMA 1999; 281:1328–9

10. Phillips DP, Ruth TE, Wagner LM. Psychology and survival. Lancet 1993; 342:1142–5

11. Kabat-Zinn J, Wheeler E, Light T, et al. Influence of a mindfulness meditation-based stress reduction intervention on rates of skin clearing in patients with moderate to severe psoriasis undergoing phototherapy (UVB) and photochemotherapy (PUVA). Psychosom Med 1998; 60:625–32

12. Derogatis LR, Abeloff MD, Melisaratos N. Psychological coping mechanisms and survival time in metastatic breast cancer. JAMA 1979; 242:1504–1508

13. Greer S. Psychological response to cancer and survival. Psychol Med 1991; 21:43–9

14. Ostermann T, Schmid W. Music therapy in the treatment of multiple sclerosis: a comprehensive literature review. Expert Rev Neurother 2006; 6:469–77

Chapter 12

1. O'Connor PW, Goodman A, Willmer-Hulme AJ, et al. Randomized multi-center trial of natalizumab in acute MS relapses: and MRI effects. Neurology 2004; 62:2038–2043

2. Wandinger KP, Wessel K, Trillenberg P, et al. Effect of high-dose methylprednisolone administration on immune functions in multiple sclerosis patients. Acta Neurol Scand 1998; 97:359–65

3. Filipovic SR, Drulovic J, Stojsavljevic N, et al. The effects of high-dose intravenous methylprednisolone on event-related potentials in patients with multiple sclerosis. J Neurol Sci 1997; 152:147–53

4. Milligan NM, Newcombe R, Compston DA. A double-blind controlled trial of high dose methylprednisolone in patients with multiple sclerosis: 1. Clinical effects. J Neurol Neurosurg Psychiatry 1987; 50:511–16

5. Beck RW, Cleary PA, Trobe JD, et al. The effect of corticosteroids for acute optic neuritis on the subsequent development of multiple sclerosis. The Optic Neuritis Study Group. N Engl J Med 1993; 329:1764–9

6. Alam SM, Kyriakides T, Lawden M, et al. Methylprednisolone in multiple sclerosis: a comparison of oral with intravenous therapy at equivalent high dose. J Neurol Neurosurg Psychiatry 1993; 56:1219–20

7. Barnes D, Hughes RA, Morris RW, et al. Randomised trial of oral and intravenous methylprednisolone in acute relapses of multiple sclerosis. Lancet 1997; 349:902–906

8. Sellebjerg F, Frederiksen JL, Nielsen PM, et al. Double-blind, randomized, placebo-controlled study of oral, high-dose methylprednisolone in attacks of MS. Neurology 1998; 51:529–34

9. Tremlett HL, Luscombe DK, Wiles CM. Use of corticosteroids in multiple sclerosis by consultant neurologists in the United Kingdom. J Neurol Neurosurg Psychiatry 1998; 65:362–5

10. Morrow SA, Stoian CA, Dmitrovic J, et al. The bioavailability of IV methylprednisolone and oral prednisone in multiple sclerosis. Neurology 2004; 63:1079–1080

11. Perumal JS, Caon C, Hreha S, et al. Oral prednisone taper following intravenous steroids fails to improve disability or recovery from relapses in multiple sclerosis. Eur J Neurol 2008; 15:677–80

12. Glass-Marmor L, Paperna T, Ben-Yosef Y, et al. Chronotherapy using corticosteroids for multiple sclerosis relapses. J Neurol Neurosurg Psychiatry 2006; 78:886–8

13. NICE. Multiple Sclerosis: Management of multiple sclerosis in primary and secondary care. London: National Institute for Clinical Excellence, 2003

14. Fog T. The long-term treatment of multiple sclerosis with corticoids. Acta Neurol Scand 1965; 41:S473–S484

15. Then Bergh F, Kumpfel T, Schumann E, et al. Monthly intravenous methylprednisolone in relapsing-remitting multiple sclerosis: reduction of enhancing lesions, T2 lesion volume and plasma prolactin concentrations. BMC Neurol 2006; 6:19

16. Goodkin DE, Kinkel RP, Weinstock-Guttman B, et al. A phase II study of IV methyl-prednisolone in secondary-progressive multiple sclerosis. Neurology 1998; 51:239–45

17. Hoffmann V, Schimrigk S, Islamova S, et al. Efficacy and safety of repeated intrathecal triamcinolone acetonide application in progressive multiple sclerosis patients. J Neurol Sci 2003; 211:81–4

18. Hoffmann V, Kuhn W, Schimrigk S, et al. Repeat intrathecal triamcinolone acetonide application is beneficial in progressive MS patients. Eur J Neurol 2006; 13:72–6

Chapter 13

1. Neighbour PA, Bloom BR. Absence of virus-induced lymphocyte suppression and interferon production in multiple sclerosis. Proc Natl Acad Sci USA 1979; 76:476–80

2. Jacobs L, O'Malley J, Freeman A, et al. Intrathecal interferon reduces exacerbations of multiple sclerosis. Science 1981; 214:1026–28

3. Knobler RL, Panitch HS, Braheny SL, et al. Clinical trial of natural alpha interferon in multiple sclerosis. Ann NY Acad Sci 1984; 436:382–8

4. The IFNB Multiple Sclerosis Study Group. Interferon beta-1b is effective in relapsing-remitting multiple sclerosis. 1. Clinical results of a multi-center, randomized, double-blind, placebo-controlled trial. Neurology 1993; 43:655–61

5. The IFNB Multiple Sclerosis Study Group and the University of British Columbia MS/MRI Analysis Group. Interferon beta-1b in the treatment of multiple sclerosis: final outcome of the randomized controlled trial. Neurology 1995; 45:1277–85

6. Richards RG. Interferon beta in multiple sclerosis. BMJ 1996; 313:1159

7. European Study Group on interferon beta-1b in secondary progressive MS. Placebo-controlled multi-centre randomised trial of interferon beta-1b in secondary progressive multiple sclerosis. Lancet 1998; 352:1491–7

8. Dubois BD, Keenan E, Porter BE, et al. Interferon beta in multiple sclerosis: experience in a British specialist multiple sclerosis centre. J Neurol Neurosurg Psychiatry 2003; 74:946–9

9. Kappos L, Clanet M, Sandberg-Wollheim M, et al. Neutralizing antibodies and efficacy of interferon beta-1a: a 4-year controlled study. Neurology 2005; 65:40–47

10. Francis GS, Rice GP, Alsop JC. Interferon beta-1a in MS: results following development of neutralizing antibodies in PRISMS. Neurology 2005; 65:48–55

11. Malucchi S, Sala A, Gilli F, et al. Neutralizing antibodies reduce the efficacy of betaIFN during multiple sclerosis. Neurology 2004; 62:2031–37

12. Hartung HP, Polman C, Bertolotto A, et al. Neutralising antibodies to interferon beta in multiple sclerosis : Expert panel report. J Neurol 2007; 254:827–37

13. Brod SA, Nguyen M, Hood Z, et al. Ingested (Oral) IFN-alpha represses TNF-alpha mRNA in relapsing-remitting multiple sclerosis. J Interferon Cytokine Res 2006; 26:150–55

14. Thorne RG, Hanson LR, Ross TM, et al. Delivery of interferon-beta to the monkey nervous system following intranasal administration. Neuroscience 2008; 152:785–97

15. D'Amico D, La Mantia L, Rigamonti A, et al. Prevalence of primary headaches in people with multiple sclerosis. Cephalalgia 2004; 24:980–84

16. Loftis JM, Hauser P. The phenomenology and treatment of interferon-induced depression. J Affect Disord 2004; 82:175–90

17. Durelli L, Bongioanni MR, Cavallo R, et al. Chronic systemic high-dose recombinant interferon alfa-2a reduces exacerbation rate, MRI signs of disease activity, and lymphocyte interferon gamma production in relapsing-remitting multiple sclerosis. Neurology 1994; 44:406–13

18. Myhr KM, Riise T, Green Lilleas FE, et al. Interferon-alpha-2a reduces MRI disease activity in relapsing-remitting multiple sclerosis. Neurology 1999; 52:1049–56

19. Tremlett HL, Yoshida EM, Oger J. Liver injury associated with the beta-interferons for MS: a comparison between the three products. Neurology 2004; 62:628–31

20. Caraccio N, Dardano A, Manfredonia F, et al. Long-term follow-up of 106 multiple sclerosis patients undergoing IFN-{beta} 1a or 1b therapy: predictive factors of thyroid disease development and duration. J Clin Endocrinol Metab 2005; 90:4133–7

21. Monzani F, Caraccio N, Dardano A, et al. Thyroid auto-immunity and dysfunction associated with type I interferon therapy. Clin Exp Med 2004; 3:199–210

22. Midgard R, Ag KE, Trondsen E, et al. Life-threatening acute pancreatitis associated with interferon beta-1a treatment in multiple sclerosis. Neurology 2005; 65:170–71

23. Tai YJ, Tam M. Fixed drug eruption with interferon-beta-1b. Australas J Dermatol 2005; 46:154–7

24. Ekstein D, Linetsky E, Abramsky O, et al. Polyneuropathy associated with interferon beta treatment in patients with multiple sclerosis. Neurology 2005; 65:456–8

25. O'Rourke KE, Hutchinson M. Stopping beta-interferon therapy in multiple sclerosis: an analysis of stopping patterns. Mult Scler 2005; 11:46–50

26. Boskovic R, Wide R, Wolpin J, et al. The reproductive effects of beta interferon therapy in pregnancy: a longitudinal cohort. Neurology 2005; 65:807–811

27. Achiron A, Barak Y, Gail M, et al. Cancer incidence in multiple sclerosis and effects of immunomodulatory treatments. Breast Cancer Res Treat 2005; 89:265–70

28. Noseworthy JH, Ebers GC, Vandervoort MK, et al. The impact of blinding on the results of a randomized, placebo-controlled multiple sclerosis clinical trial. Neurology 1994; 44:16–20

29. Filippini G, Munari L, Incorvaia B, et al. Interferons in relapsing-remitting multiple sclerosis: a systematic review. Lancet 2003; 361:545–52

30. Trojano M, Paolicelli D, Zimatore GB, et al. The IFNbeta treatment of multiple sclerosis (MS) in clinical practice: the experience at the MS Center of Bari, Italy. Neurol Sci 2005; 26 Suppl 4:s179–82

31. Pozzilli C, Prosperini L, Sbardella E, et al. Post-marketing survey on clinical response to interferon beta in relapsing multiple sclerosis: the Roman experience. Neurol Sci 2005; 26:s174–s178

32. Chaudhuri A, Behan PO. Treatment of multiple sclerosis: beyond the NICE guidelines. QJM 2005; 98:373–8

33. Ebers GC, Heigenhauser L, Daumer M, et al. Disability as an outcome in MS clinical trials. Neurology 2008; 71:624–31

34. Clanet M, Cucheratt M. Interferons in relapsing remitting MS: a systematic review comments on a meta-analysis. Int MS J 2003; 10:134–5

35. Blaylock R. Harmful Brain Effects of Interferons. Salt Lake City, Utah: Mercola Fulfillment Center, 2004

36. Patten SB, Francis G, Metz LM, et al. The relationship between depression and interferon beta-1a therapy in patients with multiple sclerosis. Mult Scler 2005; 11:175–81

37. Nortvedt MW, Riise T, Myhr KM, et al. Type 1 interferons and the quality of life of multiple sclerosis patients. Results from a clinical trial of interferon alfa-2a. Mult Scler 1999; 5:317–22

38. Simone IL, Ceccarelli A, Tortorella C, et al. Influence of interferon beta treatment on quality of life in multiple sclerosis patients. Health Qual Life Outcomes 2006; 4:96

Chapter 14

1. Schrempf W, Ziemssen T. Glatiramer acetate: mechanisms of action in multiple sclerosis. Autoimmun Rev 2007; 6:469–75

2. Horani A, Muhanna N, Pappo O, et al. The beneficial effect of glatiramer acetate (Copaxone(R)) on immune modulation of experimental hepatic fibrosis. Am J Physiol Gastrointest Liver Physiol 2006; 292:G628–38

3. Aharoni R, Teitelbaum D, Arnon R, et al. Copolymer 1 acts against the immunodominant epitope 82–100 of myelin basic protein by T-cell receptor

antagonism in addition to major histocompatibility complex blocking. Proc Natl Acad Sci USA 1999; 96:634–9

4. Aharoni R, Teitelbaum D, Leitner O, et al. Specific Th2 cells accumulate in the central nervous system of mice protected against experimental auto-immune encephalomyelitis by copolymer 1. Proc Natl Acad Sci USA 2000; 97:11472–7

5. Brenner T, Arnon R, Sela M, et al. Humoral and cellular immune responses to copolymer 1 in multiple sclerosis patients treated with Copaxone. J Neuroimmunol 2001; 115:152–60

6. Duda PW, Schmied MC, Cook SL, et al. Glatiramer acetate (Copaxone) induces degenerate, Th2-polarized immune responses in patients with multiple sclerosis. J Clin Invest 2000; 105:967–76

7. Gran B, Tranquill LR, Chen M, et al. Mechanisms of immunomodulation by glatiramer acetate. Neurology 2000; 55:1704–14

8. Miller A, Shapiro S, Gershtein R, et al. Treatment of multiple sclerosis with copolymer-1 (Copaxone): implicating mechanisms of Th1 to Th2/Th3 immune-deviation. J Neuroimmunol 1998; 92:113–21

9. Aharoni R, Herschkovitz A, Eilam R, et al. Demyelination arrest and remyelination induced by glatiramer acetate treatment of experimental auto-immune encephalo-myelitis. Proc Natl Acad Sci USA 2008; 105:11358–63

10. Hestvik A, Skorstad G, Price D, et al. Multiple sclerosis: glatiramer acetate induces anti-inflammatory T-cells in the cerebrospinal fluid. Mult Scler 2008; 14:749–58

11. Iarlori C, Gambi D, Lugaresi A, et al. Reduction of free radicals in multiple sclerosis: effect of glatiramer acetate (Copaxone(R)). Mult Scler 2008; 14:739–48

12. Kreitman RR, Blanchette F. On the horizon: possible neuro-protective role for glatiramer acetate. Mult Scler 2004; 10 Suppl 1:S81–6; discussion S86–9

13. Blanchette F, Neuhaus O. Glatiramer acetate: evidence for a dual mechanism of action. J Neurol 2008; 255 Suppl 1:26–36

14. Khan O, Shen Y, Caon C, et al. Axonal metabolic recovery and potential neuro-protective effect of glatiramer acetate in relapsing-remitting multiple sclerosis. Mult Scler 2005; 11:646–51

15. Tsai SJ. Glatiramer acetate could be a potential therapeutic agent for Parkinson's disease through its neuro-protective and anti-inflammatory effects. Med Hypotheses 2007; 69:1219–21

16. Bornstein MB, Miller A, Slagle S, et al. A pilot trial of Cop 1 in exacerbating-remitting multiple sclerosis. N Engl J Med 1987; 317:408–14

17. Bornstein MB, Miller A, Slagle S, et al. A placebo-controlled, double-blind, randomized, two-center, pilot trial of Cop 1 in chronic progressive multiple sclerosis. Neurology 1991; 41:533–9

18. Johnson KP, Brooks BR, Cohen JA, et al. Extended use of glatiramer acetate (Copaxone) is well tolerated and maintains its clinical effect on multiple sclerosis relapse rate and degree of disability. Copolymer 1 Multiple Sclerosis Study Group. Neurology 1998; 50:701–708

19. Teitelbaum D, Arnon R, Sela M. Immunomodulation of experimental auto-immune

encephalomyelitis by oral administration of copolymer 1. Proc Natl Acad Sci USA 1999; 96:3842–7

20. Mancardi GL, Sardanelli F, Parodi RC, et al. Effect of copolymer-1 on serial gadolinium-enhanced MRI in relapsing-remitting multiple sclerosis. Neurology 1998; 50:1127–33

21. Comi G, Filippi M, Wolinsky JS. European/Canadian multi-center, double-blind, randomized, placebo-controlled study of the effects of glatiramer acetate on magnetic resonance imaging-measured disease activity and burden in patients with relapsing multiple sclerosis. European/Canadian Glatiramer Acetate Study Group. Ann Neurol 2001; 49:290–97

22. Johnson KP, Brooks BR, Ford CC, et al. Sustained clinical benefits of glatiramer acetate in relapsing multiple sclerosis patients observed for 6 years. Copolymer 1 Multiple Sclerosis Study Group. Mult Scler 2000; 6:255–66

23. Baumhackl U. The search for a balance between short and long-term treatment outcomes in multiple sclerosis. J Neurol 2008; 255 Suppl 1:75–83

24. Brochet B. Long-term effects of glatiramer acetate in multiple sclerosis. Rev Neurol (Paris) 2008; 164:917–26

25. Johnson KP, Ford CC, Lisak RP, et al. Neurologic consequence of delaying glatiramer acetate therapy for multiple sclerosis: 8-year data. Acta Neurol Scand 2005; 111:42–7

26. Rovaris M, Comi G, Rocca M, et al. Long-term follow-up of patients treated with glatiramer acetate: a multi-centre, multinational extension of the European/Canadian double-blind, placebo-controlled, MRI-monitored trial. Mult Scler 2007; 13:502–508

27. La Mantia L, Milanese C, D'Amico R. Meta-analysis of clinical trials with copolymer 1 in multiple sclerosis. Eur Neurol 2000; 43:189–93

28. Sormani MP, Bruzzi P, Comi G, et al. The distribution of the magnetic resonance imaging response to glatiramer acetate in multiple sclerosis. Mult Scler 2005; 11:447–9

29. Munari L, Lovati R, Boiko A. Therapy with glatiramer acetate for multiple sclerosis. Cochrane Database Syst Rev 2004:CD004678

30. Wolinsky JS. The use of glatiramer acetate in the treatment of multiple sclerosis. Adv Neurol 2006; 98:273–92

31. Bell C, Graham J, Earnshaw S, et al. Cost-effectiveness of four immunomodulatory therapies for relapsing-remitting multiple sclerosis: a Markov model based on long-term clinical data. J Manag Care Pharm 2007; 13:245–61

32. MS Society of Canada. MS Therapy may help delay conversion from CIS to clinically definite MS. www.mssociety.ca/en/research/medmmo_20080116.htm, accessed 19 February 2008

33. Argyriou AA, Makris N. Multiple sclerosis and reproductive risks in women. Reprod Sci 2008; 15:755–64

34. Madray MM, Greene JF, Jr., Butler DF. Glatiramer acetate-associated, CD30+, primary, cutaneous, anaplastic large-cell lymphoma. Arch Neurol 2008; 65:1378–9

35. Flechter S, Kott E, Steiner-Birmanns B, et al. Copolymer 1 (glatiramer acetate) in relapsing forms of multiple sclerosis: open multi-center study of alternate-day administration. Clin Neuropharmacol 2002; 25:11–15

36. Cohen JA, Rovaris M, Goodman AD, et al. Randomized, double-blind, dose-comparison study of glatiramer acetate in relapsing-remitting MS. Neurology 2007; 68:939–44

37. Brod SA, Lindsey JW, Wolinsky JS. Combination therapy with glatiramer acetate (copolymer-1) and a type I interferon (IFN-alpha) does not improve experimental auto-immune encephalomyelitis. Ann Neurol 2000; 47:127–31

38. Vollmer T, Panitch H, Bar-Or A, et al. Glatiramer acetate after induction therapy with mitoxantrone in relapsing multiple sclerosis. Mult Scler 2008; 14:663–70

39. Gold R. Combination therapies in multiple sclerosis. J Neurol 2008; 255 Suppl 1:51–60

40. Fridkis-Hareli M, Santambrogio L, Stern JN, et al. Novel synthetic amino acid copolymers that inhibit autoantigen-specific T-cell responses and suppress experimental auto-immune encephalomyelitis. J Clin Invest 2002; 109:1635–43

41. Matsoukas J, Apostolopoulos V, Kalbacher H, et al. Design and synthesis of a novel potent myelin basic protein epitope 87–99 cyclic analogue: enhanced stability and biological properties of mimics render them a potentially new class of immunomodulators. J Med Chem 2005; 48:1470–80

42. De Stefano N, Filippi M, Confavreux C, et al. The results of two multicenter, open-label studies assessing efficacy, tolerability and safety of protiramer, a high molecular weight synthetic copolymeric mixture, in patients with relapsing-remitting multiple sclerosis. Mult Scler 2008; 15:238–43

43. Filippi M, Wolinsky JS, Comi G. Effects of oral glatiramer acetate on clinical and MRI-monitored disease activity in patients with relapsing multiple sclerosis: a multi-centre, double-blind, randomised, placebo-controlled study. Lancet Neurol 2006; 5:213–20

Chapter 15

1. Piraino PS, Yednock TA, Messersmith EK, et al. Spontaneous remyelination following prolonged inhibition of alpha(4) integrin in chronic EAE. J Neuroimmunol 2005; 167:53–63

2. Miller DH, Khan OA, Sheremata WA, et al. A controlled trial of natalizumab for relapsing multiple sclerosis. N Engl J Med 2003; 348:15–23

3. Yousry TA, Major EO, Ryschkewitsch C, et al. Evaluation of patients treated with natalizumab for progressive multifocal leukoencephalopathy. N Engl J Med 2006; 354:924–33

4. Rudick RA, Stuart WH, Calabresi PA, et al. Natalizumab plus interferon beta-1a for relapsing multiple sclerosis. N Engl J Med 2006; 354:911–23

5. Polman CH, O'Connor PW, Havrdova E, et al. A randomized, placebo-controlled trial of natalizumab for relapsing multiple sclerosis. N Engl J Med 2006; 354:899–910

6. Miller DH, Soon D, Fernando KT, et al. MRI outcomes in a placebo-controlled trial of natalizumab in relapsing MS. Neurology 2007; 68:1390–1401

7. Engelhardt B, Briskin MJ. Therapeutic targeting of alpha4-integrins in chronic inflammatory diseases: tipping the scales of risk towards benefit? Eur J Immunol 2005; 35:2268–73

8. Mullen JT, Vartanian TK, Atkins MB. Melanoma complicating treatment with natalizumab for multiple sclerosis. N Engl J Med 2008; 358:647–8

9. Schipper JP. Natalizumab in multiple sclerosis: unclear patient benefits. Ned Tijdschr Geneeskd 2007; 151:852–5

10. Vermeulen M. Still no evidence on the efficacy of immunomodulatory therapy in reducing functional impairment in multiple sclerosis. Ned Tijdschr Geneeskd 2007; 151:850–51

11. Johnson KP. Natalizumab (tysabri) treatment for relapsing multiple sclerosis. Neurologist 2007; 13:182–7

12. Hirst CL, Pace A, Pickersgill TP, et al. Campath 1-H treatment in patients with aggressive relapsing-remitting multiple sclerosis. J Neurol 2008; 255:231–8

13. Coles AJ, Compston DA, Selmaj KW, et al. Alemtuzumab vs interferon beta-1a in early multiple sclerosis. N Engl J Med 2008; 359:1786–1801

14. Millefiorini E, Gasperini C, Pozzilli C, et al. Randomized placebo-controlled trial of mitoxantrone in relapsing-remitting multiple sclerosis: 24-month clinical and MRI outcome. J Neurol 1997; 244:153–9

15. Edan G, Miller D, Clanet M, et al. Therapeutic effect of mitoxantrone combined with methylprednisolone in multiple sclerosis: a randomised multi-centre study of active disease using MRI and clinical criteria. J Neurol Neurosurg Psychiatry 1997; 62:112–18

16. Hartung HP, Gonsette R, Konig N, et al. Mitoxantrone in progressive multiple sclerosis: a placebo-controlled, double-blind, randomised, multi-centre trial. Lancet 2002; 360:2018–2025

17. Debouverie M, Taillandier L, Pittion-Vouyovitch S, et al. Clinical follow-up of 304 patients with multiple sclerosis three years after mitoxantrone treatment. Mult Scler 2007; 13:626–31

18. Martinelli BF, Rovaris M, Capra R, et al. Mitoxantrone for multiple sclerosis. Cochrane Database Syst Rev 2005:CD002127

19. Murray TJ. The cardiac effects of mitoxantrone: do the benefits in multiple sclerosis outweigh the risks? Expert Opin Drug Saf 2006; 5:265–74

20. Correale J, Rush C, Amengual A, et al. Mitoxantrone as rescue therapy in worsening relapsing-remitting MS patients receiving IFN-beta. J Neuroimmunol 2005; 162:173–83

21. Cocco E, Marchi P, Sardu C, et al. Mitoxantrone treatment in patients with early relapsing-remitting multiple sclerosis. Mult Scler 2007; 13:975–80

22. Gonsette RE. New immunosuppressants with potential implication in multiple sclerosis. J Neurol Sci 2004; 223:87–93

23. Gonsette RE. Pixantrone (BBR2778): a new immunosuppressant in multiple sclerosis with a low cardiotoxicity. J Neurol Sci 2004; 223:81–6

24. Beutler E, Sipe JC, Romine JS, et al. The treatment of chronic progressive multiple sclerosis with cladribine. Proc Natl Acad Sci USA 1996; 93:1716–20

25. Selby R, Brandwein J, O'Connor P. Safety and tolerability of subcutaneous cladribine therapy in progressive multiple sclerosis. Can J Neurol Sci 1998; 25:295–9

26. Romine JS, Sipe JC, Koziol JA, et al. A double-blind, placebo-controlled, randomized trial of cladribine in relapsing-remitting multiple sclerosis. Proc Assoc Am Physicians 1999; 111:35–44

27. Sipe JC. Cladribine for multiple sclerosis: review and current status. Expert Rev Neurother 2005; 5:721–7

28. Yahoo. Merck Serono's oral investigational treatment Cladribine tablets for multiple sclerosis significantly reduced relapse rate in two-year phase III pivotal trial. http://biz. yahoo.com/prnews/090123/3822348en public.html?.v=1, accessed February 2009

29. Likosky WH, Fireman B, Elmore R, et al. Intense immunosuppression in chronic progressive multiple sclerosis: the Kaiser study. J Neurol Neurosurg Psychiatry 1991; 54:1055–60

30. The Canadian Cooperative Multiple Sclerosis Study Group. The Canadian Cooperative trial of cyclophosphamide and plasma exchange in progressive multiple sclerosis. Lancet 1991; 337:441–6

31. Weiner HL, Mackin GA, Orav EJ, et al. Intermittent cyclophosphamide pulse therapy in progressive multiple sclerosis: final report of the Northeast Cooperative Multiple Sclerosis Treatment Group. Neurology 1993; 43:910–18

32. Smith DR, Weinstock-Guttman B, Cohen JA, et al. A randomized blinded trial of combination therapy with cyclophosphamide in patients with active multiple sclerosis on interferon beta. Mult Scler 2005; 11:573–82

33. Patti F, Reggio E, Palermo F, et al. Stabilization of rapidly worsening multiple sclerosis for 36 months in patients treated with interferon beta plus cyclophosphamide followed by interferon beta. J Neurol 2004; 251:1502–1506

34. Bittencourt PR, Gomes-da-Silva MM. Multiple sclerosis: long-term remission after a high dose of cyclophosphamide. Acta Neurol Scand 2005; 111:195–8

35. Fazekas F, Deisenhammer F, Strasser-Fuchs S, et al. Randomised placebo-controlled trial of monthly intravenous immunoglobulin therapy in relapsing-remitting multiple sclerosis. Austrian Immunoglobulin in Multiple Sclerosis Study Group. Lancet 1997; 349:589–93

36. Sorensen PS, Wanscher B, Jensen CV, et al. Intravenous immunoglobulin G reduces MRI activity in relapsing multiple sclerosis. Neurology 1998; 50:1273–81

37. Achiron A, Kishner I, Sarova-Pinhas I, et al. Intravenous immunoglobulin treatment following the first demyelinating event suggestive of multiple sclerosis: a randomized, double-blind, placebo-controlled trial. Arch Neurol 2004; 61:1515–20

38. Kalanie H, Tabatabaii SS. Combined immunoglobulin and azathioprine in multiple sclerosis. Eur Neurol 1998; 39:178–81

39. Hommes OR, Sorensen PS, Fazekas F, et al. Intravenous immunoglobulin in secondary progressive multiple sclerosis: randomised placebo-controlled trial. Lancet 2004; 364:1149–56

40. Fazekas F, Sorensen PS, Filippi M, et al. MRI results from the European Study on Intravenous Immunoglobulin in Secondary Progressive Multiple Sclerosis (ESIMS). Mult Scler 2005; 11:433–40

41. Stangel M, Gold R. High-dose intravenous immunoglobulins in the treatment of multiple sclerosis. An update. Nervenarzt 2005; 76:1267–72

42. Katz U, Kishner I, Magalashvili D, et al. Long-term safety of IVIg therapy in multiple sclerosis: 10 years experience. Autoimmunity 2006; 39:513–17
43. Pohlau D, Przuntek H, Sailer M, et al. Intravenous immunoglobulin in primary and secondary chronic progressive multiple sclerosis: a randomized placebo controlled multicentre study. Mult Scler 2007; 13:1107–17
44. Massacesi L, Parigi A, Barilaro A, et al. Efficacy of azathioprine on multiple sclerosis new brain lesions evaluated using magnetic resonance imaging. Arch Neurol 2005; 62:1843–7
45. Goodkin DE, Rudick RA, VanderBrug Medendorp S, et al. Low-dose (7.5 mg) oral methotrexate reduces the rate of progression in chronic progressive multiple sclerosis. Ann Neurol 1995; 37:30–40

Chapter 16

1. Lang TJ. Estrogen as an immunomodulator. Clin Immunol 2004; 113:224–30
2. Salemi G, Callari G, Gammino M, et al. The relapse rate of multiple sclerosis changes during pregnancy: a study. Acta Neurol Scand 2004; 110:23–6
3. Subramanian S, Matejuk A, Zamora A, et al. Oral feeding with ethinyl estradiol suppresses and treats experimental auto-immune encephalomyelitis in SJL mice and inhibits the recruitment of inflammatory cells into the central nervous system. J Immunol 2003; 170:1548–55
4. Offner H. Neuroimmunoprotective effects of estrogen and derivatives in experimental auto-immune encephalomyelitis: Therapeutic implications for multiple sclerosis. J Neurosci Res 2004; 78:603–24
5. Hernan MA, Hohol MJ, Olek MJ, et al. Oral contraceptives and the incidence of multiple sclerosis. Neurology 2000; 55:848–54
6. Alonso A, Jick SS, Olek MJ, et al. Recent use of oral contraceptives and the risk of multiple sclerosis. Arch Neurol 2005; 62:1362–5
7. Sicotte NL, Giesser BS, Tandon V, et al. Testosterone treatment in multiple sclerosis: a pilot study. Arch Neurol 2007; 64:683–8
8. Milder DG. Partial and significant reversal of progressive visual and neurological deficits in multiple sclerosis: a possible therapeutic effect. Clin Experiment Ophthalmol 2002; 30:363–6
9. Fernandez O, Guerrero M, Mayorga C, et al. Combination therapy with interferon beta-1b and azathioprine in secondary progressive multiple sclerosis. A two-year pilot study. J Neurol 2002; 249:1058–62
10. Pulicken M, Bash CN, Costello K, et al. Optimization of the safety and efficacy of interferon beta-1b and azathioprine combination therapy in multiple sclerosis. Mult Scler 2005; 11:169–74
11. Walker JE, Giri SN, Margolin SB. A double-blind, randomized, controlled study of oral pirfenidone for treatment of secondary progressive multiple sclerosis. Mult Scler 2005; 11:149–58
12. Kwiatkowska-Patzer B, Walski M, Frontczak-Baniewicz M, et al. Matrix metalloproteases activity and ultrastructural changes in the early phase of

experimental allergic encephalomyelitis. The effect of oral treatment with spinal cord hydrolisate proteins in Lewis rat. The pilot study. Folia Neuropathol 2004; 42:107–11

13. Brundula V, Rewcastle NB, Metz LM, et al. Targeting leukocyte MMPs and transmigration: minocycline as a potential therapy for multiple sclerosis. Brain 2002; 125:1297–1308

14. Metz LM, Zhang Y, Yeung M, et al. Minocycline reduces gadolinium-enhancing magnetic resonance imaging lesions in multiple sclerosis. Ann Neurol 2004; 55:756

15. Zabad RK, Metz LM, Todoruk TR, et al. The clinical response to minocycline in multiple sclerosis is accompanied by beneficial immune changes: a pilot study. Mult Scler 2007; 13:517–26

16. Zhang Y, Metz LM, Yong VW, et al. Pilot study of minocycline in relapsing-remitting multiple sclerosis. Can J Neurol Sci 2008; 35:185–91

17. Giuliani F, Fu SA, Metz LM, et al. Effective combination of minocycline and interferon-beta in a model of multiple sclerosis. J Neuroimmunol 2005; 165:83–91

18. Luccarini I, Ballerini C, Biagioli T, et al. Combined treatment with atorvastatin and minocycline suppresses severity of EAE. Exp Neurol 2008; 211:214–26

19. Zemke D, Majid A. The potential of minocycline for neuroprotection in human neurologic disease. Clin Neuropharmacol 2004; 27:293–8

20. Multiple Sclerosis Society of Canada. Acne medication may delay progress of multiple sclerosis. www.mssociety.ca/en/releases/nr_20071025.htm, accessed 17 November 2007

21. Liuzzi GM, Latronico T, Rossano R, et al. Inhibitory effect of polyunsaturated fatty acids on MMP–9 release from microglial cells: implications for complementary multiple sclerosis treatment. Neurochem Res 2007; 32:484–93

22. Horga A, Montalban X. FTY720 (fingolimod) for relapsing multiple sclerosis. Expert Rev Neurother 2008; 8:699–714

23. Agrawal YP. Low-dose naltrexone therapy in multiple sclerosis. Med Hypotheses 2005; 64:721–4

24. Smith JP, Stock H, Bingaman S, et al. Low-dose naltrexone therapy improves active Crohn's disease. Am J Gastroenterol 2007; 102:820–28

25. Gironi M, Martinelli-Boneschi F, Sacerdote P, et al. A pilot trial of low-dose naltrexone in primary progressive multiple sclerosis. Mult Scler 2008; 14:1076–83

26. Youssef S, Stuve O, Patarroyo JC, et al. The HMG-CoA reductase inhibitor, atorvastatin, promotes a Th2 bias and reverses paralysis in central nervous system auto-immune disease. Nature 2002; 420:78–84

27. Ifergan I, Wosik K, Cayrol R, et al. Statins reduce human blood-brain barrier permeability and restrict leukocyte migration: relevance to multiple sclerosis. Ann Neurol 2006; 60:45–55

28. Jenkins DJ, Kendall CW, Marchie A, et al. Effects of a dietary portfolio of cholesterol-lowering foods vs lovastatin on serum lipids and C-reactive protein. JAMA 2003; 290:502–10

29. Perras C. Sativex for the management of multiple sclerosis symptoms. Issues Emerg Health Technol 2005:1–4

30. Zajicek JP, Sanders HP, Wright DE, et al. Cannabinoids in multiple sclerosis (CAMS) study: safety and efficacy data for 12 months follow up. J Neurol Neurosurg Psychiatry 2005; 76:1664–9

31. Jackson SJ, Diemel LT, Pryce G, et al. Cannabinoids and neuro-protection in CNS inflammatory disease. J Neurol Sci 2005; 233:21–5

32. Malfitano AM, Matarese G, Bifulco M. From cannabis to endocannabinoids in multiple sclerosis: a paradigm of central nervous system autoimmune diseases. Curr Drug Targets CNS Neurol Disord 2005; 4:667–75

33. Capello E, Saccardi R, Murialdo A, et al. Intense immunosuppression followed by autologous stem cell transplantation in severe multiple sclerosis. Neurol Sci 2005; 26:s200–s203

34. Progress CfM. Goat Serum Trial. London: Coalition for Medical Progress, 2005

35. Achiron A, Lavie G, Kishner I, et al. T-cell vaccination in multiple sclerosis relapsing-remitting nonresponders patients. Clin Immunol 2004; 113:155–60

36. Loftus B, Newsom B, Montgomery M, et al. Autologous attenuated T-cell vaccine (Tovaxin(R)) dose escalation in multiple sclerosis relapsing-remitting and secondary progressive patients nonresponsive to approved immunomodulatory therapies. Clin Immunol 2009; 131:202–15

37. Stuve O, Cravens PD, Eagar TN. DNA-based vaccines: the future of multiple sclerosis therapy? Expert Rev Neurother 2008; 8:351–60

38. Garren H, Robinson WH, Krasulova E, et al. Phase 2 trial of a DNA vaccine encoding myelin basic protein for multiple sclerosis. Ann Neurol 2008; 63:611–20

39. Warren KG, Catz I, Ferenczi LZ, et al. Intravenous synthetic peptide MBP8298 delayed disease progression in an HLA Class II-defined cohort of patients with progressive multiple sclerosis: results of a 24-month double-blind placebo-controlled clinical trial and 5 years of follow-up treatment. Eur J Neurol 2006; 13:887–95

40. Schilling S, Goelz S, Linker R, et al. Fumaric acid esters are effective in chronic experimental auto-immune encephalomyelitis and suppress macrophage infiltration. Clin Exp Immunol 2006; 145:101–107

41. Schimrigk S, Brune N, Hellwig K, et al. Oral fumaric acid esters for the treatment of active multiple sclerosis: an open-label, baseline-controlled pilot study. Eur J Neurol 2006; 13:604–10

42. Kappos L, Gold R, Miller DH, et al. Efficacy and safety of oral fumarate in patients with relapsing-remitting multiple sclerosis: a multi-centre, randomised, double-blind, placebo-controlled phase IIb study. Lancet 2008; 372:1463–72

43. O'Connor PW, Li D, Freedman MS, et al. A Phase II study of the safety and efficacy of teriflunomide in multiple sclerosis with relapses. Neurology 2006; 66:894–900

Chapter 17

1. Kurtzke JF. Epidemiologic evidence for multiple sclerosis as an infection. Clin Microbiol Rev 1993; 6:382–427

2. Hammond SR, English DR, McLeod JG. The age-range of risk of developing multiple sclerosis: evidence from a migrant population in Australia. Brain 2000; 123:968–74

3. Ross RT, Cheang M. Geographic similarities between varicella and multiple sclerosis: an hypothesis on the environmental factor of multiple sclerosis. J Clin Epidemiol 1995; 48:731–7

4. Sotelo J, Ordonez G, Pineda B. Varicella-zoster virus at relapses of multiple sclerosis. J Neurol 2007; 254:493–500

5. Panitch HS. Influence of infection on exacerbations of multiple sclerosis. Ann Neurol 1994; 36:S25–S28

6. Merelli E, Bedin R, Sola P, et al. Human herpes virus 6 and human herpes virus 8 DNA sequences in brains of multiple sclerosis patients, normal adults and children. J Neurol 1997; 244:450–54

7. Challoner PB, Smith KT, Parker JD, et al. Plaque-associated expression of human herpesvirus 6 in multiple sclerosis. Proc Natl Acad Sci USA 1995; 92:7440–44

8. Soldan SS, Berti R, Salem N, et al. Association of human herpes virus 6 (HHV-6) with multiple sclerosis: increased IgM response to HHV-6 early antigen and detection of serum HHV-6 DNA. Nat Med 1997; 3:1394–7

9. Caselli E, Boni M, Bracci A, et al. Detection of antibodies directed against human herpes virus 6 U94/REP in sera of patients affected by multiple sclerosis. J Clin Microbiol 2002; 40:4131–7

10. Chapenko S, Millers A, Nora Z, et al. Correlation between HHV-6 reactivation and multiple sclerosis disease activity. J Med Virol 2003; 69:111–17

11. Opsahl ML, Kennedy PG. Early and late HHV-6 gene transcripts in multiple sclerosis lesions and normal appearing white matter. Brain 2005; 128:516–27

12. Cermelli C, Berti R, Soldan SS, et al. High frequency of human herpes-virus 6 DNA in multiple sclerosis plaques isolated by laser microdissection. J Infect Dis 2003; 187:1377–87

13. Goodman AD, Mock DJ, Powers JM, et al. Human herpesvirus 6 genome and antigen in acute multiple sclerosis lesions. J Infect Dis 2003; 187:1365–76

14. Alvarez-Lafuente R, De Las Heras V, Bartolome M, et al. Beta-interferon treatment reduces human herpes-virus-6 viral load in multiple sclerosis relapses but not in remission. Eur Neurol 2004; 52:87–91

15. Alvarez-Lafuente R, de Las Heras V, Garcia-Montojo M, et al. Human herpes-virus 6 and multiple sclerosis: relapsing-remitting versus secondary progressive. Mult Scler 2007; 13:578–83

16. Levin LI, Munger KL, Rubertone MV, et al. Multiple sclerosis and Epstein-Barr virus. JAMA 2003; 289:1533–6

17. Hollsberg P, Hansen HJ, Haahr S. Altered CD8+ T-cell responses to selected Epstein-Barr virus immunodominant epitopes in patients with multiple sclerosis. Clin Exp Immunol 2003; 132:137–43

18. Ascherio A, Munger KL, Lennette ET, et al. Epstein-Barr virus antibodies and risk of multiple sclerosis: a prospective study. JAMA 2001; 286:3083–88

19. Wagner HJ, Munger KL, Ascherio A. Plasma viral load of Epstein-Barr virus and risk of multiple sclerosis. Eur J Neurol 2004; 11:833–4

20. Sundstrom P, Juto P, Wadell G, et al. An altered immune response to Epstein-Barr virus in multiple sclerosis: a prospective study. Neurology 2004; 62:2277–82

21. Banwell B, Krupp L, Kennedy J, et al. Clinical features and viral serologies in children with multiple sclerosis: a multinational observational study. Lancet Neurol 2007; 6:773–81

22. Ramagopalan SV, Valdar W, Dyment DA, et al. Association of infectious mononucleosis with multiple sclerosis: a population-based study. Neuroepidemiology 2009; 32:257–62

23. Thacker EL, Mirzaei F, Ascherio A. Infectious mononucleosis and risk for multiple sclerosis: a meta-analysis. Ann Neurol 2006; 59:499–503

24. Posnett DN. Herpes-viruses and auto-immunity. Curr Opin Investig Drugs 2008; 9:505–14

25. Ascherio A, Munger KL. Environmental risk factors for multiple sclerosis. Part I: the role of infection. Ann Neurol 2007; 61:288–99

26. Krone B, Oeffner F, Grange JM. Is the risk of multiple sclerosis related to the 'biography' of the immune system? J Neurol 2009; 256: 1052–60

27. Perez-Cesari C, Saniger MM, Sotelo J. Frequent association of multiple sclerosis with varicella and zoster. Acta Neurol Scand 2005; 112:417–19

28. Mancuso R, Delbue S, Borghi E, et al. Increased prevalence of varicella zoster virus DNA in cerebrospinal fluid from patients with multiple sclerosis. J Med Virol 2007; 79:192–9

29. Sotelo J, Ordonez G, Pineda B. Varicella-zoster virus at relapses of multiple sclerosis. J Neurol 2007; 254:493–500

30. Sotelo J, Martinez-Palomo A, Ordonez G, et al. Varicella-zoster virus in cerebrospinal fluid at relapses of multiple sclerosis. Ann Neurol 2008; 63:303–11

31. Frattaroli J, Weidner G, Kemp C, et al. Clinical events in prostate cancer lifestyle trial: results from two years of follow-up. Urology 2008; 72:1319–23

32. Griffiths PD. Tomorrow's challenges for herpes-virus management: potential applications of valacyclovir. J Infect Dis 2002; 186:S131–7.

33. Lycke J, Svennerholm B, Hjelmquist E, et al. Acyclovir treatment of relapsing-remitting multiple sclerosis. A randomized, placebo-controlled, double-blind study. J Neurol 1996; 243:214–24

34. Friedman JE, Zabriskie JB, Plank C, et al. A randomized clinical trial of valacyclovir in multiple sclerosis. Mult Scler 2005; 11:286–95

35. Hong J, Tejada-Simon MV, Rivera VM, et al. Anti-viral properties of interferon beta treatment in patients with multiple sclerosis. Mult Scler 2002; 8:237–42

Chapter 18

1. Khan F, Pallant J. Chronic pain in multiple sclerosis: prevalence, characteristics, and impact on quality of life in an Australian community cohort. J Pain 2007; 8:614–23

2. Solaro C, Brichetto G, Battaglia MA, et al. Antiepileptic medications in multiple sclerosis: adverse effects in a three-year follow-up study. Neurol Sci 2005; 25:307–10

3. Silver M, Blum D, Grainger J, et al. Double-blind, placebo-controlled trial of lamotrigine in combination with other medications for neuropathic pain. J Pain Symptom Manage 2007; 34:446–54

4. Angell M. The Truth About the Drug Companies: How they deceive us and what to do about it. Carlton North: Scribe Publications, 2005

5. Jensen MP, Barber J, Romano JM, et al. A comparison of self-hypnosis versus progressive muscle relaxation in patients with multiple sclerosis and chronic pain. Int J Clin Exp Hypn 2009; 57:198–221

6. Shapiro H. Could n–3 polyunsaturated fatty acids reduce pathological pain by direct actions on the nervous system? Prostaglandins Leukot Essent Fatty Acids 2003; 68:219–24

7. Giovannelli M, Borriello G, Castri P, et al. Early physiotherapy after injection of botulinum toxin increases the beneficial effects on spasticity in patients with multiple sclerosis. Clin Rehabil 2007; 21:331–7

8. Siev-Ner I, Gamus D, Lerner-Geva L, et al. Reflexology treatment relieves symptoms of multiple sclerosis: a randomized controlled study. Mult Scler 2003; 9:356–61

9. Mackereth PA, Booth K, Hillier VF, et al. Reflexology and progressive muscle relaxation training for people with multiple sclerosis: a crossover trial. Complement Ther Clin Pract 2009; 15:14–21

10. Lee P, Chen R. Vitamin D as an analgesic for patients with type 2 diabetes and neuropathic pain. Arch Intern Med 2008; 168:771–2

11. Chwastiak LA, Gibbons LE, Ehde DM, et al. Fatigue and psychiatric illness in a large community sample of persons with multiple sclerosis. J Psychosom Res 2005; 59:291–8

12. Lerdal A, Gulowsen Celius E, Krupp L, et al. A prospective study of patterns of fatigue in multiple sclerosis. Eur J Neurol 2007; 14:1338–43

13. Johansson S, Ytterberg C, Hillert J, et al. A longitudinal study of variations in and predictors of fatigue in multiple sclerosis. J Neurol Neurosurg Psychiatry 2008; 79:454–7

14. Niepel G, Tench CR, Morgan PS, et al. Deep gray matter and fatigue in MS A T1 relaxation time study. J Neurol 2006; 253:896–902

15. Benedict RH, Wahlig E, Bakshi R, et al. Predicting quality of life in multiple sclerosis: accounting for physical disability, fatigue, cognition, mood disorder, personality, and behavior change. J Neurol Sci 2005; 231:29–34

16. Marrie RA, Fisher E, Miller DM, et al. Association of fatigue and brain atrophy in multiple sclerosis. J Neurol Sci 2005; 228:161–6

17. Figved N, Klevan G, Myhr KM, et al. Neuropsychiatric symptoms in patients with multiple sclerosis. Acta Psychiatr Scand 2005; 112:463–8

18. Harboe E, Greve OJ, Beyer M, et al. Fatigue is associated with cerebral white matter hyperintensities in patients with systemic lupus erythematosus. J Neurol Neurosurg Psychiatry 2007; 79:199–201

19. Tellez N, Rio J, Tintore M, et al. Fatigue in multiple sclerosis persists over time: a longitudinal study. J Neurol 2006; 253:1466–70

20. Johnson SL. The concept of fatigue in multiple sclerosis. J Neurosci Nurs 2008; 40:72–7

21. Smith MM, Arnett PA. Factors related to employment status changes in individuals with multiple sclerosis. Mult Scler 2005; 11:602–609

22. Finlayson M. Pilot study of an energy conservation education program delivered by telephone conference call to people with multiple sclerosis. NeuroRehabilitation 2005; 20:267–77

23. Mathiowetz VG, Finlayson ML, Matuska KM, et al. Randomized controlled trial of an energy conservation course for persons with multiple sclerosis. Mult Scler 2005; 11:592–601

24. Tesar N, Bandion K, Baumhackl U. Efficacy of a neuropsychological training programme for patients with multiple sclerosis: a randomised controlled trial. Wien Klin Wochenschr 2005; 117:747–54

25. van Kessel K, Moss-Morris R, Willoughby E, et al. A randomized controlled trial of cognitive behavior therapy for multiple sclerosis fatigue. Psychosom Med 2008; 70:205–13

26. Oken BS, Kishiyama S, Zajdel D, et al. Randomized controlled trial of yoga and exercise in multiple sclerosis. Neurology 2004; 62:2058–64

27. Navipour H, Madani H, Mohebbi MR, et al. Improved fatigue in individuals with multiple sclerosis after participating in a short-term self-care programme. NeuroRehabilitation 2006; 21:37–41

28. Fragoso YD, Santana DL, Pinto RC. The positive effects of a physical activity program for multiple sclerosis patients with fatigue. NeuroRehabilitation 2008; 23:153–7

29. Wingerchuk DM, Benarroch EE, O'Brien PC, et al. A randomized controlled crossover trial of aspirin for fatigue in multiple sclerosis. Neurology 2005; 64:1267–9

30. Zifko UA, Rupp M, Schwarz S, et al. Modafinil in treatment of fatigue in multiple sclerosis. Results of an open-label study. J Neurol 2002; 249:983–7

31. Rosenberg JH, Shafor R. Fatigue in multiple sclerosis: a rational approach to evaluation and treatment. Curr Neurol Neurosci Rep 2005; 5:140–46

32. Rammohan KW, Rosenberg JH, Lynn DJ, et al. Efficacy and safety of modafinil (Provigil) for the treatment of fatigue in multiple sclerosis: a two centre phase 2 study. J Neurol Neurosurg Psychiatry 2002; 72:179–83

33. Stankoff B, Waubant E, Confavreux C, et al. Modafinil for fatigue in MS: a randomized placebo-controlled double-blind study. Neurology 2005; 64:1139–43

34. Kumar R. Approved and investigational uses of modafinil: an evidence-based review. Drugs 2008; 68:1803–39

35. Fleming WE, Pollak CP. Sleep disorders in multiple sclerosis. Semin Neurol 2005; 25:64–8

36. Metz LM, Patten SB, Archibald CJ, et al. The effect of immunomodulatory treatment on multiple sclerosis fatigue. J Neurol Neurosurg Psychiatry 2004; 75:1045–47

37. Hadjimichael O, Vollmer T, Oleen-Burkey M. Fatigue characteristics in multiple sclerosis: the North American Research Committee on Multiple Sclerosis (NARCOMS) survey. Health Qual Life Outcomes 2008; 6:100

38. Ziemssen T, Hoffmann J, Apfel R, et al. Effects of glatiramer acetate on fatigue and days of absence from work in first-time treated relapsing-remitting multiple sclerosis. Health Qual Life Outcomes 2008; 6:67

39. Heesen C, Nawrath L, Reich C, et al. Fatigue in multiple sclerosis: an example of cytokine mediated sickness behaviour? J Neurol Neurosurg Psychiatry 2006; 77:34–9

40. Johnson SK, Diamond BJ, Rausch S, et al. The effect of ginkgo biloba on functional measures in multiple sclerosis: a pilot randomized controlled trial. Explore (NY) 2006; 2:19–24

41. Lovera J, Bagert B, Smoot K, et al. Ginkgo biloba for the improvement of cognitive performance in multiple sclerosis: a randomized, placebo-controlled trial. Mult Scler 2007; 13:376–85

Chapter 19

1. Kern S, Ziemssen T. Review: brain–immune communication psychoneuroimmunology of multiple sclerosis. Mult Scler 2007; 14:6–21

2. Angell M. The Truth About the Drug Companies: How they deceive us and what to do about it. Carlton North: Scribe Publications, 2005

3. Knowler WC, Barrett-Connor E, Fowler SE, et al. Reduction in the incidence of type 2 diabetes with lifestyle intervention or metformin. N Engl J Med 2002; 346:393–403

4. Smith RE, Olin BR, Madsen JW. Spitting into the wind: the irony of treating chronic disease. J Am Pharm Assoc (Wash DC) 2006; 46:397–400

5. Kappagoda CT, Ma A, Cort DA, et al. Cardiac event rate in a lifestyle modification program for patients with chronic coronary artery disease. Clin Cardiol 2006; 29:317–21

6. Fekete EM, Antoni MH, Schneiderman N. Psychosocial and behavioral interventions for chronic medical conditions. Curr Opin Psychiatry 2007; 20:152–7

7. Aronne LJ. Therapeutic options for modifying cardiometabolic risk factors. Am J Med 2007; 120:S26–34

8. Jelinek GA, Hassed CS. Managing multiple sclerosis in primary care: are we forgetting something? Qual Prim Care 2009; 17:55–61

9. Cameron-Smith D, Sinclair AJ. Trans fats in Australian fast foods. Medical Journal of Australia 2006; 185:293

10. Cabot S. Liver Cleansing Diet: Love your liver and live longer. Sydney: Women's Health Advisory Service, 1998

11. Plant J. Your Life is in Your Hands: Understanding, preventing and overcoming breast cancer. Revised edition. New York: Virgin Books, 2006

12. Campbell TC, Campbell TM. The China Study. New York: Benbella Books, 2006

13. Erasmus U. Fats That Heal, Fats That Kill. Updated and expanded edition. New York: Alive Books, 1998

14. Sabate J, Haddad E, Tanzman JS, et al. Serum lipid response to the graduated enrichment of a Step I diet with almonds: a randomized feeding trial. Am J Clin Nutr 2003; 77:1379–84

15. Jenkins DJ, Kendall CW, Marchie A, et al. Dose response of almonds on coronary heart disease risk factors: blood lipids, oxidized low-density lipoproteins, lipoprotein(a), homocysteine, and pulmonary nitric oxide: a randomized, controlled, crossover trial. Circulation 2002; 106:1327–32

16. Marchioli R, Barzi F, Bomba E, et al. Early protection against sudden death by n–3 polyunsaturated fatty acids after myocardial infarction: time-course analysis of

the results of the Gruppo Italiano per lo Studio della Sopravvivenza nell'Infarto Miocardico (GISSI)-Prevenzione. Circulation 2002; 105:1897–1903

17. Marchioli R, Schweiger C, Tavazzi L, et al. Efficacy of n–3 polyunsaturated fatty acids after myocardial infarction: results of GISSI-Prevenzione trial. Gruppo Italiano per lo Studio della Sopravvivenza nell'Infarto Miocardico. Lipids 2001; 36:S119–26

18. Arias AJ, Steinberg K, Banga A, et al. Systematic review of the efficacy of meditation techniques as treatments for medical illness. J Altern Complement Med 2006; 12:817–32

19. van der Mei IA, Ponsonby AL, Dwyer T, et al. Past exposure to sun, skin phenotype, and risk of multiple sclerosis: case-control study. BMJ 2003; 327:316

20. Munger KL, Zhang SM, O'Reilly E, et al. Vitamin D intake and incidence of multiple sclerosis. Neurology 2004; 62:60–65

21. Brown SJ. The role of vitamin D in multiple sclerosis. Ann Pharmacother 2006; 40:1158–61

22. Ramagopalan SV, Maugeri NJ, Handunnetthi L, et al. Expression of the multiple sclerosis-associated MHC class II Allele HLA-DRB1*1501 is regulated by vitamin D. PLoS Genet 2009; 5:e1000369

23. Chaudhuri A. Why we should offer routine vitamin D supplementation in pregnancy and childhood to prevent multiple sclerosis. Med Hypotheses 2005; 64:608–18

24. Willer CJ, Dyment DA, Sadovnick AD, et al. Timing of birth and risk of multiple sclerosis: population based study. BMJ 2005; 330:120

25. Russell WR. Multiple Sclerosis: Control of the disease. Oxford: Pergamon Press, 1976

26. NICE. Multiple Sclerosis: Management of multiple sclerosis in primary and secondary care. London: National Institute for Clinical Excellence, 2003

27. Milanese C, Beghi E, Giordano L, et al. A post-marketing study on immunomodulating treatments for relapsing-remitting multiple sclerosis in Lombardia: preliminary results. Neurol Sci 2005; 26 Suppl 4:s171–3

28. Haas J, Firzlaff M. Twenty-four-month comparison of immunomodulatory treatments: a retrospective open label study in 308 RRMS patients treated with beta interferons or glatiramer acetate (Copaxone). Eur J Neurol 2005; 12:425–31

29. Caon C, Din M, Ching W, et al. Clinical course after change of immunomodulating therapy in relapsing-remitting multiple sclerosis. Eur J Neurol 2006; 13:471–4

30. Carra A, Onaha P, Luetic G, et al. Therapeutic outcome three years after switching of immunomodulatory therapies in patients with relapsing-remitting multiple sclerosis in Argentina. Eur J Neurol 2008; 15:386–93

31. Gajofatto A, Bacchetti P, Grimes B, et al. Switching first-line disease-modifying therapy after failure: impact on the course of relapsing-remitting multiple sclerosis. Mult Scler 2008; 15:50–8

32. Coyle PK. Switching algorithms: from one immunomodulatory agent to another. J Neurol 2008; 255 Suppl 1:44–50

33. Castelli-Haley J, Oleen-Burkey MK, Lage MJ, et al. Glatiramer acetate versus interferon beta-1a for subcutaneous administration: Comparison of outcomes among multiple sclerosis patients. Adv Ther 2008; 25:658–73

34. Mikol DD, Barkhof F, Chang P, et al. Comparison of subcutaneous interferon beta-1a with glatiramer acetate in patients with relapsing multiple sclerosis (the REbif vs Glatiramer Acetate in Relapsing MS Disease [REGARD] study): a multi-centre, randomised, parallel, open-label trial. Lancet Neurol 2008; 7:903–914

35. Cadavid D, Wolansky LJ, Skurnick J, et al. Efficacy of treatment of MS with IFN{beta}-1b or glatiramer acetate by monthly brain MRI in the BECOME study. Neurology 2009; 72:1976–83

36. Metz LM, Patten SB, Archibald CJ, et al. The effect of immunomodulatory treatment on multiple sclerosis fatigue. J Neurol Neurosurg Psychiatry 2004; 75:1045–47

37. Baumhackl U. The search for a balance between short and long-term treatment outcomes in multiple sclerosis. J Neurol 2008; 255 Suppl 1:75–83

38. Jelinek GA, Gawler RH. 30 year follow up at pneumonectomy of a 58-year-old survivor of disseminated osteosarcoma. Med J Aust 2008; 189:663–5

39. Ornish D, Magbanua MJ, Weidner G, et al. Changes in prostate gene expression in men undergoing an intensive nutrition and lifestyle intervention. Proc Natl Acad Sci USA 2008; 105:8369–74

INDEX

Note: Key subjects are in bold. Bold numbers refer to those pages containing the major information about each entry.